D1476124

WITHDRAWN
UTSA LIBRARIES

C04731303

Folio
RA
967
.P626
1982

L132285

LIBRARY
The University of Texas
at San Antonio

hospital architecture

DAVID R. PORTER

hospital architecture

GUIDELINES FOR DESIGN AND RENOVATION

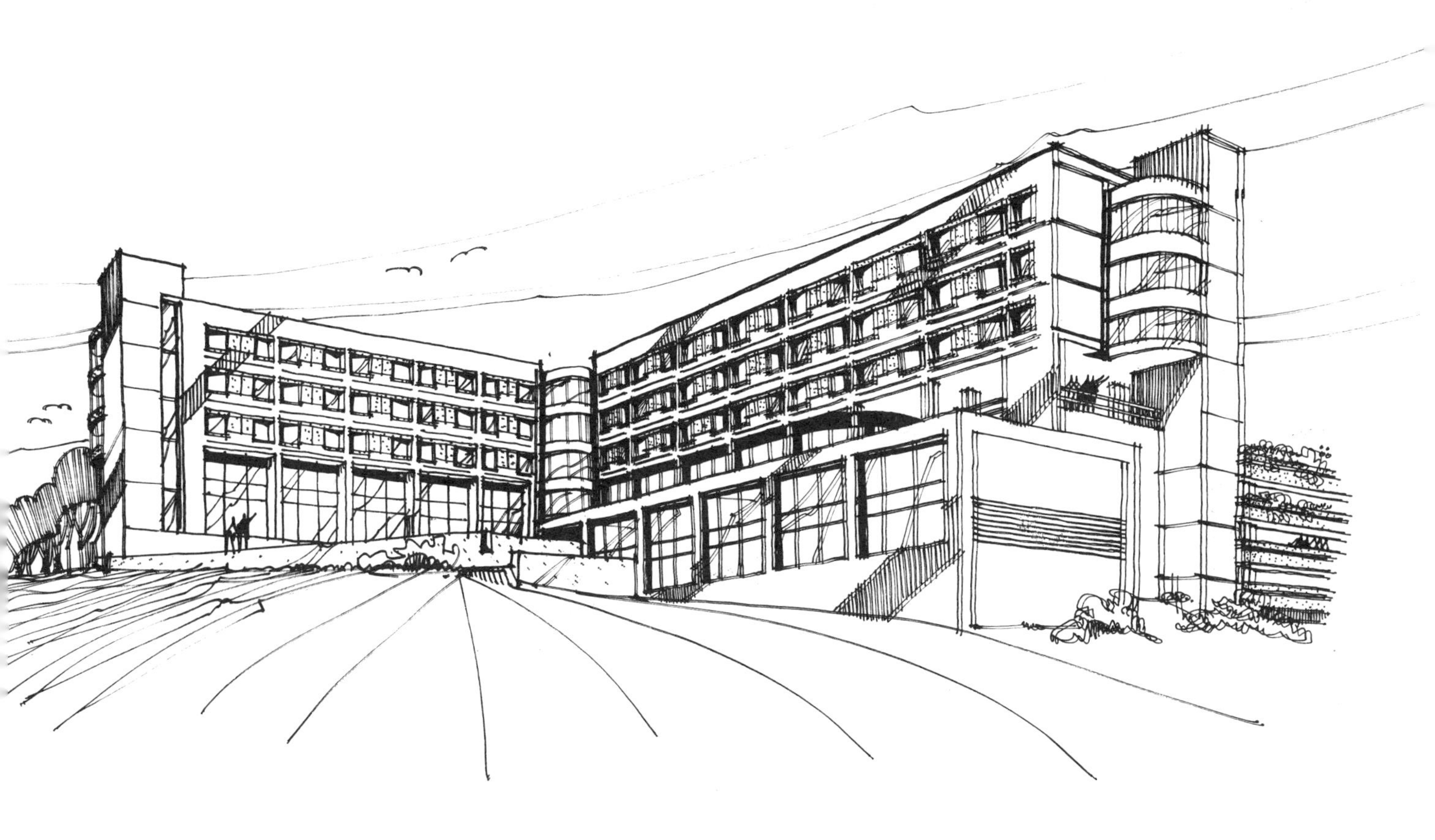

HEALTH ADMINISTRATION PRESS
ANN ARBOR, MICHIGAN
1982

To the memory of Dr. Louis Block,
the best of men.

Copyright © 1982 by the Foundation of the American College of Healthcare Executives. Printed in the United States of America. All rights reserved. This book or parts thereof may not be reproduced in any form without written permission of the publishers.

Copyright previously held by the Regents of The University of Michigan.

Library of Congress Cataloging in Publication Data

Porter, David R.
Hospital architecture.

1. Hospitals—Design and construction.
I. Title.
RA967.P626 362.1'1'0682 81-22906
ISBN 0-914904-53-1 (pbk.) AACR2

Health Administration Press
A Division of the Foundation of the
American College of Healthcare Executives
1021 E. Huron St.
Ann Arbor, MI 48104-9990
(313) 764-1380

LIBRARY
The University of Texas
At San Antonio

contents

THE ELEMENTS OF THE STRUCTURE

foreword

Currently, the role of the federal government in the planning and regulation of hospitals is in a state of transition. While it is difficult to predict the final outcome of this transition, it seems certain that the cost of health care will be a dominant concern for all hospitals throughout the 1980s.

The concern for health care costs becomes increasingly apparent as these costs continue to rise. National health care expenditures totaled $198.6 billion during the twelve months ending March 31, 1979, up 13.3 percent from a year earlier. During this same twelve-month period expenditures for hospital care were $78.3 billion, a 12.2 percent increase over the previous year. National health care expenditures now represent 9 percent of the nation's gross national product, up from 7.2 percent in 1970, with no sign of slowing down. Finally, in the twelve months ending March 31, 1979, expenditures amounted to $776 per person for health care and $164 per person for physicians' services; 12 percent of the money spent on hospital care was related to depreciation and interest charges stemming from hospital construction and other capital expenditures.

The initial thrust of federal government's involvement in containing the costs of hospital care was through health planning, which provided a basis for determining whether a proposed hospital capital project, or new service, was needed. The health planning movement originated in 1966 with the passage of Public Law 89–749, the Partnership For Health Act. This law called for the establishment of comprehensive health planning agencies on both areawide and statewide bases, and had as its primary goal the creation of a voluntary system of community planning. The law served as the major impetus for community health planning and for the interaction of hospitals with health planning agencies until 1972.

At that time Public Law 92–603, the Social Security Amendments of 1972, was passed by Congress; this act called for the establishment of professional standards review organizations to monitor the utilization of acute and, eventually, long-term care beds. In addition, it set forth a reimbursement limitation system whereby health care providers had to apply for a Certificate of Need for permission to spend $100,000 or more on capital expenditures. Failure to apply or a negative finding of need for such expenditure by the designated planning agency would lead to the loss of reimbursement dollars for depreciation and interest under government payment programs. The large-scale significance of this requirement is that it established review programs in states that had no certificate of need programs, and it encouraged states to implement such programs in order to avoid having their programs dictated by the federal government. From a hospital's perspective, this law strengthened the notion that institutional planning is important and necessary.

The major piece of health planning legislation in the 1970s was the National Health Planning and Resources Development Act of 1974 (Public Law 93–641). This law set up health systems agencies and state health planning and development agencies to be responsible for developing regional and statewide health systems plans and annual implementation plans. These plans help in evaluating and approving or disapproving specific proposals for capital expenditures submitted by hospitals and other providers under state certificate of need programs. The system has been extended through 1982 by the passage of Public Law 96–79, the Health Planning and Resources Development Amendments of 1979. These laws have formalized the health planning structure and made detailed hospital planning and design a way of life for project applicants.

Health planning agencies are working on the cost problem by attempting to discourage further investment in capital facilities and to encourage noninstitutional care. While some new forms of health care delivery are being recognized by the medical industry and the public as meaningful alternatives to hospital care, hospitals continue to play a major role in providing health care because:

—Although the rate of increase of the population is declining because of the dramatic drop in the birth rate during the 1960s and 1970s, the population is still increasing and will still need services.

—The population of the United States is growing older. In 1930 only 5.4 percent of the total population was 65 or older; in 1973, that figure had grown to over 10 percent. There are now more than 23 million people in the United States who are 65 and over; by the year 2000, this number is expected to be 32 million. Even more significant is the fact that the age cohorts of 75 and over are growing more rapidly than those 65 and over. The older the population, the more likely it is to need inpatient services.

After the Presidential elections of 1980, the federal government advocated a change in the basic approach to the containment of health care costs. The Reagan Administration judged the previous activities under the various planning laws as ineffective in cost containment and regulatory in nature. The administration advocates reliance on competitive forces in the market place to contain health costs instead of government regulation. Competitive forces contain costs in other industries and should have a role in containing costs in the health industry.

Competitive forces are less effective in the hospital field than other fields because many health programs (e.g. Medicare, Medicaid and some Blue Cross Plans) pay hospitals for the cost (or charges if lower) of services provided. The cost of services provided is determined after the fact and therefore, the full effect of declining utilization on costs is not felt by the hospital. Many observers today believe that reimbursement rules must change in order for competitive forces to be more effective in containing health care costs.

In view of these trends, statewide hospital rate setting is more likely today than ever before. Some states already set hospital rates (e.g., New York, Maryland) and cost containment in these states has been more effective than in other states.

In addition to state rate setting programs, there have been congressional discussions of changing the reimbursement principles associated with government programs such as Medicare. These discussions concern various alternatives to the reimbursement of the cost of service as determined after the fact.

One can predict that the 1980s will see continuing government involvement in attempts to contain health care costs. While it is not possible to predict with certainty what the government's initiatives will be, it is possible to make some generalized statements. It appears that in the 1980s more hospitals will have their rates set by a third party in such a way as to foster competition. In addition, there are likely to be major changes in state certificate of need legislation. While some states may eliminate certificate of need programs, many states will simply streamline their programs to make them less costly to administer. In some cases, this will result in less local input from health consumers in certificate of need programs.

What are the implications of these trends on hospital architecture and design? The increased federal reliance on competition to contain costs will obviously increase competition in the health field. This increased competition makes coordinated market research and master planning more essential now than in the past. Further, increased competition makes hospital rates a more important factor than before, and this implies the need to be cost effective in architecture and design. That is, the need for realistic projections of future utilization and cost effective designs to meet that utilization appear to be the way of the 1980s.

It is these endeavors to which David Porter has dedicated his professional life and to which he has so effectively spoken in this book. The use of this book by hospital administrators, boards, planners, consultants, architects, and engineers will lead to the design of better health care facilities. Such facilities can be defended before regulatory bodies, an important attribute now, and an even more important attribute in the future.

MANDELL BELLMORE, Ph.D.
President
Block, McGibony & Associates, Inc.

acknowledgments

I owe a great deal of gratitude to all those who have contributed their knowledge and time to this book, especially those listed below:

—Mandell Bellmore: Foreword

—Mark Gottlieb: hospital consultant

—Robert von Otto: engineering consultant

—Gerry Higgs: structural engineer

—Richard Horrworth: value management

—James W. Walters: cost and codes, long-term care

—Pamela Mason Porter: patient profile

—Barbara van Veen: Department functions

—Randolph W. Shotwell: materials handling

—Ray F. Smith: mechanical definitions

—Laique Rehman: international partner

—Elizabeth A. R. Robinson and Michael C. Martin: editors

—Perkins & Will: generous contribution of illustrations

—Henningson, Durham & Richardson: illustrations

A special thanks to my business partner, Pamela Porter. Her beauty and enthusiasm has made our working together a benefit for me and for every one of our clients.

introduction

The goal of this book is to inform the hospital administrator, board member, planner, and health care student of the process, pitfalls, and terminology of health care facility programming and design. The process of planning, building, or renovating is highly technical and, to the uninitiated, often fraught with problems. This book is intended to explain the programming and design of health care facilities in sufficient detail to establish a common language and understanding between architects and engineers on the one hand and health care administrators and planners on the other. The process of creating a new building, or altering an existing one, is described from conception to completion.

Initially, the need for thorough planning by and for the facility is considered. The plans and programs of a health care institution set its future and are the key to its survival. Long-range building concepts, including the incorporation of current structures, the mechanical energy plant, and site potential and phasing, establish the future of the physical facility for the next twenty years. Careful planning by trustees, administrators, and outside consultants can assure not only the financial viability of the institution, but also its survival *vis-a-vis* regulatory agencies. For these reasons, the first topics addressed in this book are the need for planning and the different levels of planning.

This complex process requires the integration of a wide variety of professionals into a planning team. Members of the health facilities staff and technical experts need to work together to create the new programs and structure. The issues of who should be on the planning team, what such a team does, when it is needed, and how it operates are considered. The various types of consultants needed for facility programming and design are described, as are their skills and fees. Technical planning and design services include architects and engineers (civil, structural, mechanical, and electrical) plus value management services, equipment specialists, and construction management. The bidding process is defined and appropriate construction management discussed. In addition, pricing design is presented and its value to the institution considered.

Initial planning considerations are then presented: what general physical plan is being considered; how is the current physical plant to be incorporated; what are the space requirements, cost constraints, time schedules, and codes and standards that must be included?

These efforts are then brought together in overall facility design development. Issues that cross departmental lines are now included. Traffic, transportation of patients and materials, communication flow, parking, site, and needs for adjacent space must all be incorporated into systems and processes that are designed to integrate them.

Construction of the facility requires the development of working drawings and specifications based on programming and design. The legal relationships between the client, architect and general contractor are defined. The actual construction, including changes and inspections, is the final step in the production of the building.

Throughout the process, the health facility must consider the larger community it serves and should take the time to solicit support for its efforts. Good public relations are invaluable. Groundbreaking and opening ceremonies are an excellent opportunity to reach the public.

Planning any facility for human needs must focus on the population to be served. The patients, and their characteristics and experiences in the facility, should be described and included in the design. In a healing institution, aesthetic as well as physical and emotional needs are important to the eventual patient outcome, for the layout of public areas greatly affects patient and family.

The details of operational programming for each department's needs are considered next. Utilization and planning ratios determine the site of each department, based on federal guidelines and the author's architectural and consulting experience. These requirements include not only floor space, but also relationships within the department and with other departments. In addition, departments vary in their need for equipment, spatial efficiency, and patient or staff amenities.

Interior design defines furnishing, finishes, and general appearance of the building's interior. It is especially important in public and patient areas, because there it affects the person's facility. Thoughtful interior design can also increase staff efficiency and satisfaction.

The process of creating a new facility, or a new section of a facility, is long and complex. The many steps and resources available are described here in sufficient detail to enable those not trained in architecture or construction to understand and use the programming and design process to produce the most appropriate facility for their specific needs.

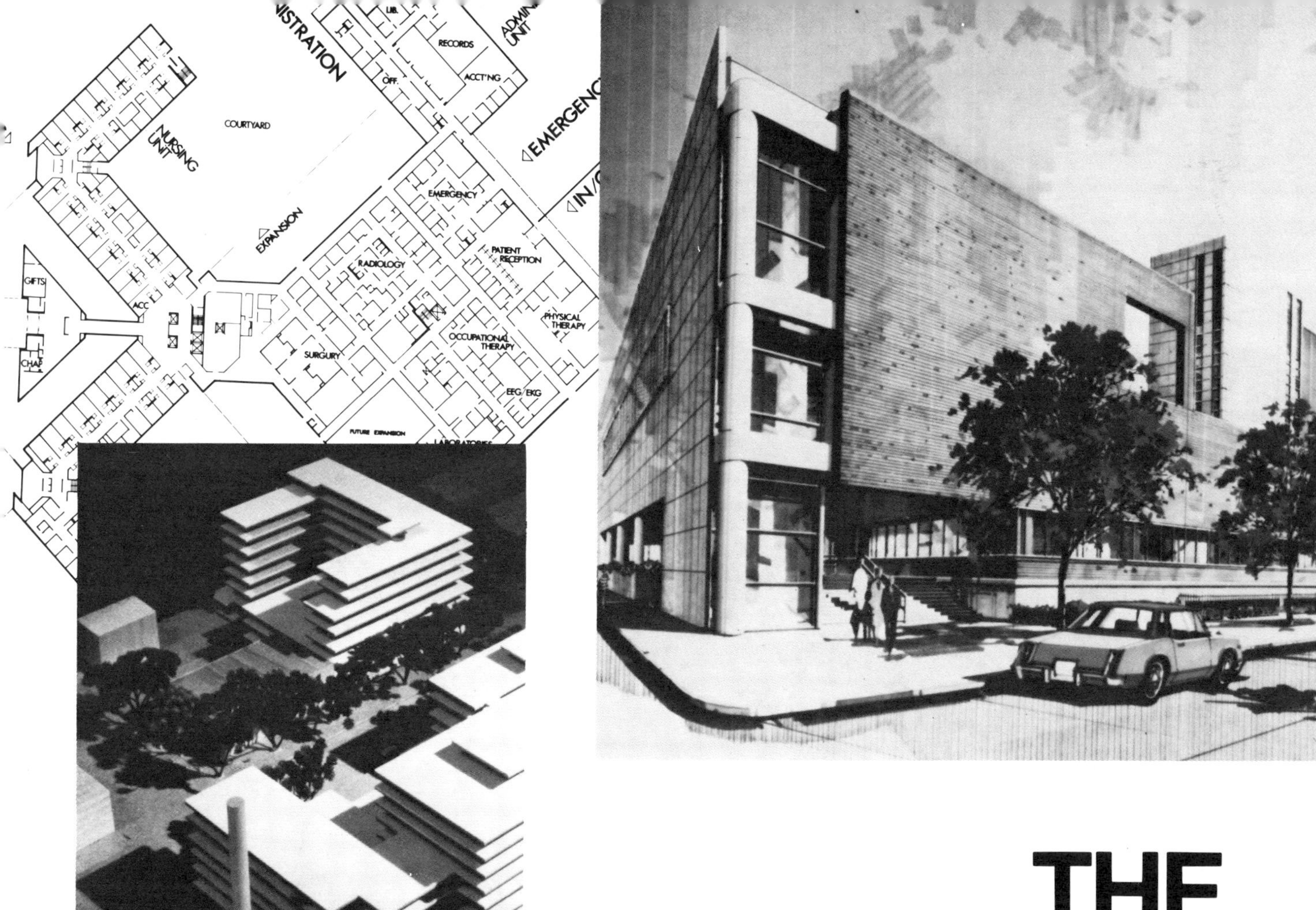

THE PROCESS:

FROM DESIGN TO DEDICATION

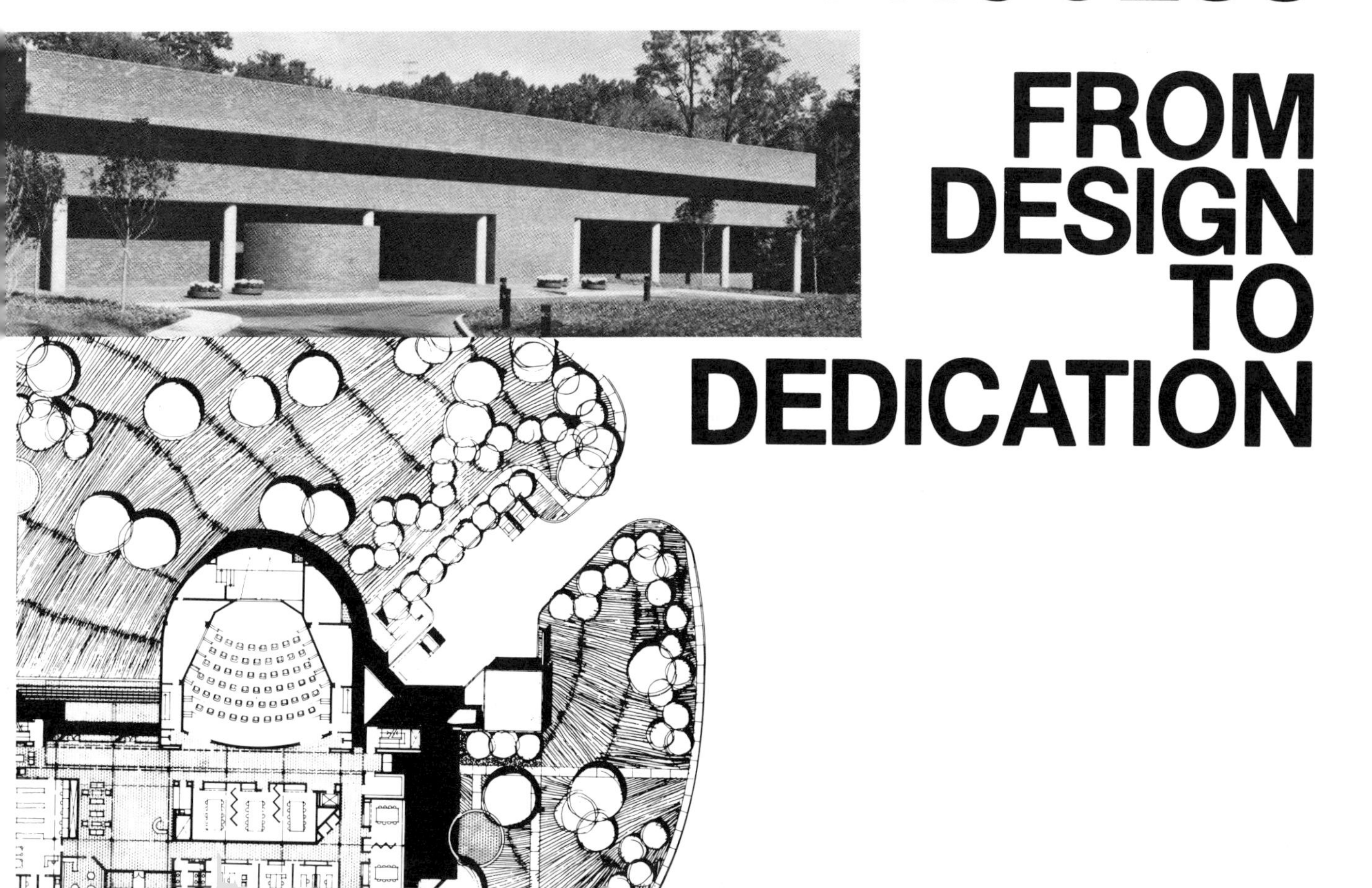

I

planning needs

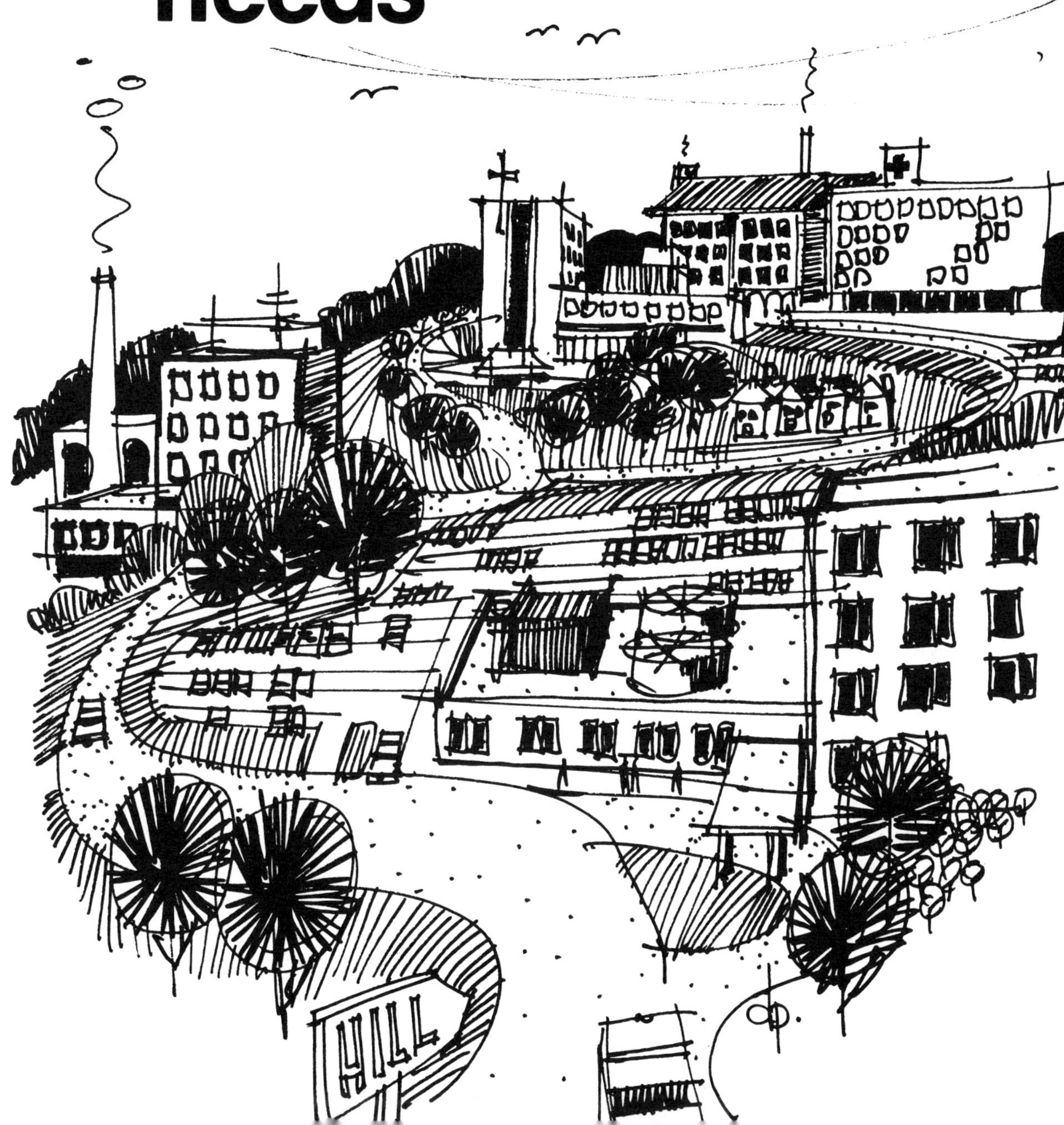

Health care administrators and planners have become the key to community health programs and facilities in the United States. Regional planning and federal controls have supplanted the local physicians and hospital boards as primary forces in determining a community's health care program. The hospital administrator has always been the operating manager of his facility, but now, because of sophisticated public and private financing, control of proprietary interest, major insurance and third-party payment controls, and reduced utilization of facilities, he has been thrust into an expanded leadership role.

The health care industry is one of the largest and most complex in the country, with a labor force to match. The health care administrator has a correspondingly complex management role: every area of social need, including housing, welfare, ecology, defense, and education, is addressed in a health care program. Although I deal here with design and construction of medical facilities, it must be noted that a strong management team is essential to the daily functioning of a facility and must be included in expansion plans.

The process of creating a new or expanded facility begins with a plan based on the institution's history, current situation, and future projections. Each hospital fills definite needs in its community. These health needs, along with the community's ability to pay for them, must be specified before the governing board can commit planning and construction monies for an appropriate facility. The plan must consider all aspects of the hospital's role:

—Regional Plan: Does the facility fit into the broad state and regional program of need? What are the public health requirements?

—Service Area: Who are the people served by the facility? Where do they work and live? What are their health needs?

—Patient Needs: What are the present family health needs? Future Needs?

—Medical Staff: What prompts a doctor to refer a patient to this facility? Where do the local doctors live and work?

—Hospital Staff: What major benefits and needs are available to attract and hold a proper number of staff? To attract and hold nurses?

—Organization: How does the chain of command and internal make-up of the organization affect the fulfillment of patient needs? What are the projected costs of department work loads?

—Physical Plant: What is the current size, location, and cost of the plant? What is its probable future use?

—Financial Feasibility: Can the patient reimbursements and other facility funds cover new construction or renovation costs?

A variety of planning studies can be executed to aid the administrator. A long-range plan and facility master plan are necessary in order for local and state regulatory agencies to grant overall approval of any specific program or space addition. The bonding underwriters that set the class of bond will also require a long-range document. The long-range plan defines the institution's role and future program goals or defines the market. The facility master plan translates the role and goals into a defined physical space plan.

The other types of studies described are unique to specific needs in further refining or implementing a long-range plan. The institute-specific plan is a shared planning effort among hospitals in a region to help define bed need per institution.

LONG-RANGE PLAN

The long-range, or master plan, covers the following areas:

—demographic study of service area

—study and definition of community health care needs and available services

—analysis of medical staff

—organizational plan

—size and physical concept

—financial feasibility

This type of study defines the present service area, or market, the socio-economic characteristics, health care inventory in the area, present scope of problems, utilization, volume, present organization, fiscal condition, building and site limitations, and medical staff analysis. These conditions are projected into the future and form the basis for a plan. The plan, which usually covers between five and ten years, is coordinated with the Health Systems Agency (HSA) region and with state

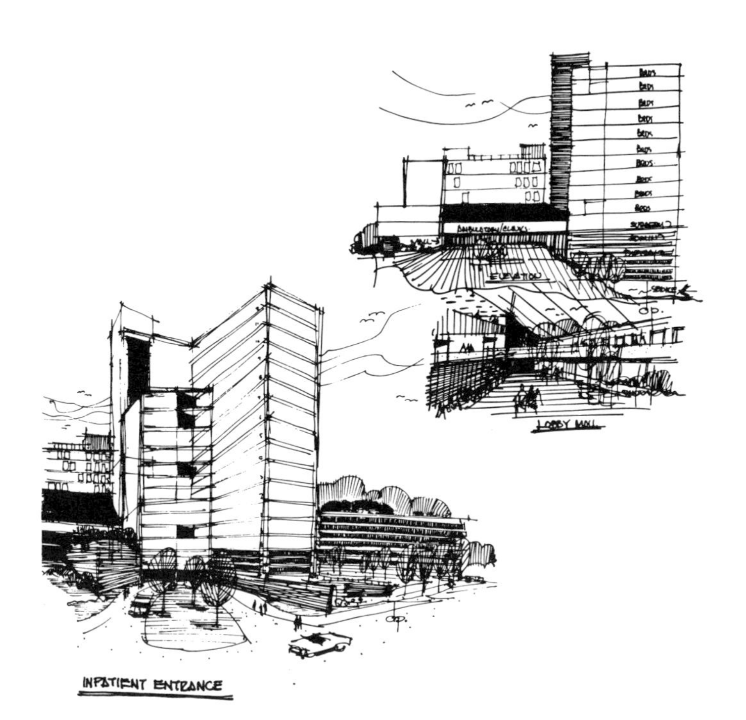

GOOD SAMARITAN HOSPITAL

CINCINNATI OHIO

FACILITY MASTER PLAN

DAVID R. PORTER -CONSULTING ARCHITECT

Robert E. von Otto consulting engineer
Gallagher/Craig&Assoc. architects
OConner and Engel&Assoc. engineers

MASTER SITE PLAN

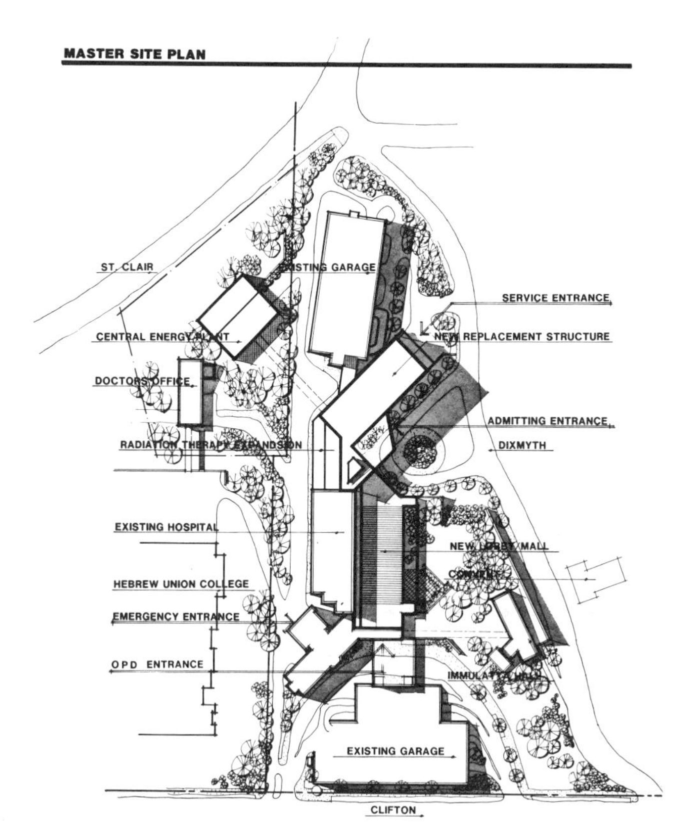

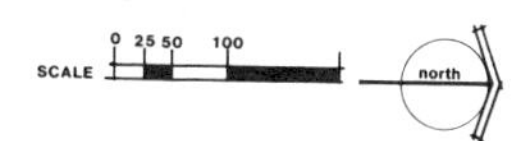

GOOD SAMARITAN HOSPITAL

CINCINNATI OHIO

FACILITY MASTER PLAN

DAVID R. PORTER -CONSULTING ARCHITECT

Robert E. von Otto consulting engineer
Gallagher/Craig&Assoc. architects
OConner and Engel&Assoc. engineers

PHASING PLAN

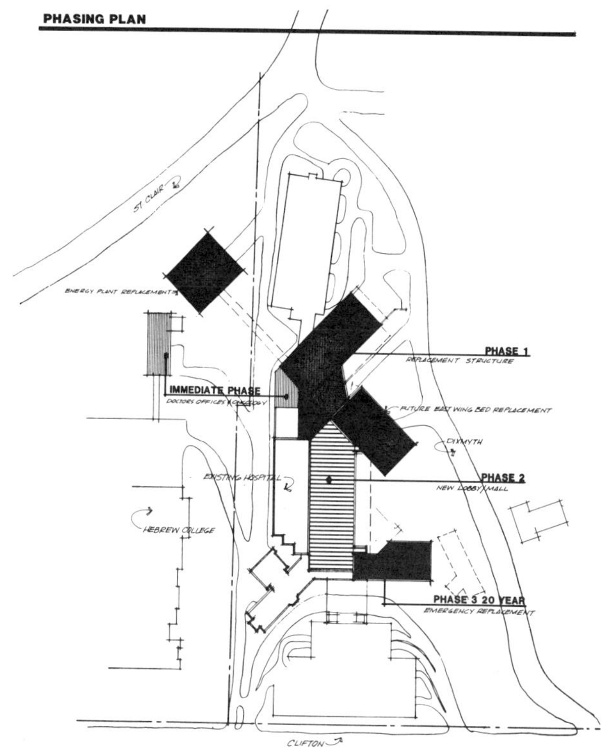

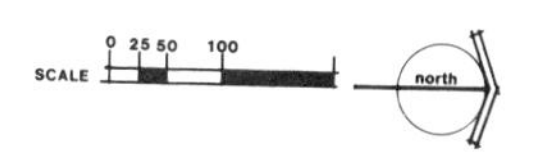

GOOD SAMARITAN HOSPITAL

CINCINNATI OHIO

FACILITY MASTER PLAN

DAVID R. PORTER -CONSULTING ARCHITECT

Robert E. von Otto consulting engineer
Gallagher/Craig&Assoc. architects
OConner and Engel&Assoc. engineers

plans; it defines the hospital's goals for the future. The financial portion of this plan is conceptual; it estimates what can be done. Although this plan is often referred to as the master plan or long-range plan, it amounts to a projection of goals, not specific plans for development.

FACILITY MASTER PLAN

The facility master plan covers the following areas:

—site analysis

—evaluation of the existing facility

—projection of facility needs

—profile of program and service utilization

—development of options

—recommended development scheme and an alternative

—energy plan based on an engineering study

— construction budget

—construction schedule

NEW BUILDING SECTION

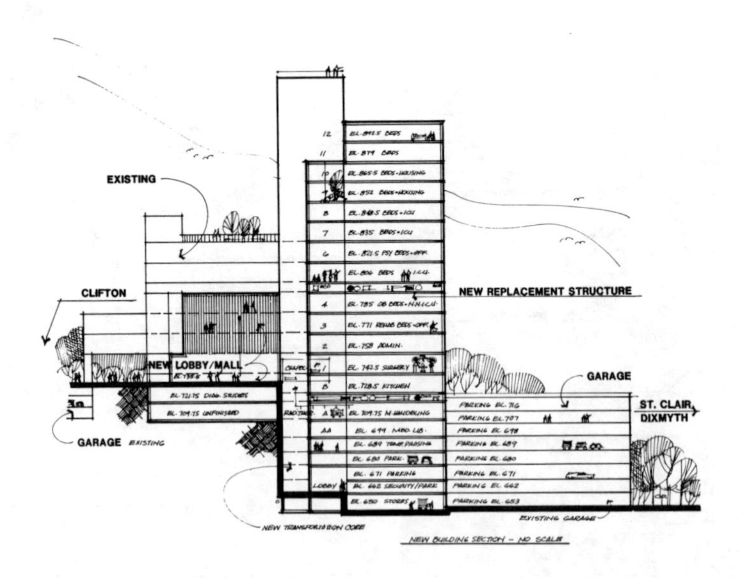

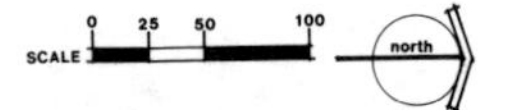

GOOD SAMARITAN HOSPITAL **CINCINNATI OHIO**

FACILITY MASTER PLAN

DAVID R. PORTER -CONSULTING ARCHITECT

Robert E. von Otto consulting engineer
Gallagher/Craig&Assoc. architects
OConner and Engel&Assoc. engineers

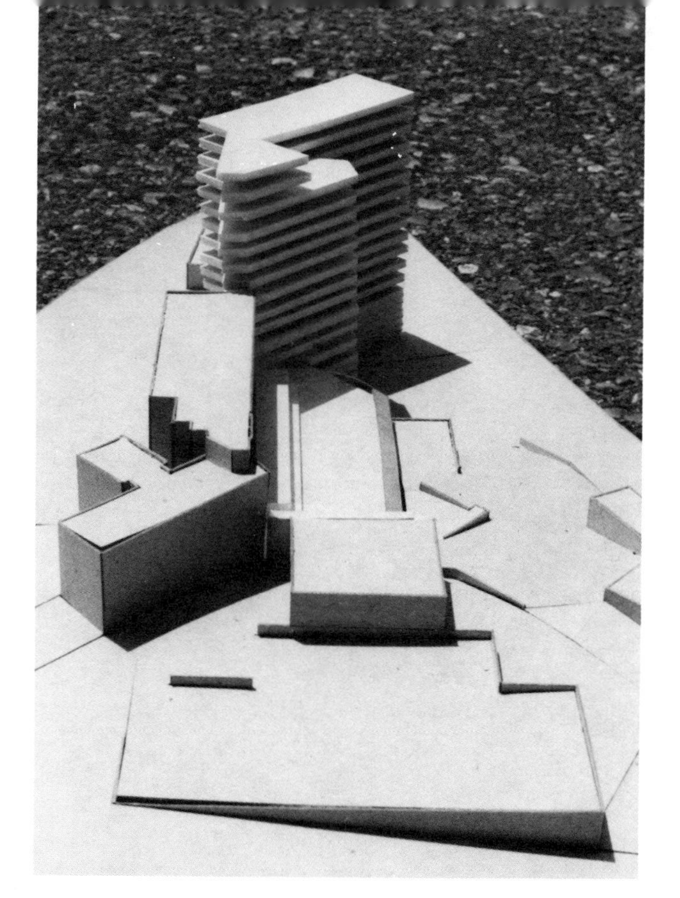

Models of existing and proposed structures.
Good Samaritan Hospital, Cincinnati, Ohio

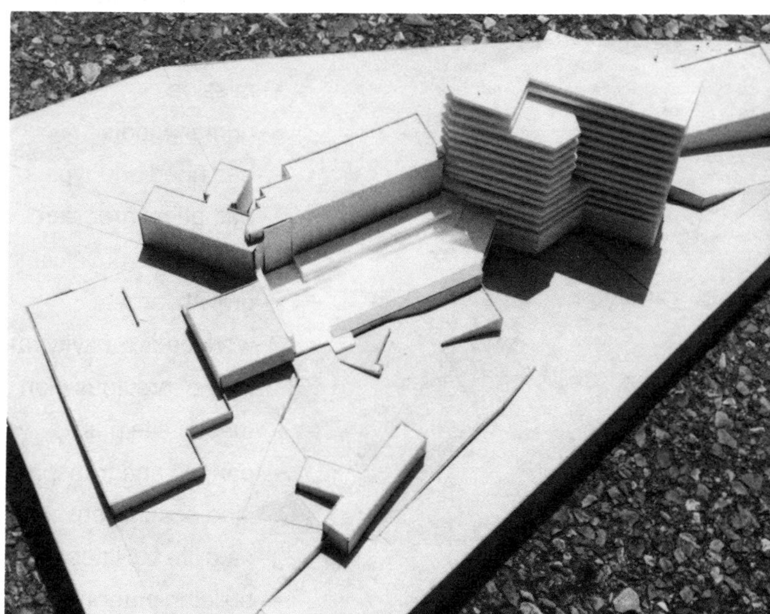

It combines program goals with site and facility needs in order to plan for several phases of construction, with a long-term facility plan of about twenty years. The facility master plan presents solutions to limitations caused by growth of programs and beds or by facility condition and age. This plan should take into account:

—the environmental character of the site and facility
—transportation and parking
—topography
—soil conditions
—building datum levels
—zoning
—building age and potential
—utilities
—energy usage and condition
—functional relationships
—space assignment
—staffing characteristics
—budget considerations

Such a plan provides a guide to all remodeling and future construction; it will be the document submitted to the planning and regulatory agencies.

The planning staff of the hospital can set up a committee which, together with consultants, will frame a statement of the hospital's role and goals. Such a statement should cover the following areas:

1) institutional roles
   —mission
   —primary goals
   —bed need and type
   —outpatient program
   —personnel (physicians and staff)
   —growth targets
   —workloads, activity ratios, and space requirements
2) review of previous plan
   —master site plan
   —parking and transportation needs
   —land acquisition
   —satellite facilities
   —building potential

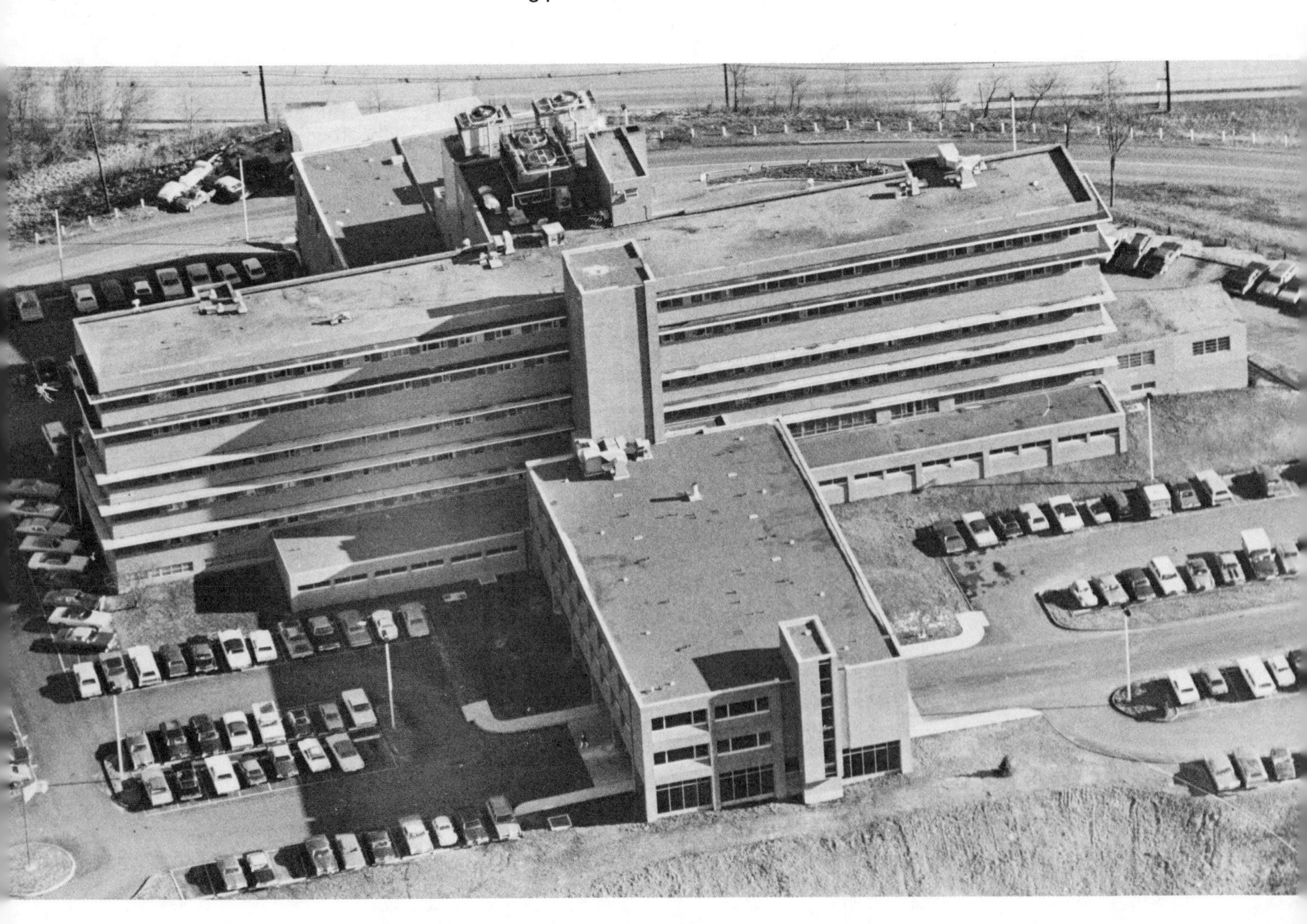

Aerial photo of existing facility.
St. Luke Hospital, Fort Thomas, Kentucky

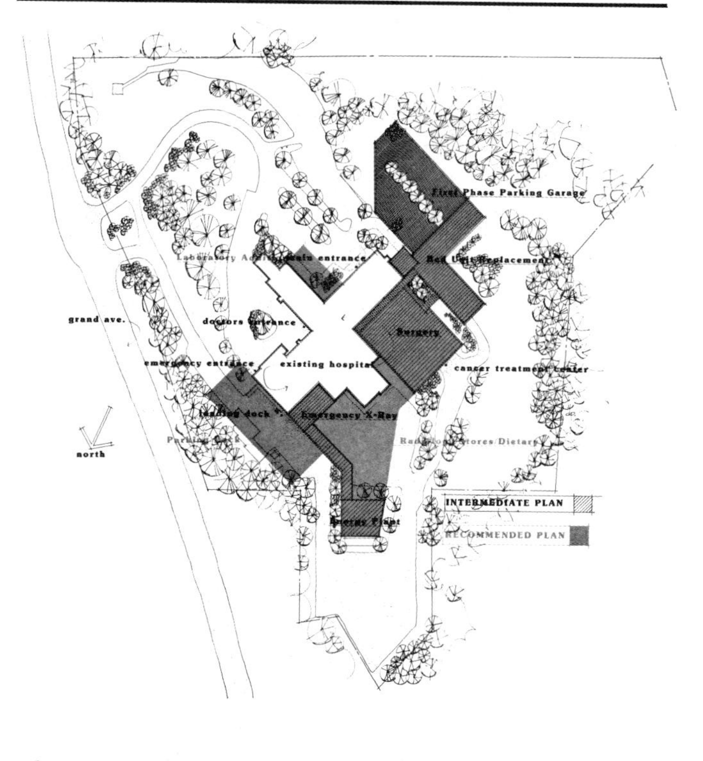

SCALE MODEL recommended phase

ST LUKE HOSPITAL
FORT THOMAS, KY
FACILITY MASTER PLAN
David R Porter - Consulting Architect
robert e von otto consulting engineer

3) regional and local regulations
 - —conformance to the code of the Joint Commission on the Accreditation of Hospitals
 - —institute-specific plan review by the HSA, if complete
 - —joint plans with nearby facilities

4) financial feasibility
 - —debt and borrowing potential
 - —building program potential

The facility master plan is a very effective tool for all physical planning and renovation. It indicates the most cost-effective way of constructing space for short-term needs. When a particular space decision is made, the hospital can see immediately what effect it will have on other departments. As goals and programs change, the master plan can be adjusted. It also predicts the need for beds, replacements, or service base adjustments and lets the HSA and other facilities know what to expect. The master plan aids in regional planning because it establishes the individual facility's markets and goals.

INSTITUTE-SPECIFIC PLAN

The institute-specific plan determines:

—market share of the planning region, defined as bed number and mix per thousand population assigned to specific hospitals

—projected utilization based upon admissions and length of stay (also included are rural, research, and teaching needs)

—site and building potential and limitations

The institute-specific plan was recommended by the Department of Health, Education, and Welfare (now the Department of Health and Human Services). It is designed to integrate the individual hospital's plans with those of other hosptials in the region. The number of hospital beds in the United States ranges from 2–5 persons per 1,000. This ratio cannot be standardized because different regions have different needs. Even the weather plays a role in bed need! The hospital must understand what possible impact this national effort can have on its plans, and be prepared to make voluntary bed adjustments.

One of the first institute-specific plans was developed for the HSA in Cincinnati. Mandell Bellmore built a computer model that defines market share by physician and consumer and by preference and county. This exciting model was reviewed by twenty-seven hospital facilities and the local hospital council. It was adjusted for differences in teaching utilization, and only nine bed exceptions (six rural and three research) were made to the model's projection of need for acute care beds. Part of the plan was directed at physical facility potential, in order to allow area hospitals to understand each others' limitations and potential. As the consulting architect, I was able to develop a rating method for physical and functional aspects of these facilities, building phasing potential, and site limitations. The potential of each of the twenty-seven hospitals was presented and approved. With the help of Bellmore's model, the region could see the twenty-year picture in construction planning and cost in relation to each hospital's bed needs. Each year the model will adjust to preferences in the market and pick up changes due to relocation and to primary, secondary, and tertiary movement.

Institute-specific plans should reduce political and consumer battles and allow sound planning to proceed.

Certificate of Need

The certificate of need, which is required by law for expenditures over $100,000–$150,000, outlines the reason a building project or funded program is needed, its probable costs, and its compliance with life safety and other codes. Much of this information is generated by the hospital when it draws up its long-range role and goals and its facility master plan. Most certificates of need cite better physical environment, patient demand, or competition for quality staff as reasons for a new program or building project.

The certificate-of-need application for equipment or physical additions must be defended in regard to projected utilization of services or beds based upon past need or actual cost of physical construction, and the ability of the facility to fund the project. The application consists of a program statement, the data presentation, the long-range goals and plan, the project plans and cost, and a financial plan. Also required are supporting documents from surrounding facilities that could be affected, coordination with the regional agency, and the published health plan.

Certificates-of-need for mergers or for tax-exempt hospitals require specific expertise in the health care field. If the objective is increased third-party reimbursement or minimum asset exposure in the event of a malpractice suit, legal counsel must also be involved. A consultant should be chosen on the basis of his experience, an interview, and discussions with previous clients.

Certificate-of-need laws have been adopted by most states, but the procedures differ. Texas has established a statewide jury-type planning system that is controlled by a judge who is not subject to pressure. The system seems to minimize time, but it is unique in the United States. Most certificates of need are submitted to regional health systems agencies. The certificates of need pass through a local committee process and hearing, an HSA staff review and recommendation, and the HSA governing board process. State approval is required next, plus a possible glance from HHS. This long process is routine, and each step must be planned for. Many biases will be tried and tested, and politics will tend to enter in. The escalation of a project's cost during this time must be anticipated. One definition of a five-year plan is, "Start today and it will take five years to occupy."

Recent amendments to the planning law, such as the Satterfield Amendment, have attempted to clear up the process by defining what policies should be applied to which applications. Too many times in the past bed reduction or hospital board makeup has been used to pressure building applications into not dealing with those subjects. In the long run, the trauma of planning is costly for the patient; all improvement should reduce political differences and implement sound needs.

A professional in-house staff and national consulting expertise are necessary in certificate-of-need applications. The cost of such personnel is less than the cost of "reinventing the wheel" each time.

Operational Planning

Operational planning determines current and projected space needs within a facility and is necessary for certificate-of-need documentation; it is the written program for an architectural project. It also takes a look at service utilization and program concepts based upon current and projected inpatient and outpatient markets. Past and present ratios of procedures per gross square foot of space are studied, projected, and compared with national guidelines. Where government guidelines may suggest a ratio of 40 to 50 tests per gross square foot, a hospital with an automated clinical laboratory may actually perform up to 100 tests per gross square foot. Staff limitations or demands for teaching can also affect these guidelines dramatically.

Operational planning studies establish a department-by-department description of needed space ratios outlining the number and type of surgeries, X-ray rooms, and outpatient services.

In the early 1970's, the National Bureau of Standards tried to formulate a typical nursing floor layout in terms of staff mix, patient care concepts, and automated materials. Patient preference varied too greatly for such standardization. Any size of nursing unit (300–600 square feet per bed) may serve best in a given situation, and no typical layout can adjust to all needs. Patient mix by service or by illness, type of energy required, staff availability, and various communications concepts can completely change a design. Each department (see Chapters VIII-XI) refers to such operational data as "planning guidelines." This information, in descriptive form, makes up the operational program.

Both health care consultants and consulting architects offer operational planning services; the planning can also be performed in-house.

Functional Planning

The health care consultant or consulting architect should *not* dictate room-by-room square footage. Operational planning comes first and defines *major* needs. The operation plan is then developed into a functional plan, which lists every room and suggests net sizes for major rooms as well as total department size.

The key to functional planning is not just a room list, but understanding that travel and adjacencies will affect operational costs for the life of the facility. The initial cost of the building is insignificant compared to the cost of running and staffing it over twenty years, sometimes eighteen to twenty times the initial cost. Therefore, no one can set the exact room sizes until concepts of space engineering and travel patterns are developed.

The architect develops cost limits per gross square footage based upon construction cost goals and program needs. The exact functions will change size depending upon column layouts, mechanical shafts, exit requirements, code standards, and space design. The essential control of functional planning is gross space. Individual functions are best listed by physical position such as number of people waiting, desk positions (based upon number of staff), and patient-staff-visitor separation and movement.

An approved functional plan is required to set construction cost, to allow the architect to proceed with the design of the building, and to assure the administrator of an approved document in case of in-house staff changes.

Materials Management Study

The cost-savings of automated materials-management systems are based upon a life-cycle analysis of manual labor versus labor time saved. A study on this issue should be contained in the long-range plan or facility master plan.

The detailed design of a materials-handling system is a composite of trips, tImes, and amounts to be automated through a physical structure. This process must be included in the design contract and should be performed by an independent consultant working with the architect or by the architect working with various manufacturers. Most manufacturers offer consulting contracts on a fee basis as part of the design effort.

Staffing Study

Personnel costs are a fact of life in this labor intensive industry. A good study of staffing can allow the facility to plan the most appropriate staffing patterns for its needs. Nursing time, mix, and management are very important in computing cost of care per patient. Various communications and paper-handling systems can affect staffing pattern and location. Each method should be studied and its state of the art investigated. Progressive management and productivity can be overstated, but staff cost greatly affects all budgets and should be given due attention. Staff planning requires a combination of the skills and knowledge of facility administration and a management consultant. It may be best performed in-house.

Equipment Planning

The planning and design of fixed equipment (that is, equipment built in to a hospital facility) is the architect's responsibility. Movable equipment (that is, equipment replaced, moved from existing locations, or simply portable equipment) is not typically the architect's responsibility, but it could be added to his work, and to his fee. Most architects recommend an equipment consultant for this service. The consultant would program, list, and specify movable items in each room during the design stage. Working closely with the architect, he would test the space needed for each item of equipment requested by the staff. This allows for full coordination of the required mechanical and electrical services, counter or floor space, and proper functioning at the bench or table level.

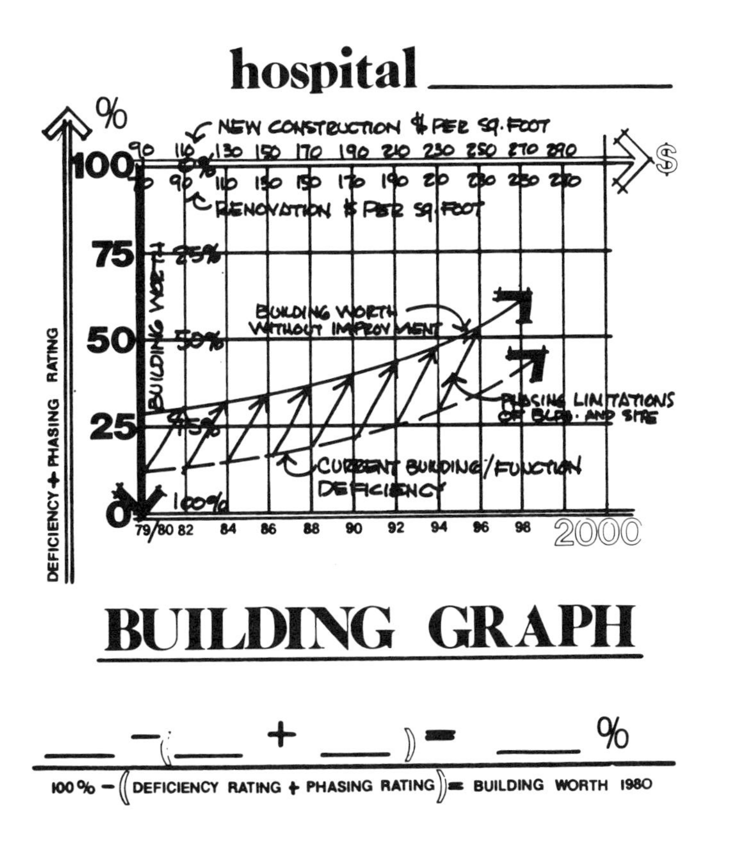

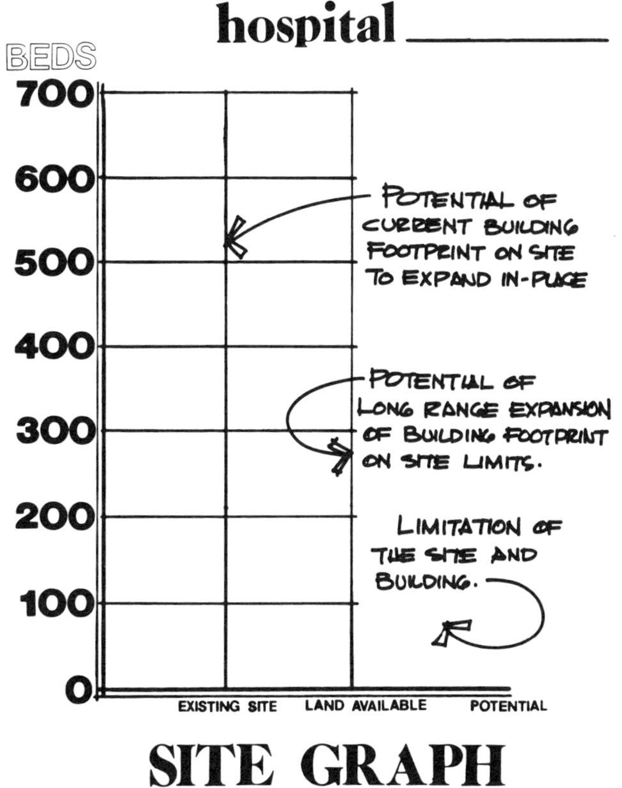

The equipment consultant deals with technical medical equipment. In contracts, the interior designer deals with furniture and accessories (see Chapter XII.) This medical equipment accounts for 10 to 15 percent of the construction cost.

Typical equipment planning includes:

—familiarization with the project
—operational analysis
— definition of material flow networks
—interviews with clients
—analysis of existing resources
—preliminary lists of equipment
—equipment workbooks
—revised list of equipment
—layout of movable equipment
—technical specifications
—bidding, procurement, and placement

Financial Feasibility Study

Major accounting firms (the "Big Eight") make financial feasibility studies their business. Experts in the hospital field know financing mechanisms and their application to a specific project. Because of the fact that a legal responsibility is assumed in the financial market, the best consultant often saves the most in time and cost. More sophistication is needed by individual facilities in this critical area. The future of even the best developed certificates of need and planning hinges on the cost picture. An aggressive and accurate financial plan is required for every project from the outset. This study determines the institution's debt capacity to fund a project and recommends the funding mechanisms available at the current and projected money market.

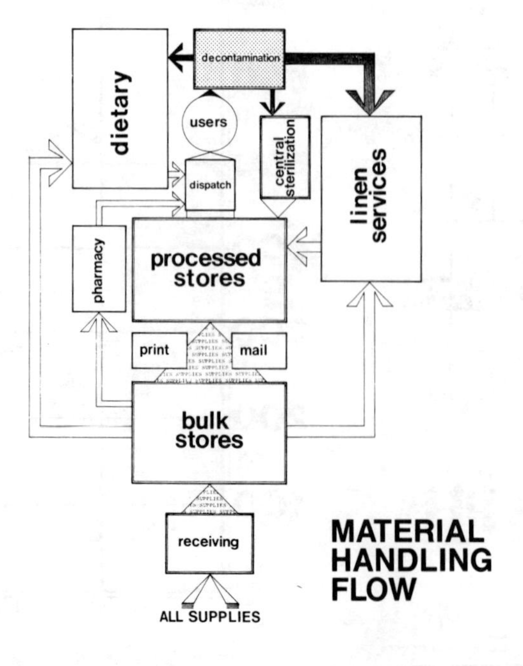

MATERIAL HANDLING FLOW

II

the design team

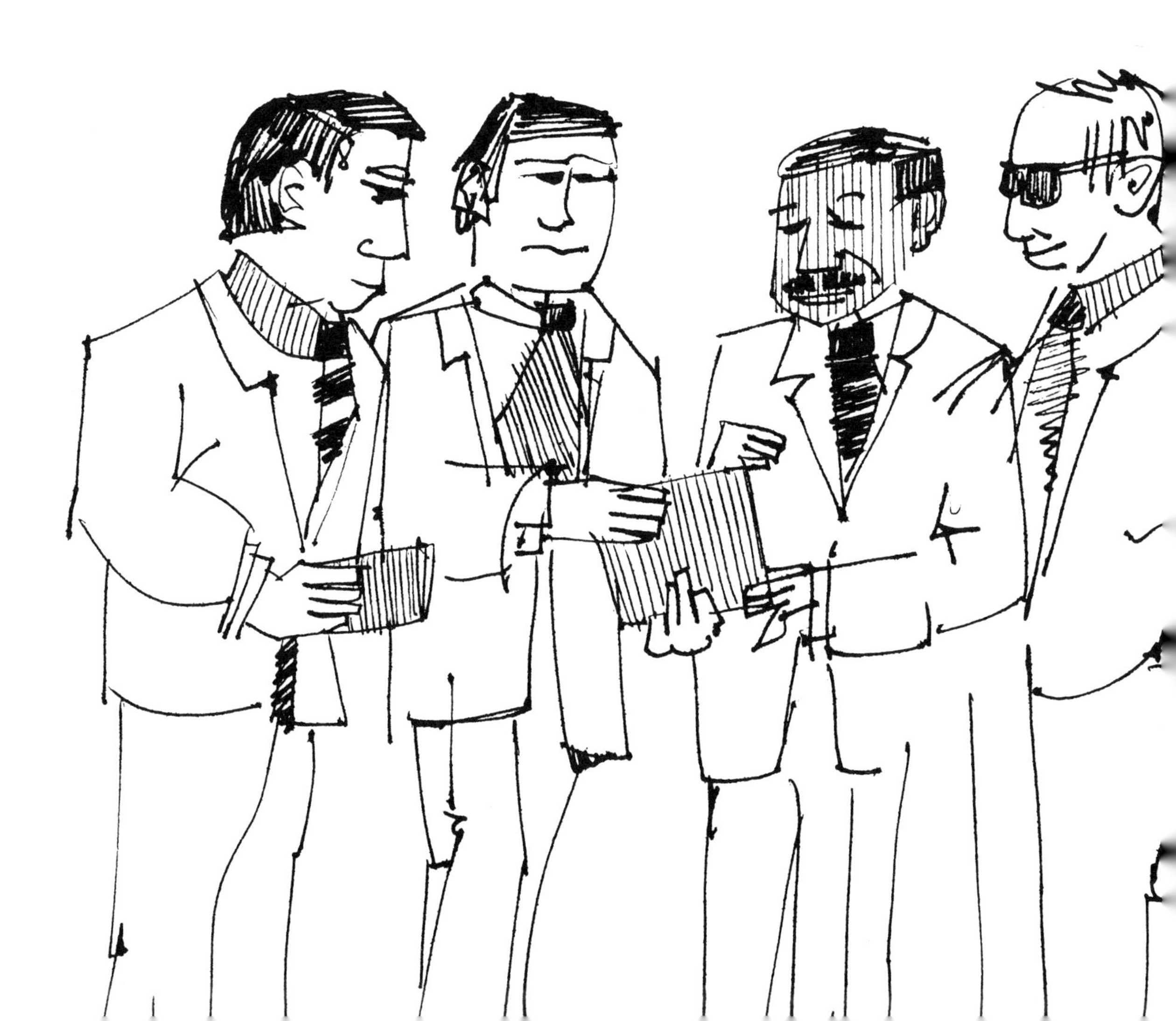

It has become impossible for the hospital administrator to deal with the government bureaucracy without expert advice. Consultants can be hired for special studies on every aspect of the hospital, from setting up a pharmacy to coping with multiple codes.

Regional planning is an excellent concept, and a local planning agency can be highly beneficial to the goals of its family of hospitals. The role each facility plays in the service area, state, region, and nation should be evaluated so that each facility is strong and unique. The hospital's medical and professional staff and administration are responsible for the needs of the people they serve. The degree to which needs are met is a function of the experience, ideas, organization, and age mix of these groups of people. The consultant draws on the expertise of people in every area of the hospital and combines this expertise with his own to come up with a plan for implementing the hospital's regional role. The consultant's recommendations focus on the total operational future of the facility, including service area market financial future, projected staff specialties, bylaw makeup, service sharing, and program projection. The consultant acts in many capacities, but his most important function is to provide an independent professional opinion and plan based on an unbiased look at the total operation. Therefore, the consultant is usually retained to develop a long-range plan.

The role of the hospital consultant and consulting architect in design and construction is that of a programmer. Once the facility's role in the community has been established, the operational and functional plans must be established. They should be based on department utilization projections and compared to national standards (see Chapter I). The consultant relates the needs and requests of the administrator and the department heads to innovations and operations that they may not be aware of.

Consultants are nationally organized, but work on individual studies commissioned by the hospitals. Fees are not regulated, and the cost of the long-range plan will vary depending on the scope of services. The size of an independent consulting firm's staff can vary from one person to thirty. Many major corporations and accounting firms are also acting as health care consultants.

Consulting fees used to be based on a percentage of construction costs; services can include role and program planning, medical staff analysis, fixed equipment recommendations, materials-handling concepts, departmental operation and staffing, and functional programming. Because of the increased sophistication in each of these subjects, and the practice of bidding professional fees as a lump sum, or price, the fee is now based upon number of hours, with full accounting backup. On a federal project, even profit is controlled with a strict auditing procedure.

Administrators may need multiple consulting and building design services at every stage of planning. Because of the amount of government control and review, as well as the very sophisticated competition for every bed, service, and cost, the hospital itself is now involved in planning. Full-time architects, health care planners, professional engineers, and market planners have become common on the hospital staff. The federal systems, such as the Veterans Administration, the National Institutes of Health, and the Department of Health and Human Services, have employed architects, engineers, and planners for years, and the larger hospitals have always needed planners on their staff. Ongoing professional engineering management contracts are also a current trend.

Hospitals still depend on outside consultants for some studies. Further, few hospitals produce their own architectural and engineering plans for new buildings and major renovations. This is also a highly developed specialty and is needed only a few times in the facility's history.

Sorting out what consulting is needed and how much of it can be done in-house is a difficult task. The various consulting and consulting architecture services described below are only the major ones available to the administrator. There is, however, an expert consultant for any subject one can think of.

General Manager
Director of Operations
Principal Designer
Principal-In-Charge
Project Manager
Project Designer
Job Captain
Site/Civil
Architectural
Mechanical
Structural
Electrical
Programming
Construction
Estimating
Interiors
Graphics
Specifications
Quality Control

Flow of project

ARCHITECTS AND ENGINEERS

It is well established that everyone is an architect, but that a professional must be hired to assume the liabilities!

The architect is the leader of the design team. As such, he must listen and evaluate the needs and desires of all parties in the hospital. He must formulate shapes, sizes, and materials that will meet the dreams of the client, the government, and, most important, the patient.

The hospital normally selects its architect through an interview procedure or by commissioning an architect who has performed satisfactory work in the past. Schedules that define reasonable fees for certain classifications of project type and volume are published. This includes all basic services, plus total engineering.

Architects

Architects usually earn their Bachelor of Architecture degree in a five-year university curriculum. Their training is based on a combination of mathematics and art. Besides standard course work in English, social studies, and science, the architect concentrates on a design sequence that outlines the theory, history, and detail of architectural design and concept. Because of his training in art and engineering, the architect emerges as a social designer, able to deal with the needs of animals, vegetables, and human beings. There are many specialties that architects can pursue. The hospital architect may be a specialist, but his design tasks include everything from animal runs to helicopter pads.

Architects' offices range from one or two to 300 or 400 employees. Some firms that include in-house engineers may employ up to 1,000 persons. Major firms often contain interior design departments, equipment consultants, construction management groups and so on.

The following four types of architectural firms are involved with health care:

1) *Engineering architect*. These firms are usually managed by engineers and offer a full scope of services. They compete at a high level and produce excellent functional buildings with an emphasis on systems management and technical detail.
2) *Design-build architect*. The design-build firm takes a project from design to finished construction, carrying out most of the engineering in-house. The fees of such firms seem lower, but are equal when compared to the combined designing, engineering, and general contracting.
3) *Local architect*. The size of a firm does not indicate its quality: the actual team from a large firm working on a major facility may only number eight to ten architects and an equal number of engineers. Local firms vary in size and earn 10–80 percent of their commissions in health care. Engineering may be done in-house or by a consultant. The practice of joint-venturing with a nationally recognized architectural firm is also common because the "prime" firm may not have much experience in health care projects.

4) *Design architects—national and international*. The national firm has either many offices throughout the country or a home base and only a few regional offices. Its health design expertise includes master planning, layout, equipment, and programming for projects ranging from university medical center planning to rural primary care centers.

(I do not prefer any particular type of firm; I have been a principal, owner, and manager in all four.)

Although architects must take a national registration examination, each state has its own licensing requirements. The architect and engineer must have this state license because of the effect that design has on public safety. Incorporation is allowed in the architectural profession, but it does not limit the liability of the individual architect. Each firm carries error and omission liability insurance to protect it in case of legal action. Error and omission is defined in each separate action, but it can be summed up as follows: "If an item is left out of the construction for any reason, then the owner has never paid for it and it should be added at his expense. If an item is installed in the construction correctly as specified and does not physically work, then the architect or engineer has erred." There are, as might be expected, many variations on this rule.

Another commonly misunderstood legal aspect of the contract should be mentioned: if the owner specifies a top dollar amount to be spent in construction, the architect shall be permitted to determine what materials, equipment, component systems, and types of construction are to be included and may adjust the scope of the project to bring it within that limit. This means that the architect must advise against, and possibly refuse, any unreasonable cost items or disproportionate program elements. This is very difficult for an architect to do since the emphasis in the project is always on what will benefit the owner.

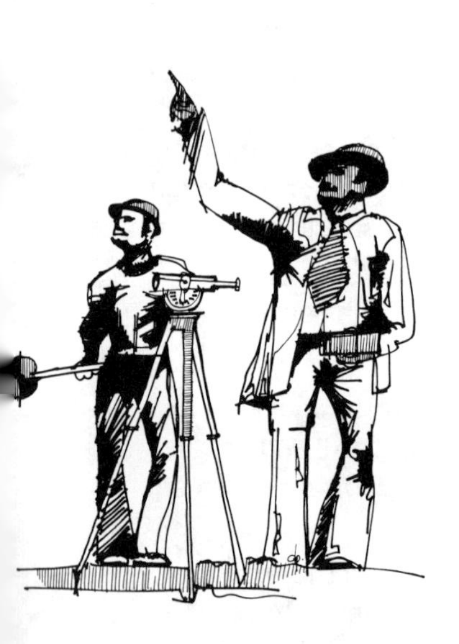

The architect, then, has a very complex role, acting as judge, artist, businessman, lawyer, accountant, and patient.

Selecting the Architect. The interview process is difficult and tiring. The list may start with ten firms and be shortened to a selected few. The selection committee may sit through four presentations a night, hearing equally good demonstrations of expertise. I have interviewed architectural firms as a city councilman and as a consultant to hospital boards, so I know the process can be grueling.

The following areas may help narrow the choice:

1) Find out which member of the firm will handle the job and evaluate his or her responses. You will be working closely with this person for years, and this is the key to a firm's selection.
2) Study the proposed team and its organization's appearance. Ask about the engineers' experiences and request a reference of complete work.
3) Check the firm's references.

4) Explain your needs and the goals of your project, such as design excellence, mechanical systems, and functional concerns, and ask questions as to how these can be met for your facility.
5) Relate the fee quoted to the larger cost of construction and efficient operation of the facility. Do not pick the lowest fee just because it is low. Once a fee is verbalized, it greatly influences a committee. However, this fee amounts to only 6–8 percent of the total amount you will spend for construction; money is not saved if the building operation does not work. Each 1-½ years of operations will cost as much as the initial construction. It is important to *trust* in your selection.

Engineers

By definition, engineers apply the physical laws of science for the benefit of mankind. The scope of engineering work is enlarged by the scientist's increasing understanding of our physical world.

Civil Engineers. Historically, engineers who worked on non-military projects became known as civil engineers. Three main divisions of civil engineering exist today.

1) Transportation, whether by land (including railroads, highways, and rapid transit), water (including canals, port and harbor improvements, and improvements to navigation such as lighthouses), or air (airports)
2) Structures, including buildings and bridges
3) Sanitation, including the collection, treatment, and distribution of potable water, as well as the collection, treatment, and disposal of waste water such as storm water and polluted water

Civil engineers contribute their talents to hospital construction in three areas:

(i)—site planning

(ii)—structural design

(iii)—construction

Site planning is the art and science of arranging the uses of land. The site planner designates these uses in detail by selecting and analyzing a site, forming a land-use plan, organizing vehicular and pedestrian traffic, developing a visual form and materials concept, readjusting the existing landform by design grading, providing proper drainage, and, finally, developing the construction details necessary to carry out the project. Although he may determine the overall uses of a site, this is not always the case. The site planner, does, however, arrange to accommodate the activities the client has specified. These components must relate to each other, to the

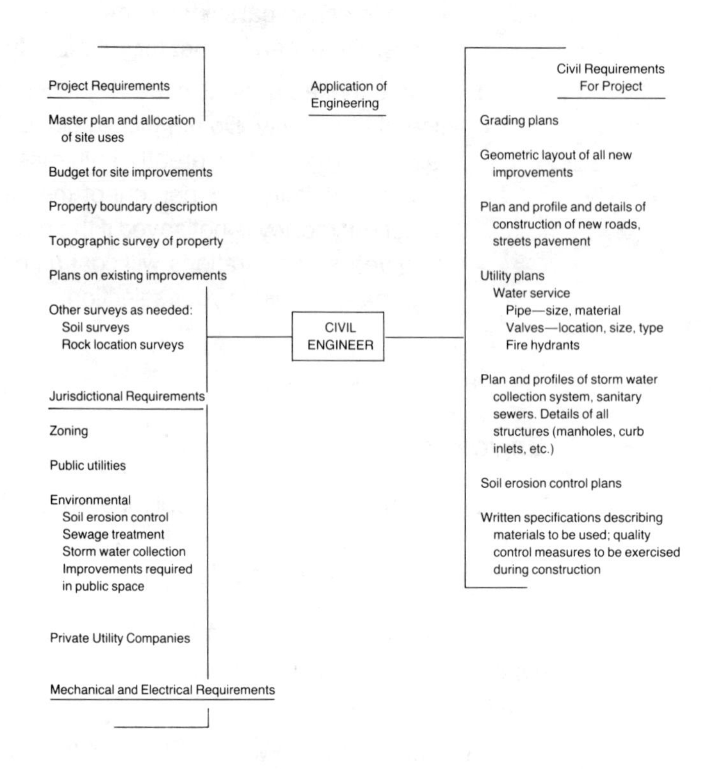

site, and to structures and activities on adjacent sites for, whether the site is large or small, it must be viewed as part ot the total environment. Site planning is done professionally by landscape and other architects, planners, and engineers.

Structural design of buildings involves determining how the entire building and its parts are to resist the loads to which they will be subjected, and communicating this information to the builder.

Civil engineers are leaders in the construction industry. The construction contractor's work will probably be under the control of a civil engineer employed by the contractor. (Since this book deals primarily with the design of hospital facilities, I will not elaborate on the civil engineer's construction role.)

Civil engineers have earned a Bachelor of Science degree in civil engineering and may have earned advanced degrees in one of its specialties. Engineers who design facilities to be used by the public are required to be registered by the state in which they practice. Requirements for registration vary, but typically include the bachelor's degree or equivalent experience (generally four or five years of design responsibility) and successful completion of a written examination. The engineer responsible for the preparation of drawings describing construction requirements must place his seal of registration on them. Registered engineers are referred to as "professional engineers" and use the initials "P.E." after their names.

How is the civil engineer's work done, and how can he help the hospital administrator optimize the facilities being designed? Regardless of who allocates the available space for buildings, access roads, parking, and open space, the location and design of features outside the building is vital to their function. The role of the civil engineer in the site-planning process is frequently to define precisely the location of all new features and to design new roads, parking, and water and drainage utilities. The hospital administrator should provide information from the master plan with regard to allocation of site uses and economic constraints. He is usually called upon to provide plans showing existing site improvements, property boundary description, topographic survey, and any other special surveys dictated by a particular site.

In developing the site plans, the engineer applies good practice to the requirements of the hospital, architect, jurisdiction, private utilities, and other engineering disciplines. He will want to balance the earthwork so there will be no need to haul earth to or from the site. He will design drainage so that normal flows are self-cleaning. The materials he specifies will be compatible with those already in use, to minimize maintenance. His solutions will be aimed at long-run economy, considering first cost, maintenance costs, and operating costs.

Frequently, the budget for new construction will not allow the higher first costs that design for long-run economy dictates. In this event, it is incumbent upon the engineer to present alternatives and their relative costs so an intelligent decision can be made. For example, paving is a significant part of site development cost that is often compromised. Anticipated traffic loading, soil and weather conditions may indicate the need for a total pavement thickness of ten inches, but only eight inches can be purchased with the money available for construction. The engineer may advise that maintenance costs will be significantly higher with eight-inch pavement, and that two inches of pavement will be required after several years' use anyway. Thus, the cost of paving could be much higher if only eight inches are originally constructed.

The engineer's work is not completed once the construction contractor is selected. The engineer must then represent the owner to see that the work required by the contract is furnished both in quantity and quality. Independent testing laboratories are required to run various on-site tests of the work to evaluate its quality. Sometimes the engineer may carry out these tests himself, but usually the contractor is required to furnish them. He may obtain them on a least-cost basis. Although this arrangement may be satisfactory, I think it is preferable for testing to be done by an independent laboratory, paid directly by the hospital, in order to avoid possible conflicts of interest.

Structural Engineers. The structural engineer's role is that of providing the optimum support for the building. On any large building project, several structural engineers and draftsmen may work under the direction of the structural engineer primarily responsible for the work. Coordinating structural work with the architect and other engineers is absolutely essential in hospital projects. The structural engineer, like any other professional, must keep himself informed on the latest technology in order to render the best service to his clients.

How does the structural engineer work? With increasing frequency, engineers are turning to computers for help. A mathematical model of a proposed building can be described to a computer, various loading conditions can be applied, and the computer will indicate changes that need to be made. The speed of the computer allows for a greater number of preliminary investigations. For all the advantages of computers, however, the structural engineer must still decide on the structural system to be used.

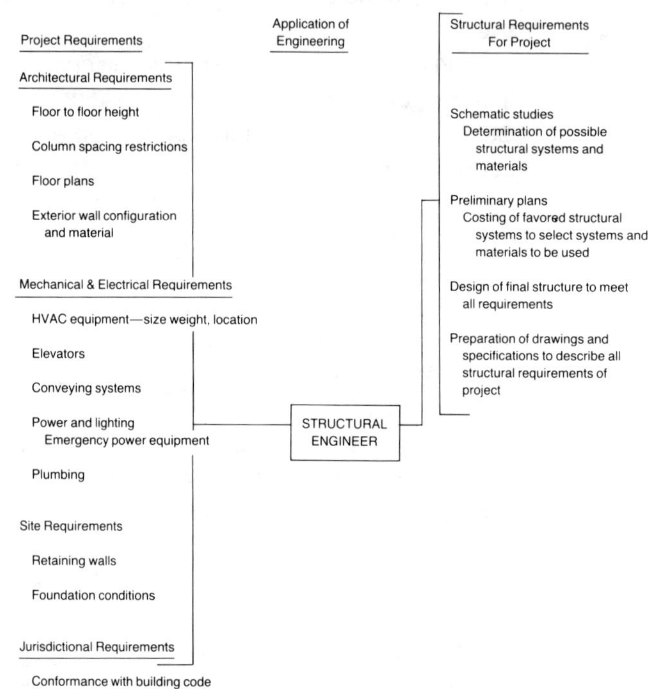

A scientific approach is employed by the engineer. First, all structural systems that meet the major requirements of the project are considered. The question of frame versus bearing wall system will probably be resolved at this point. Assuming that a frame system is indicated, the structural engineer, with the architect, then determines the column pattern that will suit the architectural requirements. Using this pattern, studies are made, with or without computer assistance, to suggest the most economical framing schemes utilizing structural steel and reinforced concrete. Preliminary plans are drawn up for these schemes so that costs can be determined. The most economical one is then selected. It is in this preliminary stage of design that the structural engineer can effect the most savings.

The supporting capability of the soil on which the building will rest is a principal factor in determining the structural system to be used and the cost of foundations. The structural engineer will advise that a soils engineer be engaged to conduct a boring and testing program and recommend the most suitable type of foundation. A skillful soils engineer may save thousands of dollars in unnecessary foundation cost.

Once the structural system has been selected, the engineer designs the building in detail, working from the top down. The design of structures is something of a chicken-and-egg problem. Given the same loading, the size and method of attachment of members in a frame has a significant effect on the load each individual member carries. Conversely, the size and method of attachment of an individual member in a frame is a function of its individual loading. Consequently, framing members are sized (based on assumed loading), the method of attachment is determined, and the frame is analyzed to check the assumed loading. Changes are made when necessary. This trial and error approach is simplified greatly by accurate judgment in the selection of original member sizes and attachments.

All of the structural engineer's judgment, design, and analysis is of little value until it is communicated by drawings and specifications. Clear, neat, and complete drawings and specifications have a beneficial effect on the cost of construction by lowering the risks of construction contractor error.

Being certain that the owner gets the quantity and quality in construction that he pays for is the reason for inspections and testing during construction. Daily inspection of a large project is desirable. It may be available from the construction manager, an inspector may be hired by the owner, or the architect or engineer may be hired to provide this service. In any case, both the architect and the engineer need to be on the job to review construction with the contractor and inspectors to make certain that the requirements of the contract are being met, to provide interpretation of their plans and specifications when required, and to provide direction when changed conditions are encountered or when the owner desires changes not included in the contract.

Mechanical and Electrical Engineers. The task of the mechanical engineer is to study the conservation of energy and apply it in the most efficient and economical way. The plumbing engineer is responsible for the processed water and the liquid waste of the entire structure. The electric power designer must be aware of the public utility supply and rates so that an economical power distribution and an emergency supply is obtained. A lighting designer is a key member of an engineering staff since he enhances all spaces through lighting and affects the mood and correct optical levels of the entire hospital staff. Let us review some of the problems that face mechanical engineers as the basic structure is being designed.

A building or a space is a thermal container. Within it an air-conditioned environment for human comfort is to be maintained, regardless of season or climate. Thermal considerations in the construction of a building shell include:

—thin panel versus massive wall

—insulation and glass and wall shading

—partial versus total glazing

—double glazing

—roof construction

All of these constitute the outdoor design conditions. These factors, along with the internal space load of lights, motors, people and special heat-producing equipment (such as sterilizers and hot plates) are required to calculate the air-conditioning load. It must be emphasized that an estimate of the actual cooling–heating load is essential before an air-conditioning system and equipment are selected. Knowledge of advances in the technology of solar space conditioning, recycled waste, total energy generation, and alternative fuels is the responsibility of the modern engineer. Since half the cost of a building is spent on engineering system construction, it is vital to apply life-cycle analysis and value management and engineering concept.

Each hospital presents a unique problem. There is no universal solution to the selection of a system even after the problem is defined, the physical circumstances evaluated, and the actual load of heating and cooling requirements established. The engineer must have an appreciation of the structure, its thermal capacity behavior, and the capabilities of the contemplated system. He must fully understand the interaction of the space with external and internal thermal loads and select a system that will effectively cancel these loads. It should be mutually agreed by all concerned that the equipment installed, the control of the system, and the building must be integrated in order to be successful.

After having established the requirements for blending the air-conditioning system into the basic structure, the architect-engineer team must consider the thermal load. They must devise a structure that is architecturally and acoustically acceptable and pleasing, and that incorporates all possible forethought to minimize the air conditioning load. Orienting the building in regard to sunlight and shade is essential. Heat gained from the sun through 150 square feet of unshaded glass facing west is 12,000 Btu (requiring one ton of cooling) as against 1200 Btu (requiring .10 ton of cooling) for 150 square feet of unshaded glass facing north. The total thermal load has a bearing on the space required for air-conditioning equipment and for transmission and distribution of the heating-cooling medium.

Systems Building. The objective of systems building is to lower cost by standardizing mechanical, electrical, and structural systems in a way that reduces on-site labor costs. Such systems are particularly effective where a large number of repetitive spaces are needed, for example, in schools, apartments, and offices. The integration of mechanical, electrical, and structural systems requires the involvement of the manufacturer in design. These integrated systems become building blocks. A variety of sizes of buildings can be constructed simply be changing the number and arrangement of the blocks.

Systems building might be applied to the repetitive portions of a hospital, such as the typical patient rooms, but the present state of the art makes them less practical for most other areas of the hospital.

The professional mechanical and electrical engineer is trained, during his formal education, in many types of engineering studies, from space to underseas design. A young engineer will specialize in a field and, once he has graduated, develop his expertise. Building systems engineering involves both a mechanical and electrical specialty and can be further broken down into the following areas:

—heating, ventiliation and air conditioning

—plumbing and process piping

—energy application

—control monitoring systems

—communications

—electric power distribution

—electric lighting design

Setting Fees and Bidding

The basic percentage fee is based on the total construction cost of a project; it is higher if the project is smaller, because major services are the same for any size project. Over the past years, percentage fees have not risen along with the cost of living index because they are adjusted by a percentage applied to an escalating construction cost index.

A fixed fee, or per diem fee, is also common to the profession, and is usually based on an hourly rate of $20–$100, depending on the status of the individual working on the project.

In the early 1970s, Maryland began bidding architects' and engineers' fees as a lump sum price. This price is based on a set of plans, or scope, that defines square footage and on a construction cost estimate. The architect calculates the number of hours necessary to complete the project and multiplies them by a direct cost loading factor, an overhead (general and administrative cost) loading factor, and a profit factor to obtain his lump sum price. Travel and related expenses may be directly reimbursable or included in the cost. This type of bidding violated the professional ethics of architects, but it is now widely used by government and private industry.

Competition has driven architectural and engineering fees down over the past few years by about 10–15 percent. The total fee seems enormous, but, if broken down by the duration of the project and by services included, the architect's profits are found to be similar to those of any other professional. Included in the architect's lump sum fee are the following:

—mechanical and electrical engineering

—structural engineering

—civil engineering and landscape design

—travel and printing cost

The American Institute of Architects' standard contract has been tried and tested over many years, and it defines well the basic services of an architect.

The two methods of obtaining a construction price are competitive bidding and negotiated bids. In competitive biddings the owner advertises for general construction prices (including mechanical, electrical, site, and architectural) or separate major work (general, mechanical, and electrical). Competitive bids are received and the lowest bid is awarded the contract. In the negotiated (or cost-plus-materials) bid, a single contractor is selected. He works to a budget, charging for his time, overhead, profit and materials.

VALUE MANAGEMENT

The newest member of the design team is the value manager. His role is to see that all other members of the design team are satisfied with their products in the structure, use, cost, and schedule. Generally, few members of the team are satisfied. Too often the client is heard to say, "Well, it is not really what I expected or what I wanted."

This condition of dissatisfaction is slowly changing with the help of value management and the value manager. The value manager creates circumstances during the design phase that result in a hospital that satisfies all members of the design team. He works methodically and continually to be sure that the knowledge and views of each member are heard and used even as the design is in process. He sees the client as a learner who, as time passes, increases his understanding of what he wants. The value manager ensures that these views are clarified and brought to the designer's attention in ways that the designer can respond to within the limits of schedule and budget. The designers are also learning that their latest and best notions can be used by the client only if he can understand their value for his hospital project.

How can one ensure that all information is communicated quickly, absorbed readily, and acted upon? By hiring a value manager. He ensures early continuing clarification of values, purposes, wants, and actions. The value manager performs the following functions:

—understanding the client's expectations

—understanding the constraints on the clients

—understanding the expectations and limitations of the architect, engineer, and construction manager

—helping the design team communicate their expectations and needs to one another

—helping the architect and engineer make changes and stay within schedule and budget

—monitoring and reporting issues that seem likely to delay design or cause dissatisfaction among members of the design team

—preparing and conducting special problem solving sessions to clarify values and objectives, improve design, maintain or lower total cost, maintain or shorten schedule, improve life cycle costs, and improve energy design and costs

—employing the methods and procedures of all problem-solving systems, including value engineering, value clarification, design-to-cost, Kepner-Tregoe, and Delphi

All of the value manager activities are intended to bring about the best possible value in design excellence, cost, and schedule.

Value management methodologies may be divided into five areas:

—information collection and interpretation

—problem identification

—alternative creation

—alternative selection

—implementation to the satisfaction of the design team

Information collection and interpretation methods include Delphi forecasting, descriptive surveys, interviews (both to teach and to learn), programmed group exchanges (value verification and clarification), and review of scope, criteria, drawings, and specifications. The aspirations of the client and designer are compared to expectations, and the understandings of each designer are presented to ensure that all members of the team keep the purposes and objectives of the others before them.

In identifying problems, the value manager uses the above methods as well as cost models, energy models, and checklists to highlight at the earliest stages those areas that can be handled before they become major problems in design excellence, cost, or schedule.

Special techniques are used to compare such things as square feet of usable space per patient, percent of interstitial space actually used for mechanical-electrical functions, floor to ceiling heights, structural design of similar structures in similar conditions, and transportation distances and time. Special procedures are also used to ease adaptation to new ideas from the client and from the architect and engineer. All things are reviewed from the standpoint that they can be done if . . . , rather than from the standpoint that they cannot be done because . . .

Those methodologies that are drawn from value engineering need special mention. Value engineering is a set of concepts and methods used to adjust designs to acquire the best total value. Using definition and analysis of function, value engineering is aimed at achieving the lowest total cost commensurate with design excellence. Specific methods include function analysis, brainstorming sessions, matrix comparisons, and analysis of life-cycle costs.

The value manager employs all of these methods and ensures that the work is thorough, successful, and in line with the wishes of the design team. He pays his way in the design team by facilitating cooperation and understanding and by identifying potential areas of delay, design problems, and cost improvements. He acts upon all of the above as approved by the design team.

For example, suppose a hospital design is budgeted for $40 million. The designer reports a year later that it will cost over $50 million to build. The value manager collects a team of mixed disciplines, including the architect and client representatives, and conducts a value engineering session. This follows an architectural review. Ways are found to bring the cost in line with needed functions without reducing the scope of the hospital.

The value manager is technical expert and as such is subordinate to the team. He is a manager, problem-solving leader, counselor, coordinator, and monitor. It is his job to make sure that all members of the design team are pleased with the result of their labors.

CONSTRUCTION MANAGEMENT

Construction management of hospital projects began in the 1960s. By now, approximately two-thirds of all projects include a constructions manager for saving time. The ideas that originated in construction for developers were applied to hospital projects and are now promoted in most government construction. For example, the practice of fast-tracking was first applied to speculative projects, such as apartment construction, in order to avoid price escalation. Fast-tracking involves beginning the foundation construction before the final building design is finished. It forced architects and engineers to complete their design and drawings before the total calculations and thought processes were concluded. Architects felt threatened because someone else now controlled their schedules and the process of design. Mechanical engineers could not accept design from the first floor up in order to offer advanced packages that might be built and bought sooner. The intended purpose of construction management had to be cleared up because negative attitudes were being formed between the construction manager, the architect and the engineer.

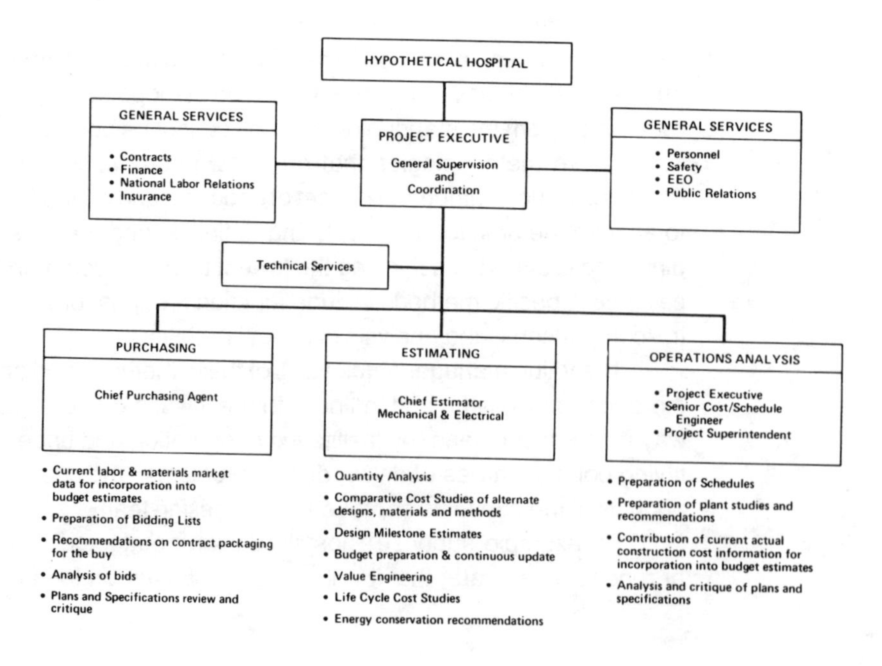

Clearly, these attitudes did not benefit the owner. Through experience and sometimes difficult contract trauma, most of the problems have been resolved, and the initial concept of saving money now approaches reality.

The advantages of including a construction manager (or project executive) early in the design phase can be great. For example, the construction manager is familiar with:

—current building systems that are available on the regional market at a competitive price

—current labor and industrial prices, enabling him to establish a proper estimate in the specific area

—sub-contracting trades that can advise on detail

—specification review

—cost consulting and scheduling

—value engineering

—studies of life-cycle cost

—energy cost and conservation

—management

—inspections

—insurance programming

—permits

—samples and testing

—shop drawing coordination

This knowledge, if applied in the design phase, can lead to cost improvements, time savings, and fewer change orders. The expected contingencies now budgeted and used should be reducible. The construction manager can also supply a guaranteed price, or upset cost of construction, that will not be exceeded. If this approach is used to set a client's budget, it is possible to set incentives for faster completion or for other means of reducing costs. The client may insist on all of the savings in these systems or time, but that only produces a very conservative price upset. The ideal method would be to bid the upsets based upon a pricing set, or scope set, of drawings, and then using a previously agreed upon formula, divide the savings between client and contractor, in some agreed-upon percentage.

Most construction managers only produce the general condition items in the construction of a project, manage the sub-contracts and overall project schedule, and do not directly build any of the project with their own labor forces. However, most are also general contractors and can perform construction if required. Many architect-engineer firms and a few accounting firms offer construction management services. The design-build firm incorporates construction management as an automatic step in its process.

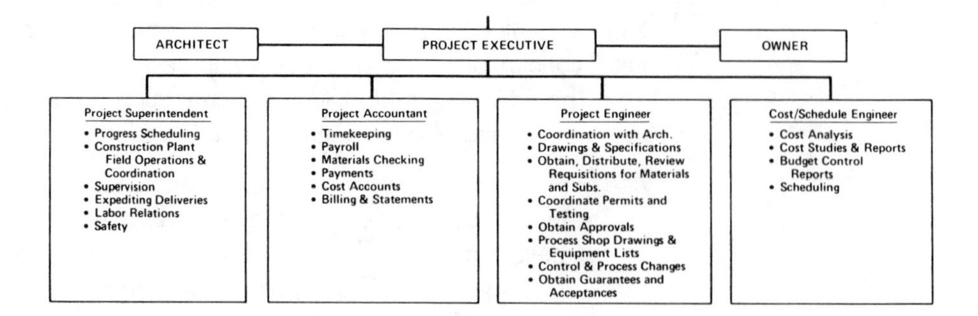

Organization Chart, Construction Phase

The construction manager's responsibilities in the concept and schematic phase of design include:

—preparing project cost model and budget

—preparing preliminary project master schedule

—conducting a visit to the site

—reviewing concept phase with architect and engineer and agreeing upon it

In the preliminary design phase, the construction manager:

—updates master schedule and cost model

—sets up preliminary construction schedule, including staging

—finds alternative systems and evaluates cost

—analyzes systems requested

The construction document phase involves:

—updating master schedule and cost model

—recommending package documents for possible fast-track construction

—reviewing specification development and construction details

—supplying a guaranteed maximum price

—identifying long-lead items and phasing concerns and performing value engineering

The bidding and construction phase requires the construction manager to prepare the bid list, release bid packages to selected bidders, receive bids, review bids, and recommend an award of work. He manages general conditions on the site, including start-up and overall supervision, and supplies voluntary alternatives submitted by the bidding contractors. The construction manager receives the contractor's proposed manufacturers and provides recommendations on them to the client, architect, and engineer. Based on data provided by the contractor, the construction manager, architect, and engineer assess substitutions and recommend changes to the client. Based on the client's reactions, the construction manager advises the contractors of approvals and rejections of submitted manufacturers.

Organization Chart, Job Site

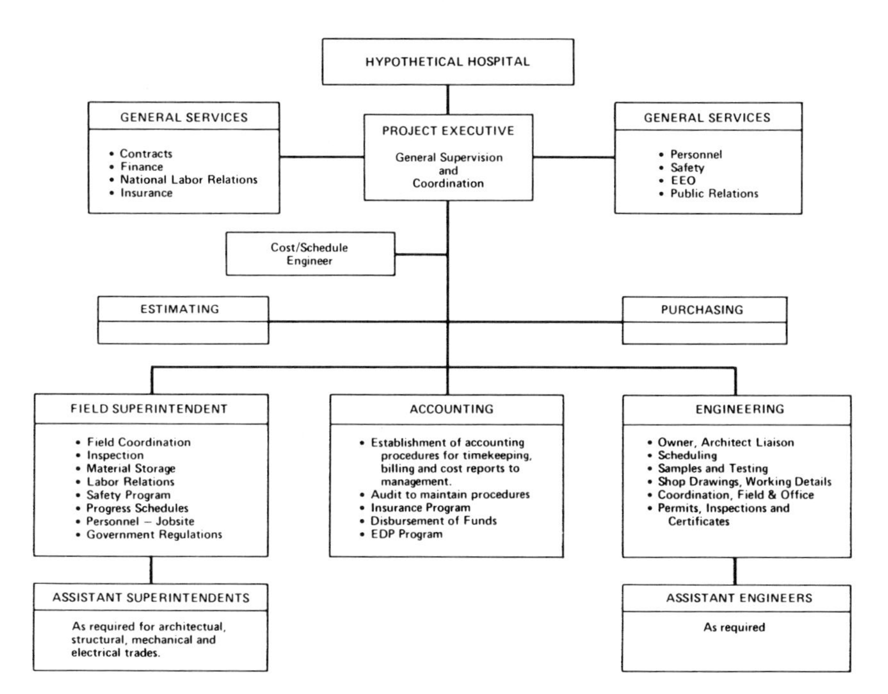

Shop drawings and equipment cuts from the subcontractors are sent to the construction manager for review and approval. The construction manager will return unacceptable drawings and cuts to the contractors. Approved work is sent to the architect and engineer for approval. Toward the end of construction, the construction manager is responsible for drawing up a certificate of substantial completion. This process includes:

—a punch list of incomplete work prepared in conjunction with architects and engineers

—after completion of the punch list by the contractor, a conference with representatives of the client and architect-engineer firm to confirm completion

—issuance by the architect of a certificate of substantial completion, with attached list of incomplete or unacceptable work

—after acceptance of the certificate of substantial completion by the client, construction manager, and architect-engineer, the firm beginning of the guarantee period, with client occupying and assuming responsibility for building spaces identified in the certificate of substantial completion

—confirmation that the work has been completed and processing, in concert with the architect-engineer firm, the final payment application

—with the client's acceptance of the certificate of final payment, the project is completed

When necessary, the construction manager can arrange for additional work that is not within the trade contract, but that is within the scope of work, and the guaranteed maximum price of the project.

Pricing Design. The introduction of a construction manager to the hospital planning team has broken with tradition, as described earlier. With someone else to talk to subcontractors, review construction details in an office, and get the advice of the men who will actually work on the job, the architect can go back to his original profession as a designer who defines quality, quantity, and form. Architects should not dictate every final construction technique or they will become inhibited in their ability to create things "that can't be built." The difference between theory and actual cost of a design must be worked out between a creative designer and an expert craftsman. Trying to be both can eliminate creative, economical design.

Pricing design is that interchange between craftsman and designer that can produce the most creative economics for the client. Rather than final details, outlines are prepared and discussed. Once this interchange has produced the desired approach, the details are sketched in and specified for quality and quantity only. The final shop drawing submitted by the contractor keeps this interchange alive, and a design can be reviewed up until the moment before it is manufactured. This approach is applied to every item and then details are sketched for each room in the hospital. For the first time, the administrator can review every item in a room at once. The benefits are immense: the administrator can make budget and design decisions by having one simple document in his hands. Other benefits of pricing design are listed below:

—guaranteed price can be reached sooner because drafted detailed drawings are not required

—the design professional can make all form, quality, and quantity recommendations for each room thus benefiting patient and staff and encouraging innovation

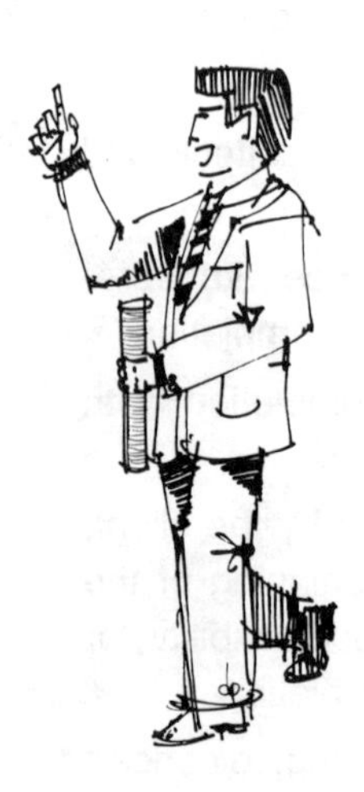

—the contractor can estimate the job more easily with the freedom of an open line to discuss each item

—details can be changed quickly

—federal and local review time is shorter because of the nature of the smaller document

As stated before, the ideas of construction management and pricing are not new, but they must be understood in order to work. The pressures for social and economic change that now bear on every health care institution can be offset by a creative approach to construction and design. Voluntary effort (VE) that applies to hospitals to reduce health care costs also applies to the architectural, engineering, and construction manager's professions.

CONCLUSION

I have talked a lot about team makeup and the importance of understanding and integrity among its members. The reason that it is so important may be clear, but I would like to stress it. The planning team represents the patient, staff, and hospital

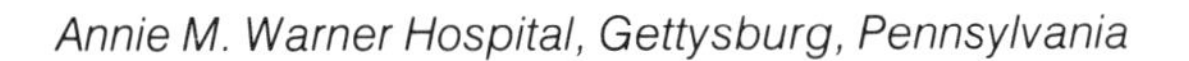

Annie M. Warner Hospital, Gettysburg, Pennsylvania

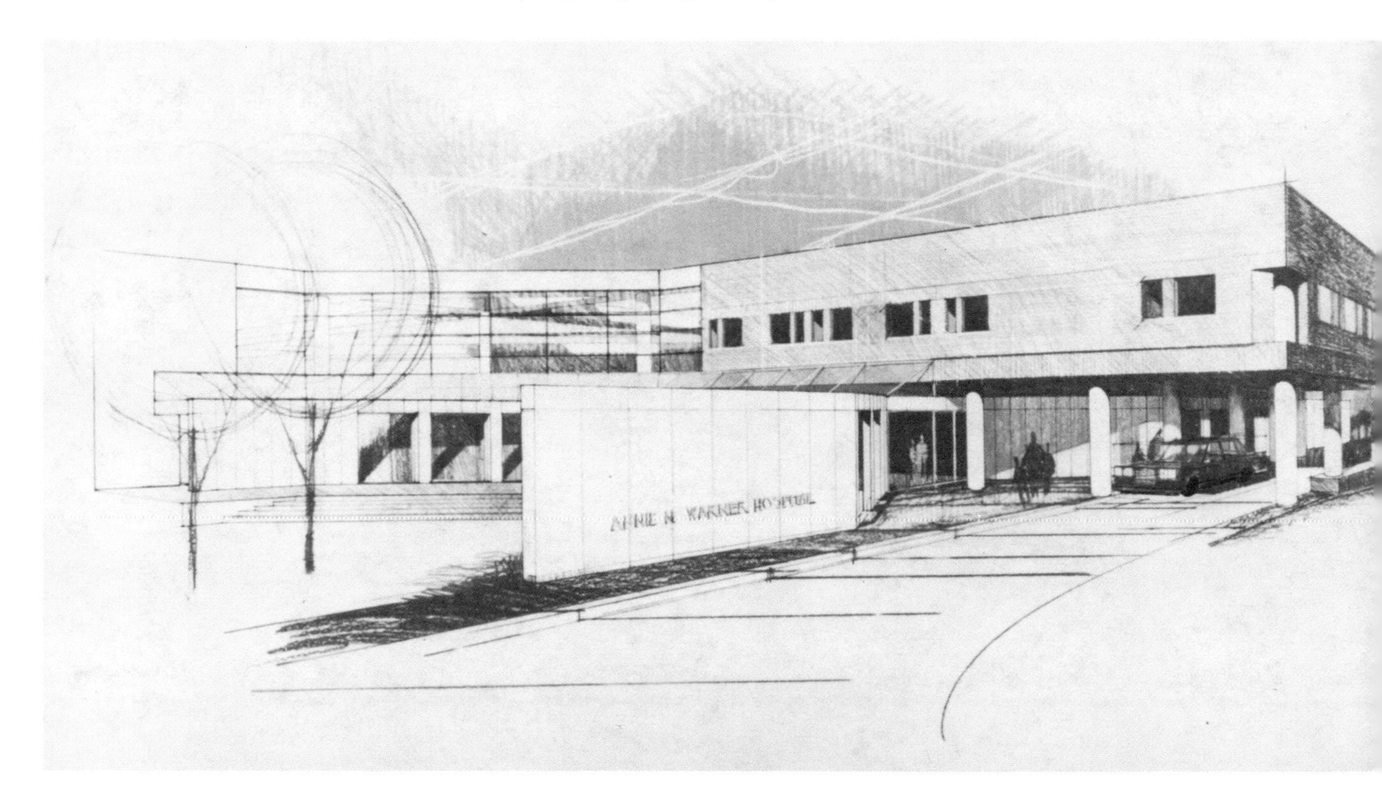

board, which is accountable to the public. The decisions and recommendations of the team are presented to and approved by the hospital planning committee and the board, but the ideas formulated by the team will affect thousands of patients in the future. This makes it absolutely necessary to choose a first-rate team in order that a mediocre project not be the final result.

III

design scope and fees

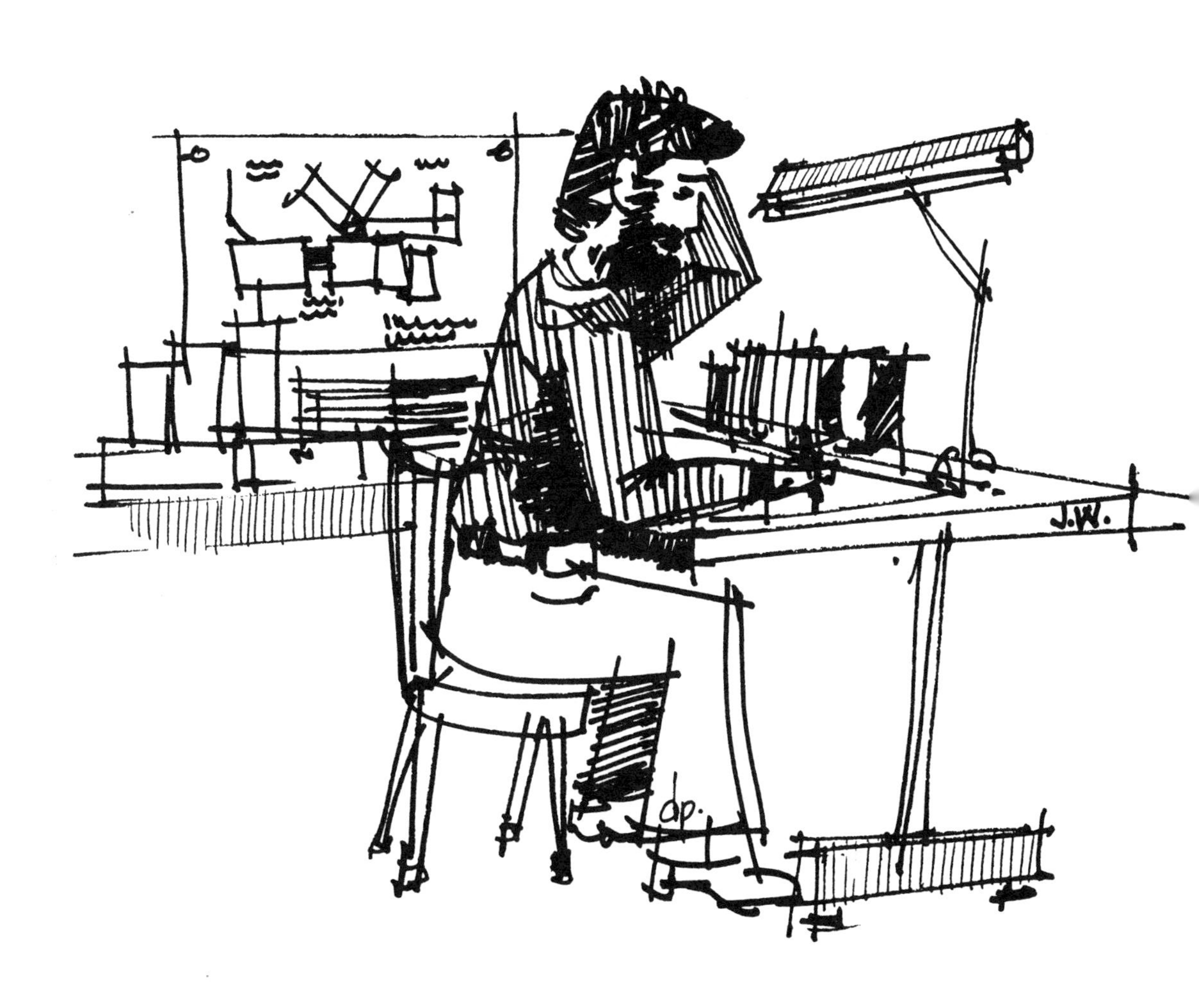

Once the need for a project is determined a game plan must be established, that is, an understanding by the entire team of the scope of ideas contemplated for the project. At this point the hospital consultant and administrator have been working on the projected and current need of the community; a facility master plan has been approved, in principal, by the local HSA; a financial study of the hospital has been completed; and an architect and engineers have now been added to fill out the team. The hospital is paying for a full team of professionals.

It is at this time that understandings must be shared through brainstorming sessions or value seminars. The architect and engineers should be on board before the certificate of need is submitted. A major part of the changes that will be produced in physical form will now be made. Irreversible cost determinations that develop now must be escalated to a schedule for the future. Each member of the team will have ideas to offer, and holding group sessions at this time will be the key to success. If no such meetings are held major conflicts can develop between the members.

ENGINEERING PLAN

When cost overruns occur in the transition from programming to building, it is usually because there is no clear engineering plan. At all phases of planning the engineering system's needs or desires must be identified. To do otherwise would be like buying a car without buying the motor.

An engineering plan may be only an engineering study with system description and loads. Existing mechanical and electrical systems for every facility should be studied. Existing mechanical systems that should be studied include:

—domestic water

—sanitary storm sewers

—natural gas piping

—oxygen

—surgical vacuum

—nitrous oxide

—compressed air

—deionized water

—fire protection

—steam

—condensate return and boiler feed water

—fuel oil

—diesel oil

—heating, ventilating, and air conditioning

—chilled water

—central monitoring of mechanical systems

The following electrical systems should be checked:

—power supply

—emergency power

—telephones

—fire alarm and detection

—doctors' in-and-out register

—radio paging

—television antenna

—loudspeaker paging

—intercom

—patient-nurses call

—clocks

—surveillance, entry, and holdup alarms

—physiological monitoring

—watchman's tour

—power distribution

—motor control centers

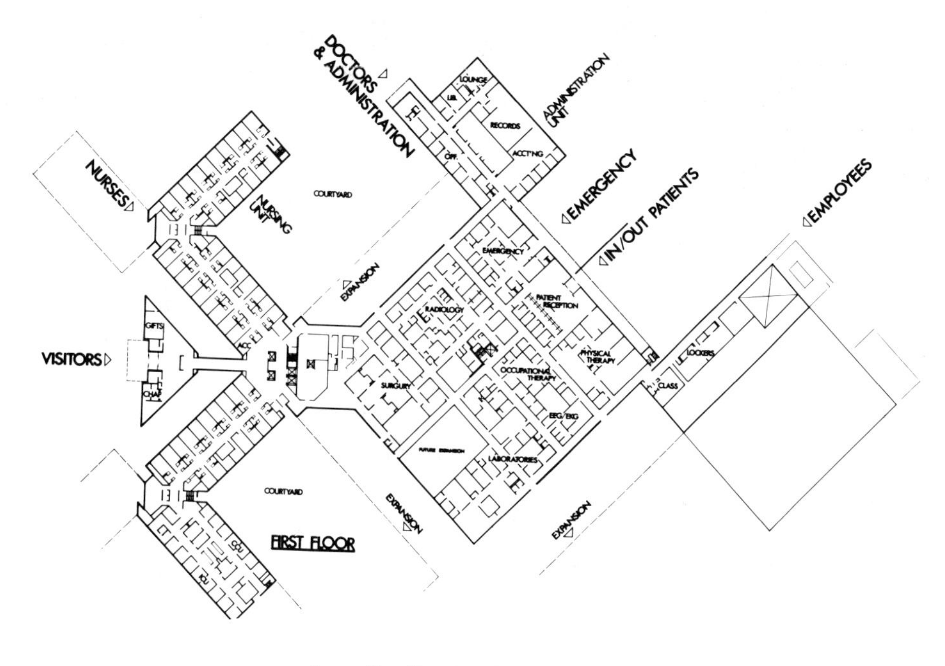

—secondary distribution feeders

—branch circuit wiring

—receptacles

—lighting

Envelope and Systems Building. The envelope is the building structure, skin, and mechanical systems. The way in which treatment is carried out, how teaching is done, and when research is done are dependent on systems and space. The envelope defines this space for twenty to eighty years.

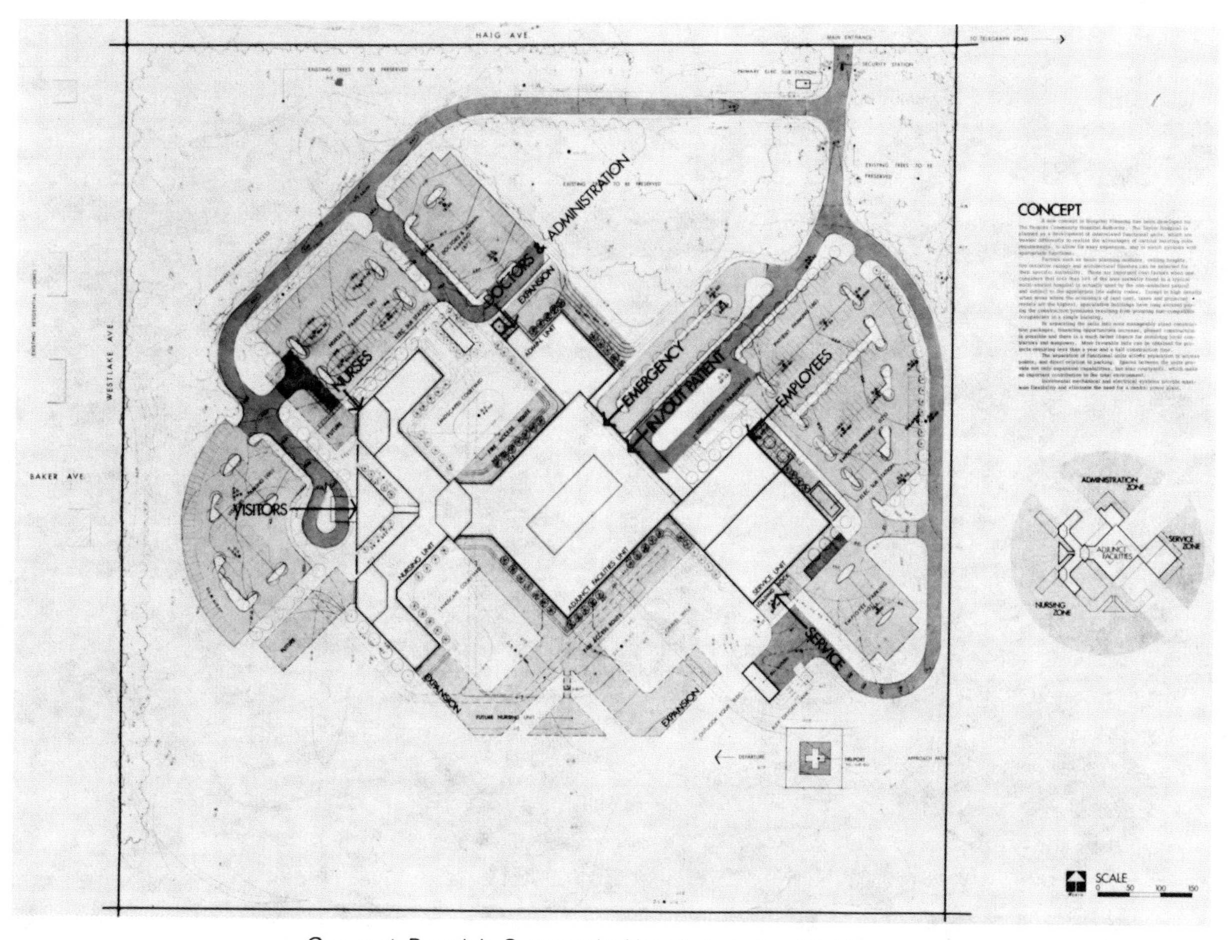

Concept. People's Community Hospital, Taylor, Michigan

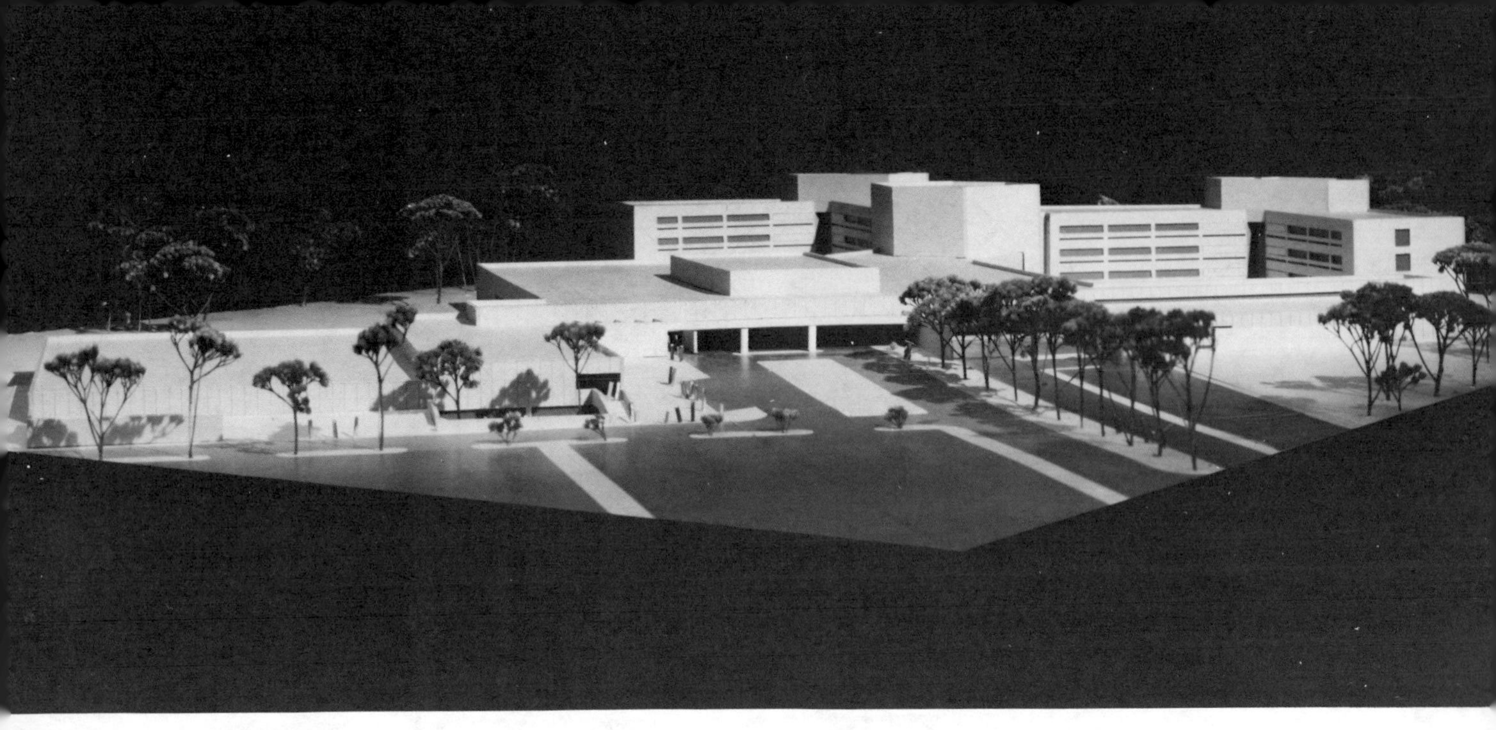

People's Community Hospital, Taylor, Michigan

Flexible space was often referred to in the 1970s, but without being well defined. The planning team must know what is being developed.

Systems building, discussed in Chapter II, takes into account the special training needed to design a particular facility. A method of monitoring, reducing maintenance, supplying gases, plumbing, and carrying materials must be worked out. This applies to any size facility and should be considered in the planning process. A good program states the mission of services and systems, as well as the broader mission of beds and service to the community.

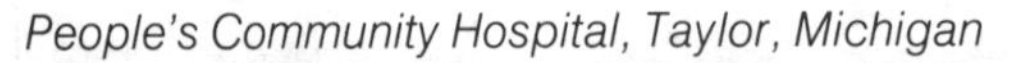

People's Community Hospital, Taylor, Michigan

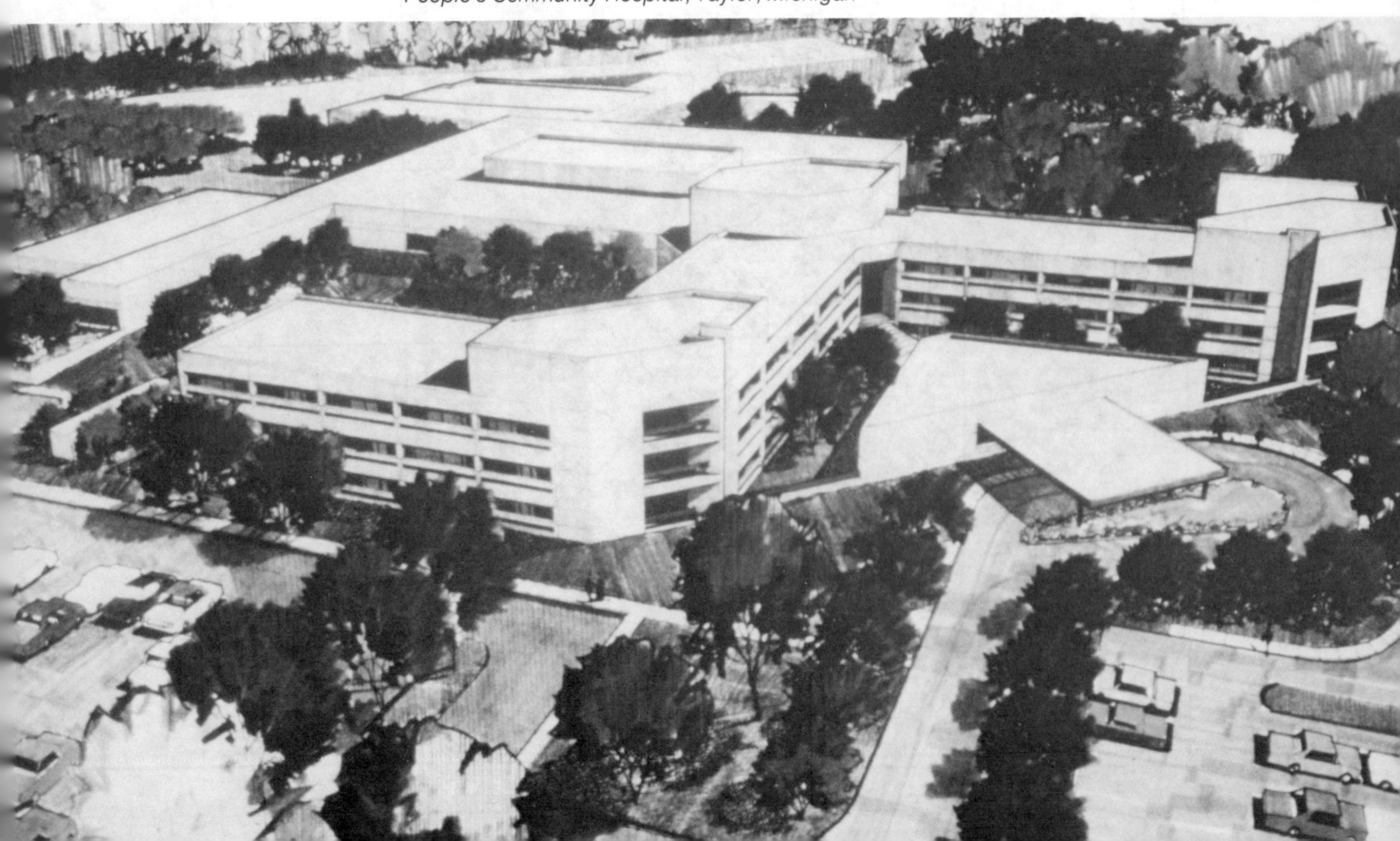

Energy Plan

The energy plan affects the long range and yearly operational cost of a hospital. It documents energy efficiency against current and projected fuel costs. The initial decision on what equipment to buy is studied against the equipment's life cycle costs (that is, when it will pay for itself and how much it will save). Solar energy, total energy, recycled energy, energy efficiency, recoverable energy, and potential energy can become feasible in the future, and these should not be ignored in the programming phase.

Operational Program

The operational program is a document that outlines the critical staffing patterns, department utilization and locations, and major functional elements that will affect hospital operation in the future (see Table 3.1). A program is written for each building project and is a part of the documentation required when a certificate of need is submitted. There is no standard operational program, and each is produced in a different way. The program should be written by the consultant who worked on the project scope or by the consulting architect who completed the facility master plan. The hospital administrator has a tremendous influence on this document and could write it himself if he had enough time.

Table 3.1 Sample Operational Program

Surgery is located on the third floor of the south wing. The existing department contains 22,842 gross square feet (g.s.f.).

Current Utilization	*1976*	*1977*	*1978*	*1979*	*1990*	*2000*
Cysto	1,467	1,122	1,277	1,358		
Major	5,991	6,144	5,549	4,741		
Minor	4,452	4,562	4,717	5,657		
Total	12,000	11,828	11,543	11,756	12,000	—
Outpatient included in above Totals	1,493	1,519	1,528	1,669	1,700/2,000	

1980 Space Requirement

11,756 procedures ÷ 1,000 per room = 12 rooms (plus 2 cystos)

12 rooms x 1,700 = 20,400 g.s.f.

11,756 procedures ÷ 20,400 g.s.f. = .576 procedures 1 g.s.f. (.33–.50 federal standard)

Continued

Table 3.1 Continued

1990 Projection

12,000 procedures ÷ 900 to 1000 per room/yr = 12–13 rooms (plus 2 cystos)
13 rooms x 1,700 = 22,666 g.s.f. = .52 procedures/g.s.f.

Planning ratio = 45 g.s.f. per bed x 750 beds = 33,750 g.s.f.
12,000 procedures ÷ 33,750 g.s.f. = .35 procedures/g.s.f.

Conclusion

40 g.s.f. per bed x 750 beds = 30,000 g.s.f.
12,000 procedures (12 rooms) ÷ g.s.f. = .4 procedures/g.s.f.

1990 Projection with Same-day Surgery Removed from the Suite

By moving the same-day surgery out of the OR suite, the length of each procedure will increase. Four to six procedures per day per room will drop to 3–5 and 900 procedures per room per year.

A bed reduction will occur in the medical-surgical service, with the medical patient days increasing and surgical patient days decreasing.

A proper forecast would be approximately 10,000 procedures per year at 900 procedures per room.

Space Requirement

10,000 procedures ÷ 900 per room = 11 rooms (plus 2 cysto)
11 rooms @ 1,900 g.s.f. = 20,900 g.s.f.
10,000 procedures ÷ 20,900 g.s.f. - .47 procedures/g.s.f.
500 bed equiv. x 40 g.s.f. per bed = 20,000 g.s.f.

2000 Projection

With advancement of medical technology and increasing same-day surgery technique, the 1990 projection should be adequate in function. Smaller equipment plus advance communications will not increase the future surgical suite.

Comments

The current surgery contains 12 operating rooms plus two cysto rooms. In 1979, only 10 rooms were open.

OR 1 Pediatrics
OR 2 Dual track lights—general
OR 3 ENT
OR 4 Eye
OR 5 Neuro
OR 6 Ortho

Table 3.1 Continued

OR 7 Ortho
OR 8 Overflow
OR 9 General
OR 10 Vascular
OR 11 General/Gyn
OR 12 Open heart

Most rooms except OR 10 are tight on space and undersized.

Storage within the OR suite is minimal. The doctors' locker area and nurses' locker rooms are inadequate in size and do not interchange from outside the suite into a substerile corridor. All traffic is through the main door into the suite.

At this time, packs and instruments are processed within the OR suite. Storage is within the corridors.

Recovery only holds 16 carts, or a total of 10 beds; 16 are needed.

The existing OR schedule is now from 7:45 am to 5:30 pm, with 4 to 6 procedures per room per day. The outpatient, or same-day, surgery will be removed from the suite this year, as the length of more complicated surgery is increasing and there are rooms needed for this reason.

Patient waiting is now in the hallway entrance to the suite. Crowded conditions and lack of privacy make this situation unacceptable.

The suite does not contain space for anesthesia carts and office area.

The soiled holding room and decontamination areas are inadequate. The mechanical system within surgery is inadequate. No individual room control is possible, with changeover from heating to cooling necessary.

The current surgery square footage now contains the neurology department space.

Recommendation

The existing surgery suite should be replaced and increased in size. A modern environmental system, adequate storage, proper room sizes, and support space must be designed. The patient holding, nursing control, and family waiting areas are high priorities in a new suite. Open heart procedures may require two rooms in the future.

Writing the operational program will spur the creative ideas of the planning team and it is absolutely necessary that their knowledge be involved. Although the architect and engineers do not write the final document, their ability to visualize design for the consultant and administrator is important. As many meetings as necessary should be held, for there is no benefit to reducing the time spent during this creative period.

The following are goals of an operational program:

—to study departmental operations in regard to existing and projected number of patients, visitors, staff, beds, tests, and procedures and to update the facility master plan each year

—to interview staff in order to establish personal and departmental needs

—to revise needs and operations in light of new national hospital standards and programs

Many times operational and functional programming (that is, a room–by–room list of needs) is combined in an effort to determine the facility's size for cost-estimating. It is important that input to the architectural design is begun before a final room–by–room size is decided; otherwise, the talents of a team member to create new space in order to meet unanticipated needs could be lost. Only after the team talks, writes, and draws its ideas can a functional program defining the exact size of the project be presented.

Once the operational program has been approved and the interdepartmental functional elements are being discussed, the entire facility must be brought together as a single design. The creation of the hospital design centers around the architect and engineers with input from the consulting team. Although designers can create exciting shapes and forms, the scope of a hospital concept has certain limitations. At the same time, no standard design can ever be used for all hospitals. Because a hospital is as complex as a city, individualized design is necessary. The economics of hospital construction indicate that more modular approaches must be developed around building systems, but the hospital operation itself eliminates a pat approach.

SPACE PROGRAM

Table 3.2 presents a list of hospital departments and can guide one in trying to visualize the size of each department in the total design. The list is for a primary and a secondary community hospital. It would be different for a tertiary or a teaching facility or one oriented toward ambulatory care. In Chapters VIII-IX, on department planning, more exact operational ratios and functional listings are presented.

Table 3.2. Space Requirements For Non-teaching General Hospitals

Area	Gross Sq. Ft. Per Bed
Administration	34
Archives	10
Ambulatory	
Emergency	15

Continued

Table 3.2 Continued

Area	Gross Sq. Ft. Per Bed
Outpatient	10
Lab substation	2
Social Services	1
Admissions and discharge	2
Auxiliary	4
Cashier	2
Clinical laboratory, pathology	35
Chapel	2
Delivery suite	13
Diagnostic radiology	40
Dietary	30
Employee facilities	9
Education, auditorium	10
Human functions	0
Inhalation therapy	2
EKG	2
EEG	1
Speech and hearing	1
Housekeeping	5
Materials management	5
Central stores	35
Central supply	12
Purchasing	2
Laundry	12
Medical records	9

Continued

Table 3.2 Continued

Area	Gross Sq. Ft. Per Bed
Medical staff facilities	3
Engineering and maintenance	60
Nuclear medicine	5
Nursery	7
Personnel	4
Pharmacy	7
Public spaces	15
Pulmonary function	3
Radiation therapy	10
Rehabilitation	
Occupational therapy	4
Physical therapy	12
Surgery	45
Subtotal*	480
Circulation	150
Nursing Units** ***	420
Total*	1,050***

*Base units are 600 to 800 gross square feet per bed.
**Inpatient bed units are 400 to 450 gross square feet per bed.
***Range of 950 to 1250 square feet per bed.
The base is defined as all departments plus circulation except the nursing units.
With intensive care, long-term care, rehabilitation, and psychiatric beds at 500 gross feet per bed.

The *total area* of a hospital is expressed in gross square feet within a hospital. *Net area* is the usable floor area of a space. *Gross area* of the building is the total enclosure as measured by, and including, the outside walls; it is the sum of the net areas and the nonassignable areas. Nonassignable areas include wall and partition thicknesses, vertical and horizontal circulation, and mechanical shafts. To convert net square feet to gross square feet, a multiple of 1.5–1.8 is usually used.

In programming and planning a hospital, most architects and consulting architects use gross square footage per department plus circulation in order to properly size the real volume and cost of a proposed design. (In this text, all departmental needs and planning ratios are given in gross square feet. These numbers represent the needs of primary and secondary general community hospitals. A teaching, or tertiary, facility will usually require 20–30 percent more space because of specialty research and teaching space required within each department as well as separate expanded programs.)

PHASING AND EXPANSION

The conversion of planning to capital improvements is carried out through phasing. Very seldom can all the needs and goals of a facility be met in one project or expenditure. In fact, expansion may be limited by the projected patient-day cost or by an HSA.

Expansion is usually controlled by the amount and type of land available. The number of entrances to a building and its footprint (the area of land covered by it at ground level) must be able to cope with an increasing barrage of people and cars. Future additions must be able to meet interior and exterior needs. To accomplish footprint growth, a phasing plan must be developed in the conceptual stage that defines future potential additions or any movement of either beds or the ancillary department base. This plan would also outline future spending needs and a budget. A long-range plan must include future expansion phasing or it will be obsolete. In addition, each phase must stand alone, as if no other were ever to be built, for hospital departments cannot close to accommodate construction. This is also important in the engineering plan as relocating an entire engineering system is very expensive.

ADDITIONAL SERVICES

There is an expert to be found on any conceivable subject: this is doubly true in hospital programs. The client must, therefore, actively determine the extent of additional services that must be employed to complete the project.

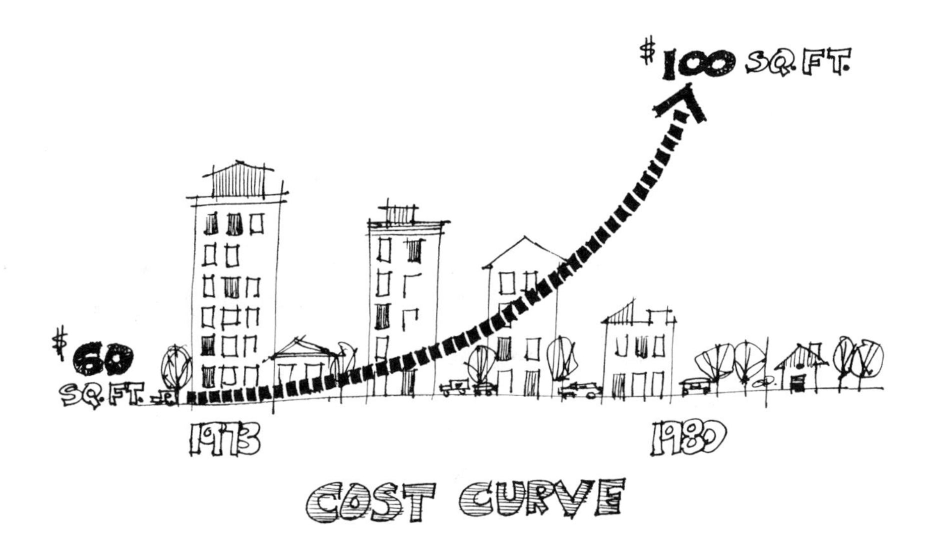

The basic contract for architectural services has been defined for only the basic services. In the following list, basic services are noted as B, and extensive additional services that may be necessary and cost extra are noted as A.

1) Hospital Consultant or Consulting Architect:

—develop long-range plan and recommendations	A
—study role	A
—medical staff questionnaire	A
—facility master plan	A
—certificate of need	A
—financial feasibility	A
—operational program	A
—personnel study	A
—equipment consulting	A
—materials-handling study	A
—patient profile	A
—fund raising	A

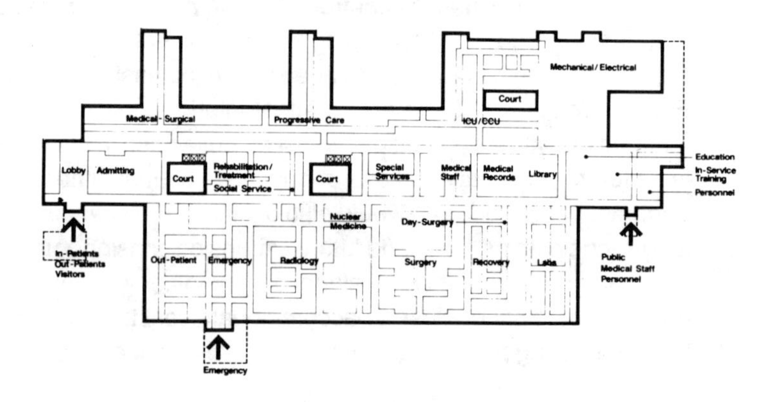

Schematic floor plan.
Medical Center of Beaver County, Pennsylvania

2) Hospital Architect:

—schematic design phase	B
—unit construction estimating	B
—design development	B
—construction documents	B
—normal engineering services	B
—specifications	B
—representative of client during construction	A or B
—periodic inspection	B
—extensive inspection	A
—architectural rendering	A or B
—scale models	A or B
—special analysis of client's needs	A
—site evaluations	A or B
—design services for future facilities	A or B
—measured drawings or investigation of existing facilities	A
—preparing documents for alternate bids	A
—detailed estimates	A
—inventories of existing material or equipment	A

—changes in drawings beyond architect's control	A
—change orders	A
—consultation on replacing work damaged by fire or other causes during construction	A
—services necessary through default of contractor	A
—reproducible records drawings	A
—operating manuals for equipment	A
—inspection past construction time	A
—serving as or briefing an expert witness for public hearing or legal proceedings	A
—extra engineering studies (energy or existing conditions)	A
—certified land survey	A
—test borings	A
—soils engineer	A
—laboratory tests (mechanical, electrical structural, chemical)	A
—legal and accounting services	A
—reproduction costs above specified amounts	A
—value management	A
—value engineering	A or B
3) Interiors:	
—interior design	A
—furniture procurement	A
—existing inventory	A

Rendering. Children's Memorial Hospital, Chicago, Illinois

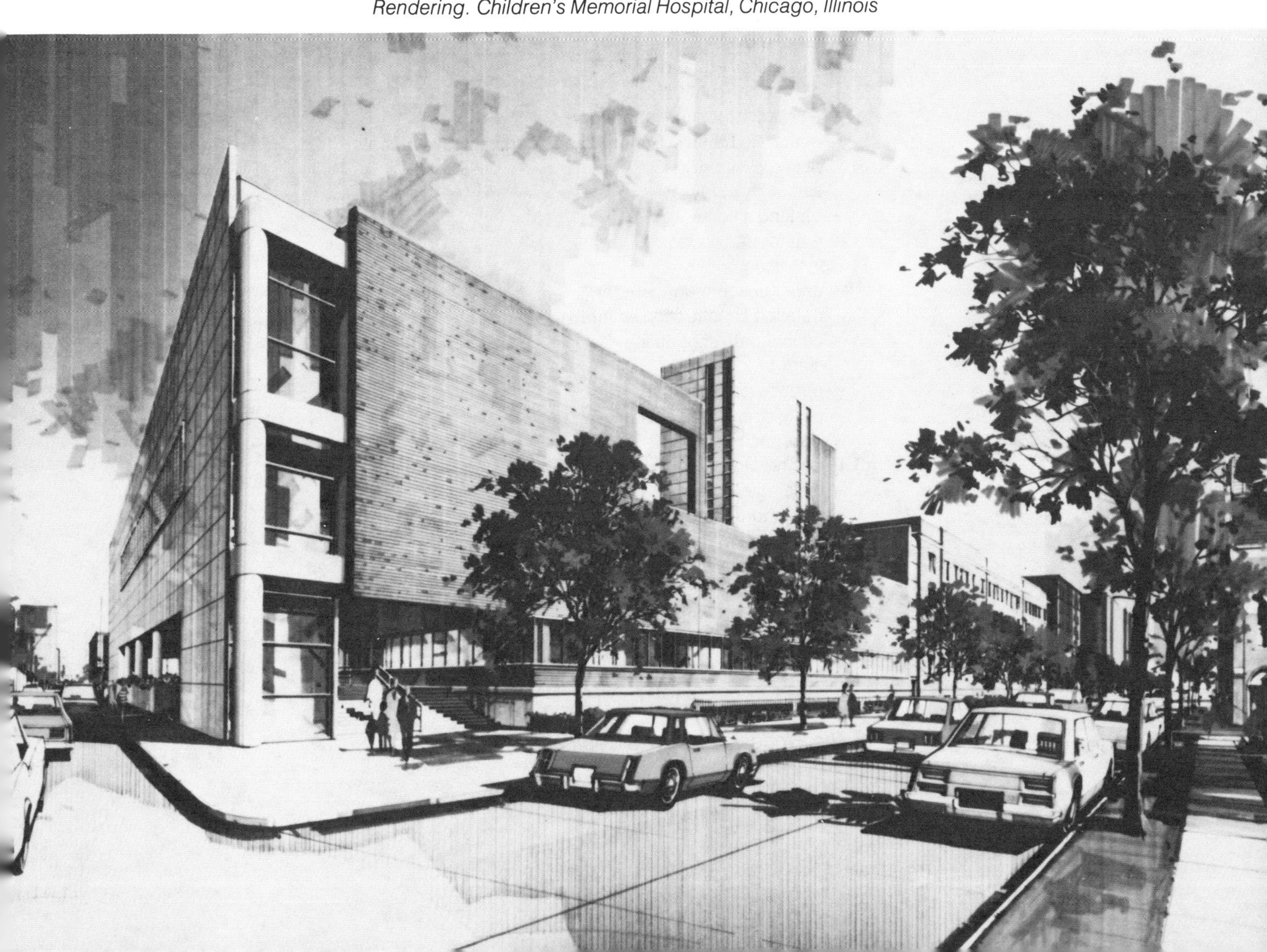

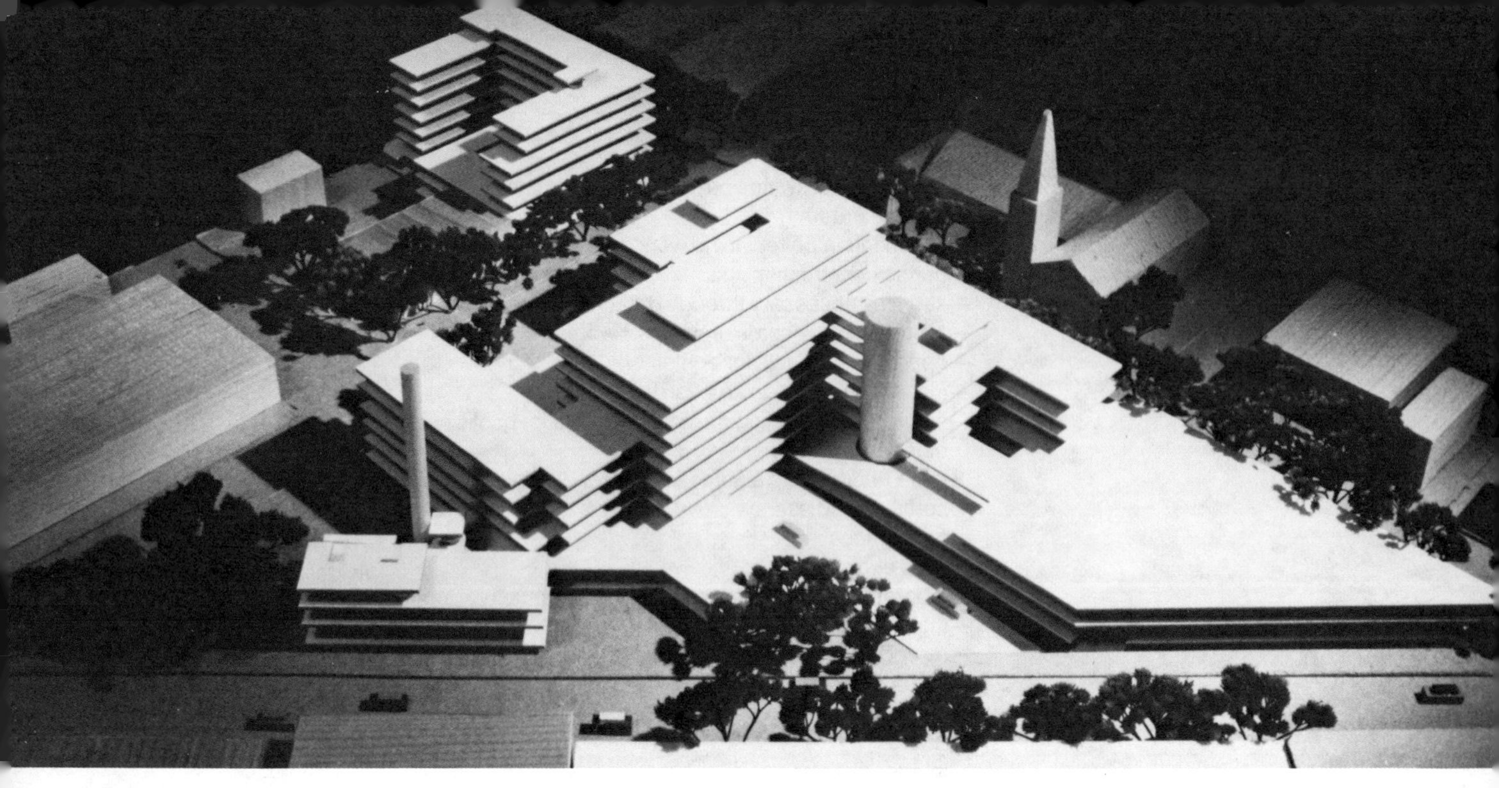

Model.
Children's Memorial Hospital,
Chicago, Illinois

4) Graphics:	
—corporate program	A
—corporate logo	A
—wall graphics	A
5) Equipment design:	
—list of movable equipment	A
—list of fixed equipment	B
—dietary consultation	A or B
—equipment-testing laboratory	A
—materials-handling (linen, trash, food, supplies, people)	A
6) Civil engineering:	
—site utility study	A or B
—parking study	A or B
—master traffic plan	A
7) Construction:	
—construction management	A
—detailed construction estimating	A
—critical-path scheduling	A
—clerk-of-the-works	A
—permits and bonds	A or B
—utility companies liaison	A or B
—insurance	A
8) Public relations:	
—building program	A
—groundbreaking ceremony	A
—employee manual	A
—photography	A
9) Manufacturing:	
—program requirement studies	A
—simulated computer studies	A

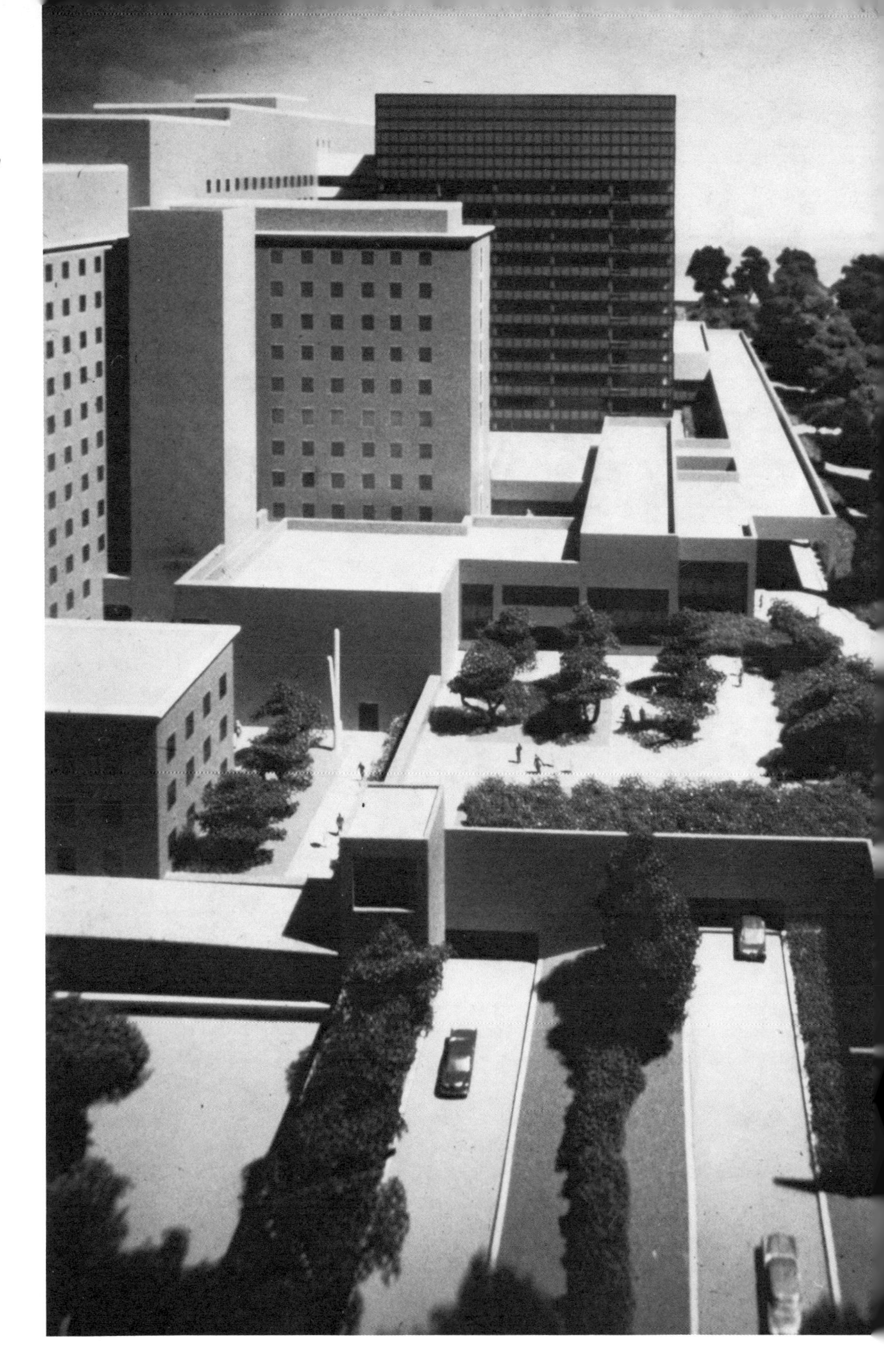

Art work photo.
National Institute of Health
Ambulatory Care
Research Facility,
Washington, D.C.

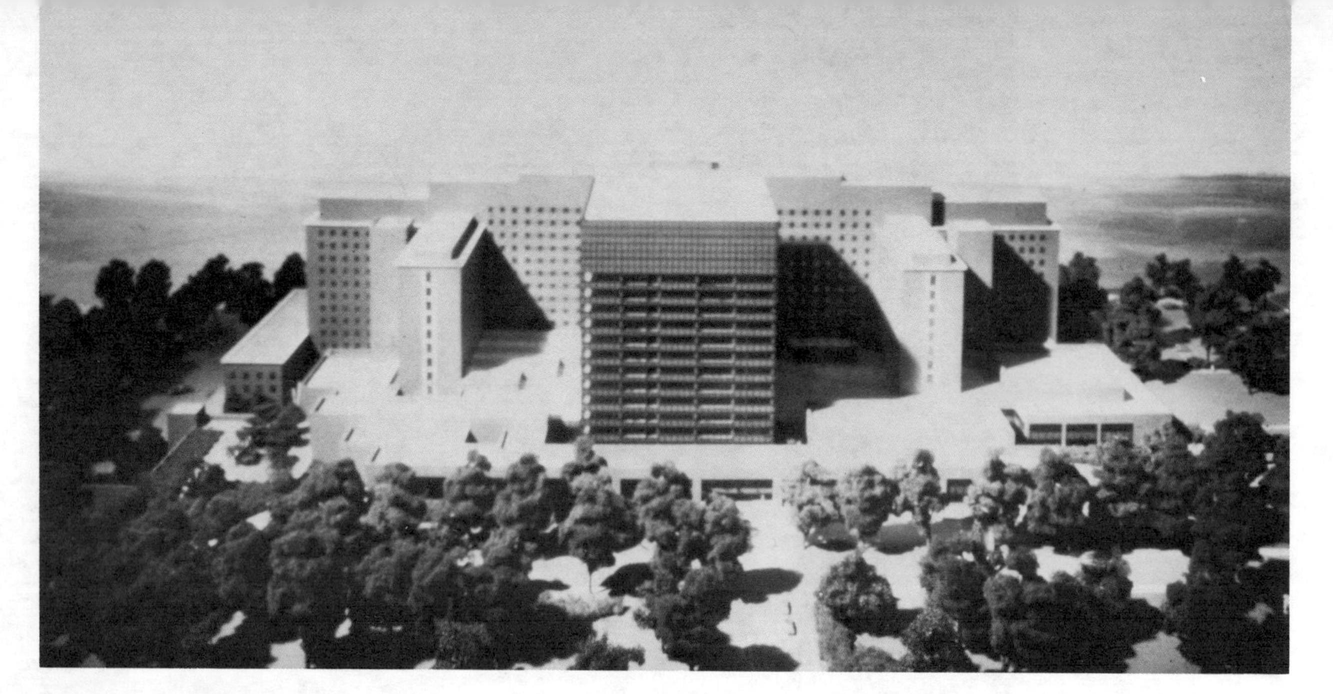

National Institute of Health
Ambulatory Care Research Facility,
Washington, D.C.

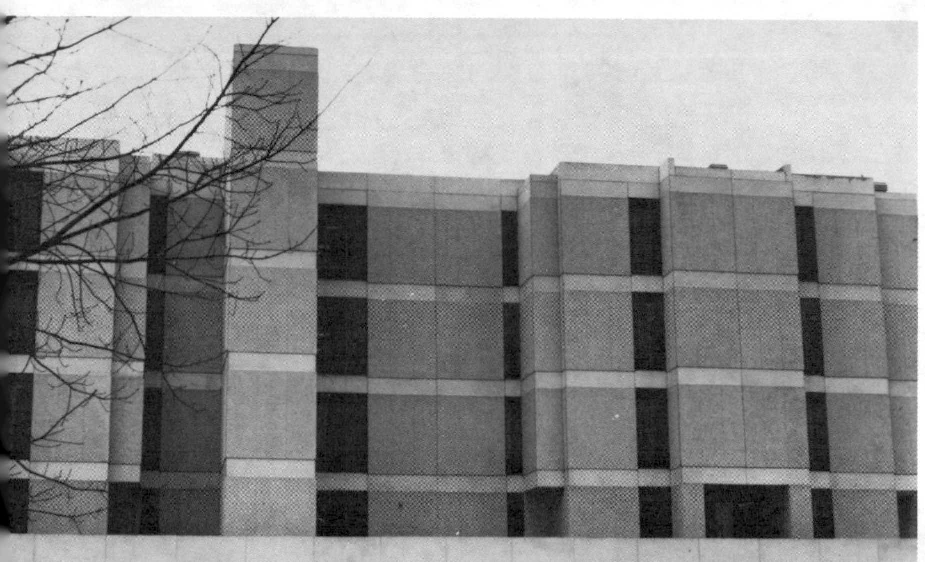

Public release photo.
Washington Hospital Center
Intensive Care Unit, Washington, D.C.

Public release photo.
Washington Hospital Center
Outpatient Facility, Washington, D.C.

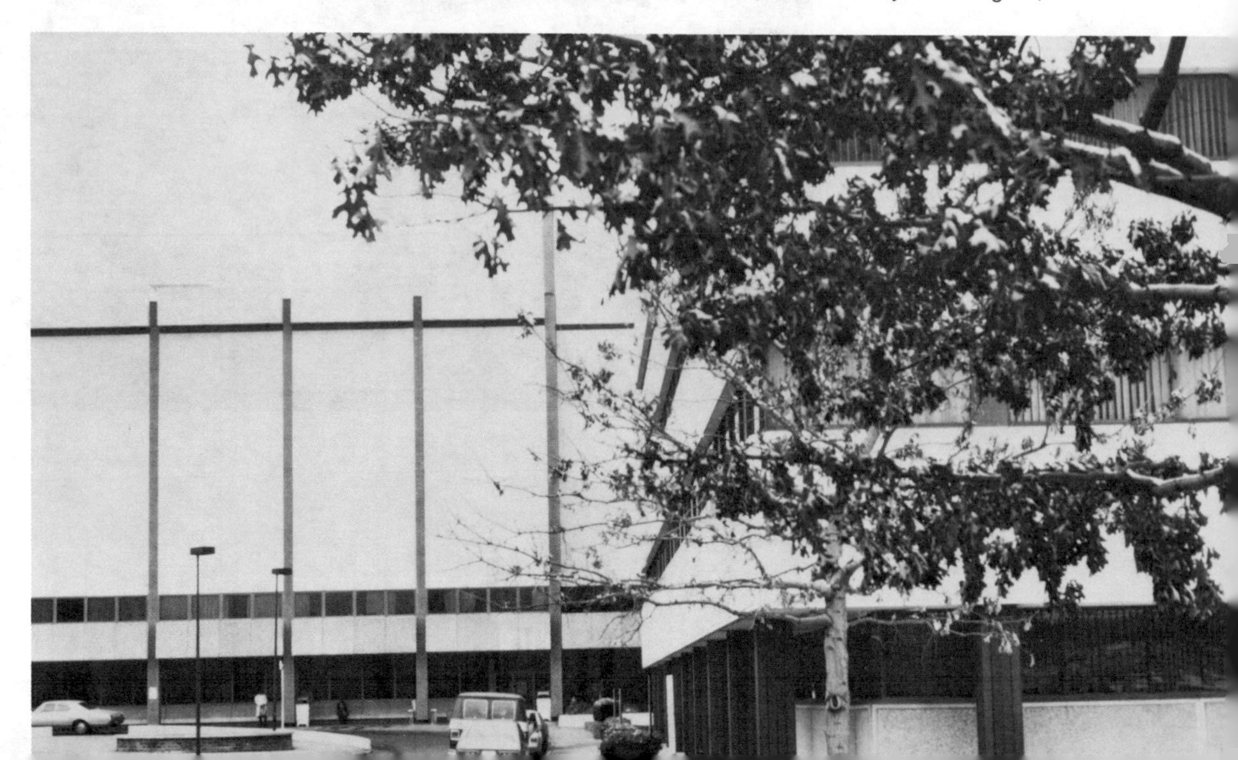

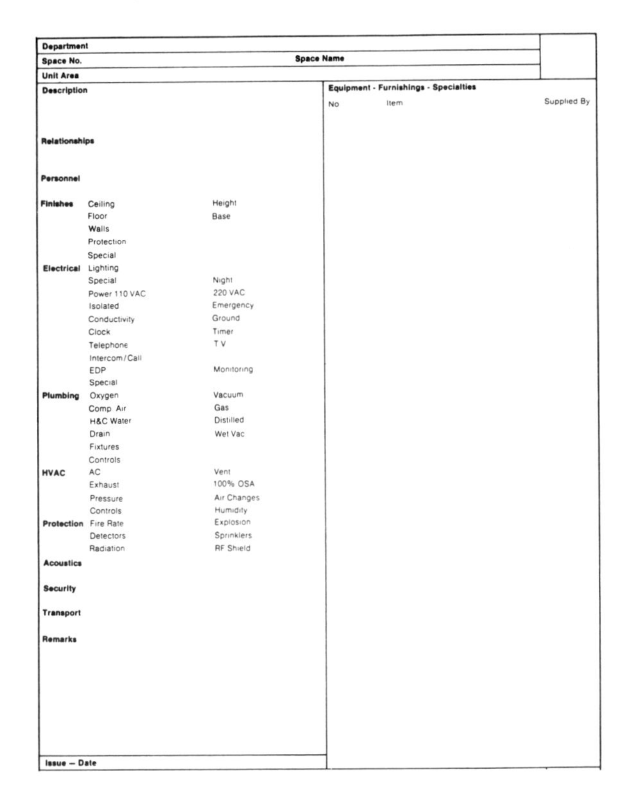

Department
Space No. Space Name
Unit Area
Description
Relationships
Personnel
Finishes Ceiling Height
Floor Base
Walls
Protection
Special
Electrical Lighting
Special Night
Power 110 VAC 220 VAC
Isolated Emergency
Conductivity Ground
Clock Timer
Telephone T V
Intercom/Call
EDP Monitoring
Special
Plumbing Oxygen Vacuum
Comp Air Gas
H&C Water Distilled
Drain Wet Vac
Fixtures
Controls
HVAC AC Vent
Exhaust 100% OSA
Pressure Air Changes
Controls Humidity
Protection Fire Rate Explosion
Detectors Sprinklers
Radiation RF Shield
Acoustics
Security
Transport
Remarks
Issue — Date

Equipment - Furnishings - Specialties
No Item Supplied By

Furnishings and equipment survey

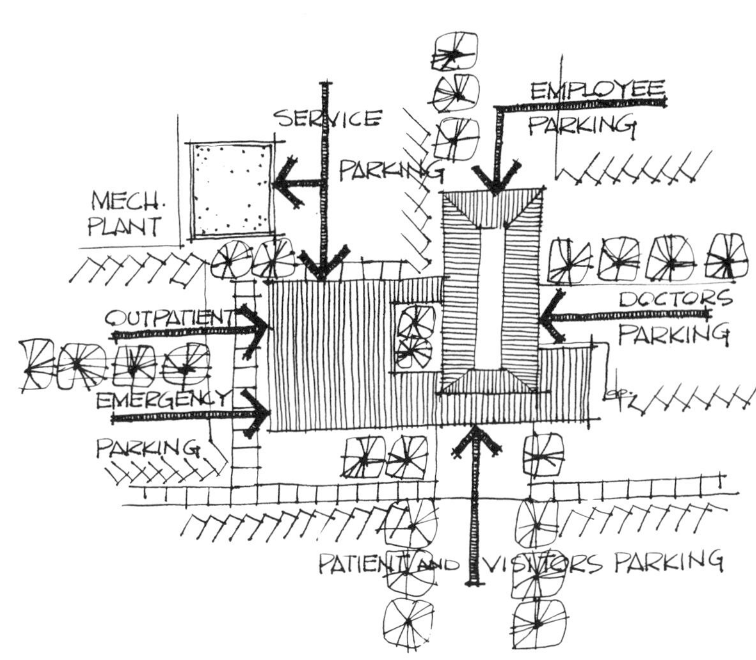

Master traffic plan

This list illustrates the numerous variations available, variations that can amount to an additional 20 percent of the construction cost. An example of a total project construction budget with fees is shown in Tables 3.3–3.6. This budget does not include the legal, accounting, and hospital administration time involved in putting a project together.

Table 3.3 Estimated Construction Costs of Hospital Wing

Department	*Net Area*	x	*Ratio of Gross Area to Net Area*	=	*Estimated Gross Area*	x	*Relative Cost Factor*	x	*Estimated Average Cost Per Square Foot ($)*	=	*Estimated Construction Cost ($ million)*
Surgery	5,300		1.6		8,500		1.90		100		1.615
Nursing	9,650		1.4		13,500		1.10		100		1.485
Business	3,700		1.3		4,800		0.9		100		0.432
General stores	5,500		1.2		6,600		0.75		100		0.495
Mechanical, electrical	4,200		1.1		4,600		0.70		100		0.323
Total*					33,400						4.340

* Average Square Footage Cost = $129.94 per square foot

Table 3.4 Sample Schematic Phase Estimate

Description	Value ($)	Percent of Total Cost
Building		
General condition	848,520	10.14
Foundation	348,200	4.16
Structure	1,228,580	14.68
Exterior enclosure	581,330	6.95
Architectural finishes	1,493,370	17.84
Specialties	95,500	1.14
Vertical transportation	202,830	2.43
Plumbing and fire protection	701,470	8.38
Heating, ventilation, and air conditioning	1,405,470	16.78
Electrical	1,046,290	12.49
Subtotal	7,951,560	94.99
Equipment	420,880	5.01
Total building	8,372,440	100.00
Site development	433,210	
Subtotal	8,805,640	
Design contingency (10%)	880,560	
Subtotal	9,696,200	
Escalation to bid date (5%)	484,800	
Total construction	10,171,000	

Table 3.5 Sample Cost Estimate at the Design Development Stage

			Labor and Materials	
Description	Quantity	Unit*	Cost ($)	Estimate ($)
Exterior Walls				
Face brick	118	M	900.00	106,200
Precast concrete panels	1,550	SF	15.00	23,250
Double-faced precast panels	575	SF	30.00	17,250
Double-faced precast panels and insulation	960	SF	32.00	30,720
Drywall backup: ½″ insulation, 6″ studs, 6″ batts	14,400	SF	2.60	37,440
⅝″ gypsum board (to drywall backup) taped	10,500	SF	0.40	4,200
Concrete masonry unit backup	3,800	SF	3.00	11,400
8″ concrete masonry unit & parapet	1,850	SF	3.00	5,550
Alum. & glass windows & entrance frame	5,300	SF	25.00	132,500

Continued

Table 3.5 continued

Description	Quantity	Unit*	Labor and Materials Cost ($)	Estimate ($)
X-cost alum. & glass door leaves & howe	13	EA	500.00	6,500
Precast coping	1,030	LF	10.00	10,300
Rollup receiving door	120	SF	25.00	3,000
Lintels, flashing, caulking, etc.		LS		5,000
Scaffolding	25,000	SF	0.50	12,500
Expansion joints, tie in, etc.		LS		2,500
Total				408,310
Partitions				
Concrete masonry unit walls	5,100	SF	3.00	15,300
Drywall—3-5/8″ stud, 1 layer 5/8″ ea. side	46,000	SF	2.50	115,000
Drywall—2-1/2″ stud, 2 layer 1/2″ ea. side	20,000	SF	3.00	60,000
Furred gypsum board	10,800	SF	1.50	16,200
Furred columns	5,000	SF	2.00	10,000
Alum. & glass @ doors, etc	300	SF	20.00	6,000
X-cost alum. & glass doors leaves, etc.	7	EA	400.00	2,800
Glazed ICU/CCU walls	840	SF	15.00	12,600
Single doors, frame, howe	211	EA	500.00	105,500
Double doors, frame, howe	80	PR	800.00	64,000
Bifold units	9	EA	175.00	1,575
Misc. lintels, etc.		LS		2,000
Scaffolding	88,000	SF	0.25	22,000
Total				432,975

*The following abbreviations are used: M, one hundred; SF, square feet; EA, each; LF, linear foot; LS, line size; PR, pair.

The hospital administrator should inform himself and his building committee of the vast possibilities that exist when developing a budget and should use professional services to his advantage. One of the most important aspects in a construction program is the administrator's ability to find and use professional services. When used properly, these services will more than pay for themselves in time saved and decisions made.

Table 3.6 An Example of a Project's Construction Budget Over Three to Four Years

Aspect of Project	*Cost ($ thousands)*
Construction (escalated to midpoint of construction)	*18,000*
Alternatives (including allowance for dietary)	*2,000*
Total construction	*20,000*
Consultant's fee (from $25,000 to $150,000)	*100*
Contingency (5%)	*1,000*
Architect's and engineer's fees (7%)	*1,470*
Movable equipment (17%, including interiors)	*3,400*
Cost consultants' fees	*28*
Dietary consultant (4% of equipment)	*20*
Interior and movable equipment fees	*340*
Graphics fee	*45*
Soil borings	*10*
Site survey	*5*
Clerk-of-the-works	*70*
Total project construction	*26,488*
Interest and financing cost during construction	*9,360*
Total project cost	*35,848*

COSTS

The final aspect of the game plan developed by the planning team is cost. It has been shown how operational costs are affected by design. No matter how much space is added above the amount programmed, it will be occupied by people and equipment and "empty" space will be used.

It must be stressed that every square foot of a hospital can become costly to the patient and therefore must be controlled. At this time, the cost per square foot of hospitals in the Washington, D.C. area ranges from $85.00 to $200.00. This range is greatly affected by the fixed equipment, physical finishes, and quality of installed systems. The 1981 average of approximately $110.00 to $140.00 per square foot for new construction will escalate 12–15 percent per year until building industry restraints can be formulated. This average cost is for construction only and does not include contingencies, fees, equipment costs, and financing costs.

Discussion of realistic costs sets the mood for all further progress. There are many ways to estimate cost, as will be shown later, but the key issue here is the dollars that the planners can project to build their concept. This will control the direction of the consultant, architect, and especially the administrator.

The responsibility for establishing a construction budget and developing a project that fits within that budget is shared by the client and the professional consultants on the project team. The budget (money available) and the cost (money required) should be reviewed, compared and made to match at scheduled intervals during the project. These reviews should be an integral part of the approval mechanism established by project directors at the beginning of the job.

While the design professions have experienced highly publicized difficulties in the management of construction costs, the importance and difficulty of establishing and maintaining a construction budget have not been given sufficient attention. Before work begins, designers should be given, or should help to develop, an approved construction cost ceiling, together with a clear statement of the project's functional, aesthetic, and quality requirements. Planning a project involves thousands of decisions or choices that affect cost: a designer who is not working within clearly specified limits must rely solely on his own sense of value, which may not be appropriate for the project and the client. Costs for hospital construction have been inflating at the rate of 12–15 percent through year 1981. This inflation may soon reach well over 20 percent per year.

The construction budget is usually established by subtracting all other costs, such as consultants, from the total projected cost. The difficulties of budgeting for construction usually arise from uncertainties about the availability or the cost of obtaining the required funds. It is not uncommon for planning and design to begin before sources of funding are finalized.

Where uncertainties remain, it is in the best interests of all concerned for the client, with the help of financial and design consultants, to make the necessary assumptions and establish a specific upper limit on construction cost. As the project and uncertainties are reduced the status of the construction budget should be monitored and adjusted.

Cost estimates must be made and revised regularly from the conception of the program until the bid documents are at least half complete. Each time the construction cost is estimated, the project budget and associated project costs should also be updated for comparison. Discrepancies between projected budgets and costs should be resolved through the joint efforts of the client and the consultants before design work proceeds.

Cost estimating techniques are determined by the type of information used to describe the project and by the estimator. The accuracy of the estimate improves as the project becomes more specifically defined. In the earliest stages, experienced professionals can employ rule-of-thumb guidelines, such as cost per bed, but the use of such techniques is extremely hazardous. Construction cost projections are not useful until they are based on reliable projections of space requirements. Construction cost estimates for a typical project might occur as the last step of each of the following tasks:

—preliminary space program by department

—final space program by room

—preliminary schematic design (definition of building mass and department locations only)

—final schematic design

—design development

—contract document 50 percent complete

Estimates made after the contract documents are more than half finished serve little practical purpose, since decisions made then have little impact on projected cost. Furthermore, any changes made beyond the midpoint that would significantly alter the construction cost would also disrupt the project delivery schedule.

Construction cost estimates for the early phases (through preliminary schematic design) are made by projecting the probable cost per square foot of either the entire project or the project components. Additions to and renovations of existing hospitals should be analyzed to determine the amount of space to be provided for each function or department. Designers and consultants who specialize in this type of project have learned to estimate the relative construction costs of hospital functions with considerable confidence.

In Table 3.3 a new wing is proposed to provide facilities for a surgical suite, a thirty-six bed nursing unit, business offices, and general stores. The project is described to the estimator by a program narrative and a net area program. The estimator must provide gross to net area conversion ratios, as well as the relative cost-per-square-foot factors for each function. The relative cost factor method illustrated here requires the estimator to first determine what the average cost per square foot of a full new hospital of comparable quality would be in the proposed location. This can be obtained from published construction-cost indexes and data from other projects bid recently in the area. If this turns out to be about $130 per square foot, construction costs are estimated to be $4.34 million (see Table 3.4).

At the end of the schematic design stage, the project will be sufficiently well defined to permit more detailed cost estimates based on the actual quantities of materials or systems shown by the plans and outline specifications. Table 3.5 shows such estimates. By the time the design development is completed, all of the building systems and components will be described in sufficient detail for a full quantity takeoff to be prepared in much the same way a contractor prepares his bid (Table 3.6). Further estimates during contract document production consist of simply adjusting individual elements of the design development estimate as minor changes occur and greater detail is provided.

Hospital consultants and architects have traditionally prepared estimates for their own plans and designs, but it is increasingly common for estimating to be done by a cost consultant. This consultant is usually either a professional construction estimator or the construction manager for the project. In either case, the expertise of the cost consultant should be called upon whenever the project must be tailored to fit the current budget.

Two of the most costly items in a construction cost estimate are time and uncertainty. Time is taken into account by escalation: an inflation factor is incorporated in the estimate to adjust prices of labor and materials to the levels expected at the time bids will be received. At a 13 percent escalation rate, a large project that might not be bid for three years after the first program-based estimate is made would cost almost 40 percent more than the current dollar estimate. Uncertainty is accounted for in the construction cost estimates by including contingencies. The bid contingency is carried in the cost estimate to cover the unpredictability of responses when bids are invited. Five percent is used as a bid contingency, but 10 percent is more realistic and considerably safer. In addition, a design contingency of 10 percent should be added to the early estimates to allow for unanticipated costs that might be necessary to satisfy all of the conditions and criteria of the building program. This design contingency can be progressively reduced to zero as the construction documents near completion since all significant costs will have been identified.

Another valuable means of managing the inevitable risk of the construction marketplace is to identify alternatives in the contract documents. Prices are quoted on the basic project (base bid), and the additional cost of the alternative is identified separately. The client can then choose to delete the alternative from the project if sufficient funds are not available. There can be several alternatives in a single bid package. They should not include any items that are critical to the success of the project, and they should add up to a least 5 percent of the estimated cost. Specifying alternatives will probably create more work for the designers who will expect to be paid for the additional services.

Cost of Money

The cost of money is a key factor for any building program. At this time, a program borrowing $5 million for construction at an interest rate which may run as high as 20 percent will pay up to $2 million in interest payments over a three-year building program and financing cost. Construction costs will average 50–60 percent of the total project cost. The remainder goes for fees, contingencies, and financing costs.

FEES

The client must anticipate the total fees and cost of a building program in order to prepare a realistic estimate for all time and costs. The certificate-of-need process has suffered a black eye because of cost overruns so often applied for after the fact. With limits set by states and HSAs for patient-day cost, and with cost containment critical to program development, the cost of construction must be most carefully considered.

Consulting Fees

There is no standard for consulting fees. Each study is costed out against a similar effort and is based upon work days times overhead plus profit. Travel costs and living expenses on the road are usually directly reimbursable and are in addition to the fee.

Studies for long-range plans vary from $25,000 to $200,000 in fees and expenses, depending on the scope of services to be performed. Facility master plans are also based upon the defined scope of services. For example, fees for a 400-bed facility would range from $25,000 to $100,000; fees for a 800-bed facility or medical center would cost $75,000 to $200,000. These fees include the cost of the supporting team of health care consultants, consulting architects, and consulting engineers.

Architect-Engineer Fees

Basic services for new construction are commonly split into two separate fees:

—schematics, design development, and contract documents

—design inspection of construction

Total services range from 6 to 8 percent of the construction estimate plus contingency. If split, the fee packages for basic services can be estimated as follows: design accounts for 5.5 to 6 percent of construction, or about $5–$6 per square foot; inspection accounts for 1.2–2 percent of construction, or 20–31 percent of the total services fee. Because of the restraints placed on budgets, many states and clients now put professional design fees up for bid and negotiate a single price (lump-sum fee) that is not based on construction costs.

The architect-engineer firm that submits a single-price bid must base this on a well defined scope of work that describes the project. Man-effort hours are calculated, and then overhead (direct and indirect) and profit are applied. A fixed effort is based upon an exact schedule. If the client's scope (size or building program) changes, the architect must negotiate a change in fee based on a 2.6–3.0 multiplier of salary, and range from $20 to $100 per hour.

Structural, mechanical, electrical, and civil engineering fees are included in the basic services or lump sum fees mentioned above and are paid by the architect. These fees are approximately as follows:

—Structural engineers receive 7–14 percent of total fee.

—Mechanical and electrical engineers get 25–35 percent of the total fee (or 5–6 percent of the estimated construction cost of the mechanical and engineering work).

—Civil engineers charge 1.5–2 percent of the total fee (the engineering systems within a hospital make up 50–60 percent of the total construction cost).

—Cost estimating is usually done for 2–3 percent of the total fee.

Because of the existing conditions and complex, detailed work, renovation fees are always higher than those for new construction: from 8 to 10 percent of the estimated construction price is standard.

Additional Fees

Fees for interior design equal 10–15 percent of the interior furnishings cost. A fee of $.75–$1.00 per square foot of space is typical. The cost of interior furnishings can be estimated at 5 percent of the construction costs.

Fees for consulting on movable equipment equal 6–7 percent of the cost of the movable equipment. The movable equipment constitutes 15–17 percent of estimated construction costs. For example:

—Graphic design will cost about $.25 per square foot.

—Professional renderings will cost $1,500–$5,000 each.

—Scale models cost $500–$15,000 each.

—Topography and site surveys run $2,000–$15,000 depending on the size of the site.

—Fees for soils testing vary with the number of test holes and range from $15,000–$50,000.

—Value management will cost .1–.3 percent of the total cost of construction.

—The dietary consultant will charge 5–6 percent of equipment costs.

—The clerk-of-the-works charges $25,000–$40,000 per year of construction.

—A materials-handling study runs $15,000–$50,000, based upon size and scope.

—As-built drawings cost $20–$30 per hour and require 30–50 hours per sheet.

—Construction management charges are 3–6 percent of the total estimated construction costs.

—An engineering audit or study will cost $15,000–$30,000, depending on scope.

—Per-diem costs range from $250–$1,000.

SCHEDULE

The next step in formulating a project is a discussion of schedule. The only thing that can be predicted is the change in seasons, and even that has a large plus or minus factor. Defining a design and construction schedule is the first step the administrator takes in committing and involving his entire staff. It will be up to him to set up numerous meetings, reviews, committees, trips, board reviews, and operation phasing once construction starts. The schedule will depend on financing, zoning, state approval, environmental approval, local approval, certificate-of-need approval, community approval, and the tremendous amount of time spent with the design team. Construction becomes as time consuming for the administrator as any other hospital department. The money the hospital spends on construction will be the largest single contract that the administrator handles, and this can cause unanticipated pressure. An awareness of schedule for such an undertaking can only be gained through experience and knowledge of the construction field. A review by an associate would be helpful at this time since a construction project will probably occupy three to four years of time and thought.

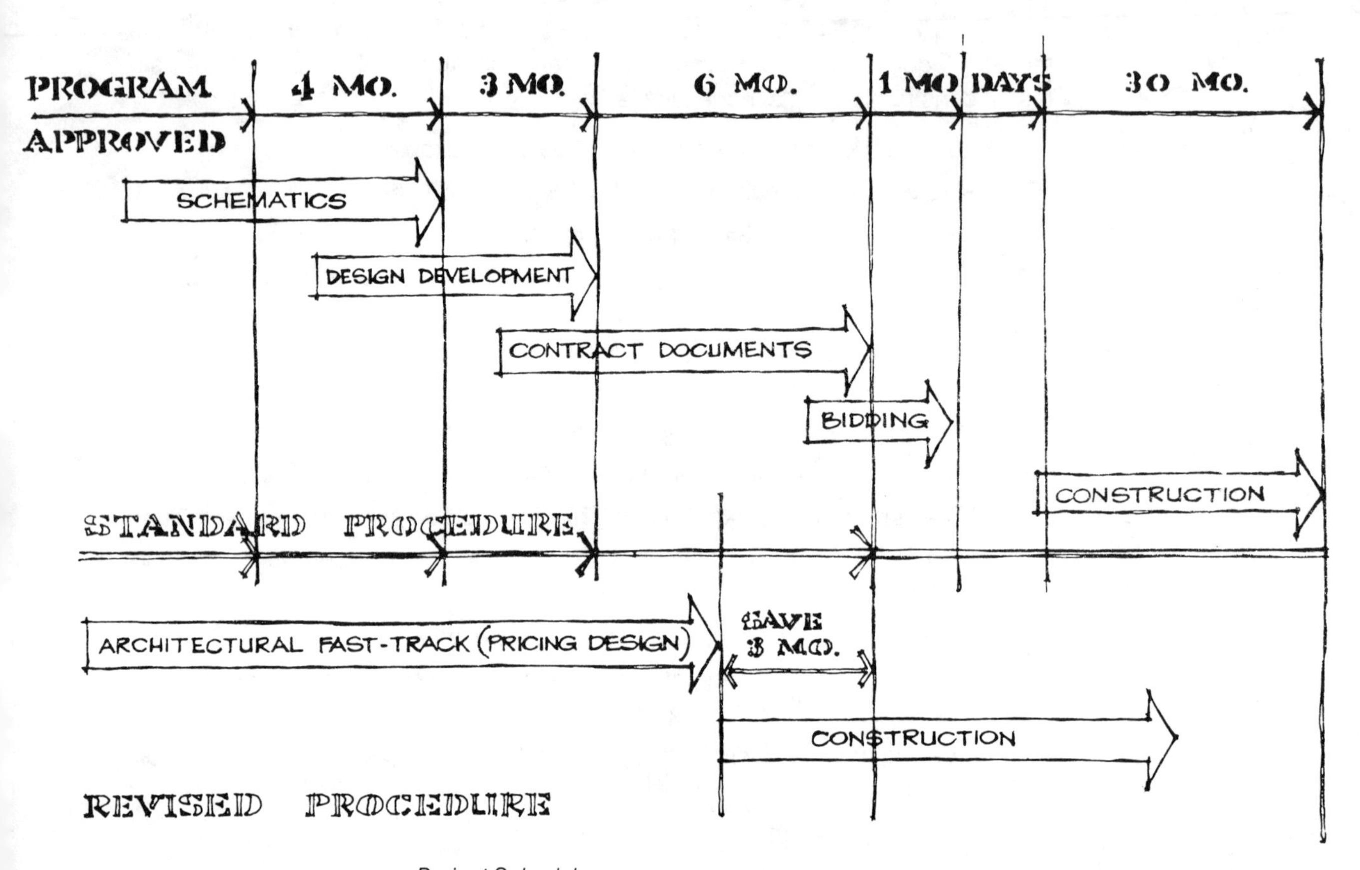

Project Schedule

There are many services geared toward schedule-estimating and time-scheduling. Bar graphs and critical-path scheduling can be used to predict each step, but each step involves so many possibilities that it is very difficult to define a typical schedule.

Review of the proposed project with every possible authority and interest group at this stage cannot be over-emphasized. Before the project goes into a design-development stage or is approved by the staff, all reviews should be completed. With the new certificate-of-need legislation, all projects over $100,000 to $150,000 will have to be approved before private or public financing can be obtained.

A listing of specific steps to take in the review process is impossible but it is possible to tell you that missing a key review can be disastrous. The following list is only a beginning:

—health systems agencies
—state planning review
—city planning
—zoning
—public health department
—environmental impact review
—historic register or historic zoning review
—federal codes
—HHS regional office
—state codes
—local codes
—community review
—public transportation
—public utilities
—board review
—committee review
—financial review

The team of consultants, architects, and engineers will assist in, and in many cases handle, the total review. Each area, however, involves important people in the health field, and the greatest amount of social, or diplomatic, time will be spent here.

A final part of the administrator's work in setting up the project schedule is that of total payment and cash flow. All of the professionals involved in basic services, additional services, construction contracts, and projected operational budgets are interested in cash flow. From the schedules developed, each area of cost flow can be projected. It is important to all members of the team that there be an even flow. It is the duty of the administrator to accomplish this. Payment schedules will be defined in the contracts of the consultants, architects, engineers, and contractors. A master plan should be drawn up to insure a monthly cash flow.

CODES AND STANDARDS

Codes apply in two areas: public health and safety, and minimum legal requirements. The hospital architect and engineers must have a working knowledge and specific reference to various building codes and health design standards. Various national and state building codes apply to each location and type of building. Municipal government usually adopts a national or state code and then forms its own zoning and building construction code. Zoning codes relate to the type and occupancy of the building and specify building setbacks: e.g., parking requirement, lot coverage, height maximums, and use classification.

The National Life Safety Code outlines specific building type requirements: smoke control; fire rating separation for walls, doors, and exit stairs; smoke and fuel contribution standards for all interior materials; and all safety-related requirements.

The facility classification, fire and exit review, and safety standards must be reviewed and approved by the city and state before construction can proceed. A building construction permit and approved occupancy certificate must be obtained in the construction process. The property and improvements are then recorded into the city or county plats.

A review by various federal agencies and the Public Health Department is also necessary in order to comply with health and safety standards. All health facilities that receive Medicare and Medicaid reimbursement must meet federal requirements for design and construction. Various national codes that apply to the handicapped and to staff operational safety must also be reviewed in order to conform. Barrier-free standards, Occupational Safety and Health Administration codes, and aids for the blind are a must in health care design.

The hospital must undergo national review for licensing and accreditation. This review is conducted by the Joint Commission on the Accreditation of Hospitals, an independent review commission. The Joint Commission review involves facility compliance with national standards and administration standards, and a quality review.

Major codes for health care design are: (i) the Life Safety code (National Fire Protection Association, Code 101) and all other NFPA fire codes; (ii) technical handbook for Facilities Engineering and Construction Manual, Part 4, Facilities Design and Construction (architectural section 412, Design of Barrier-Free Facilities); and (iii) minimum requirements of construction and equipment for hospital and medical facilities, HEW Public Health Service, Health Resources Administration, DHEW publication (HRA) 79-14500. If the hospital structure is deficient in any of these major areas of safety, fire, minimum function, barrier-free access, and public health standards, the facility may lose accreditation or be determined not in conformance either in part or totally. Nonconformance implies that the deficiencies will be brought up to code. The ultimate threat is loss of accreditation.

IV

the design elements

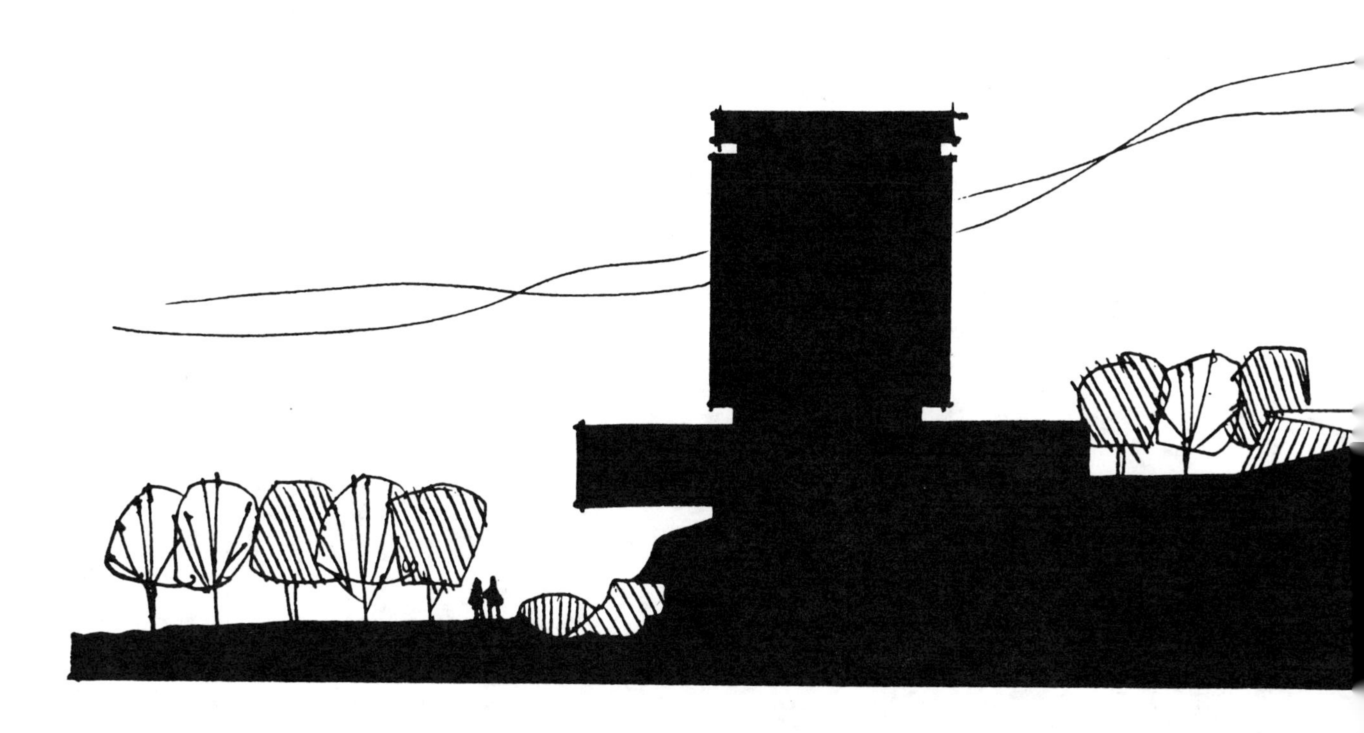

The design of any given hospital must take into consideration a myriad of factors. In general, however, these factors fall into two categories: those features and problems which are common to all hospitals (though specific solutions vary), and those features and problems related to the specific philosophies and objectives of a given facility.

COMMON FACTORS

Factors common to all modern hospitals include:

—design standards

—the elements in the architectural and engineering design process

—long-range facility plans

—structural systems

—functional adjacencies

—traffic and transportation

—site and parking (including external traffic patterns and entrances)

—material handling systems

—electronic systems

—engineering systems

—heating, ventilation, air conditioning and electrical system

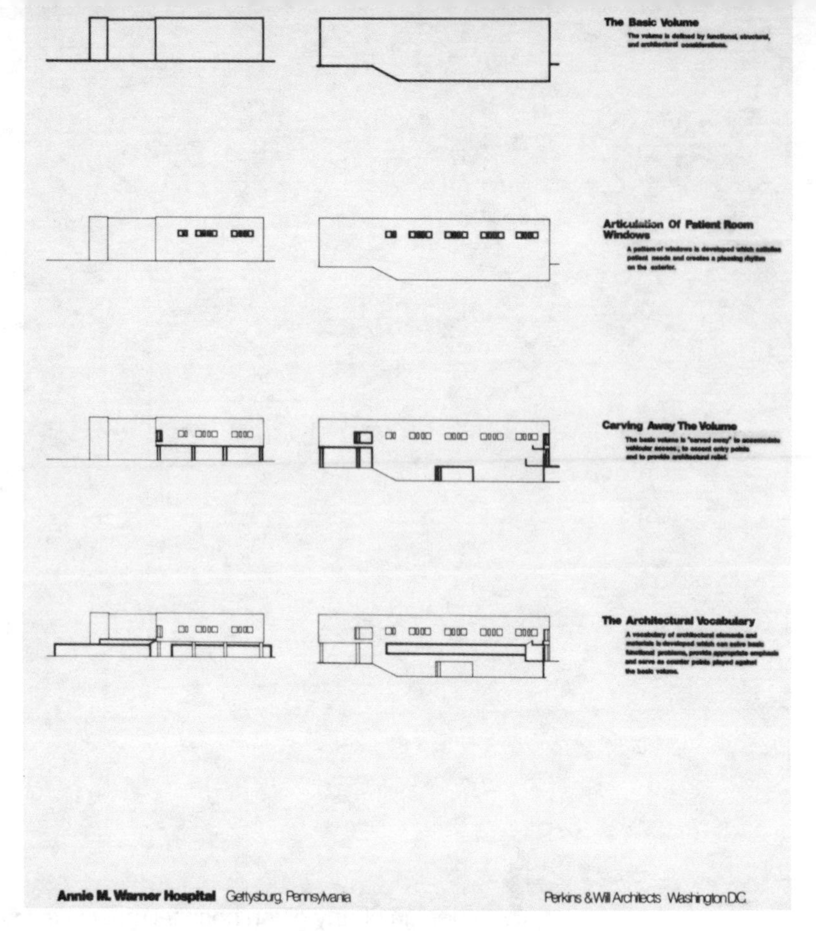

Annie M. Warner Hospital, Gettysburg, Pennsylvania

The hospital architect is bound by restrictions and codes that are absolutely necessary for public safety. Everyone agrees that the vast number of requirements must someday be coordinated and changed, but those who try to beat the intent of the codes are irresponsible.

The federal government's standards are listed in the Department of Health, Education, and Welfare's Public Health Service document "General Standards of Construction and Equipment for Hospital and Medical Facilities" which covers the steps involved in design and outlines minimum standards of size, program, fire safety, and engineering systems, as well as various trade and safety codes that control all areas of hospital construction. These federal standards should be a minimum guide for all hospital projects. The building design must also meet all building codes, ordinances, and regulations enforced by the city, county, or state. Where these do not exist, one of the national building codes will be in effect.

It is impossible to expect the hospital administrator and board to be familiar with all of the codes required in designing and building a structure. Meeting the national and local standards required of hospital operation is itself a full-time effort. However, the administrator should try to review the federal minimum standards and insist that his architect and engineer observe them.

Another area of concern to the architect and to the hospital administrator is that of human standards. The architect is responsible for size, space, and furniture—for every height, shape, weight, and mood of the human body. Ramsey and Sleeper's

Architectural Graphic Standards and various publications on design for the handicapped are valuable for the administrator in understanding the design solutions of the architect.

Elements in the Design Process

The most important thing the architect brings to a project is design talent. Design affects the dignity of the patient, the efficiency and comfort of the staff, and the reputation of the hospital. It applies to the function as well as the form of a building. Architectural and engineering design play an equal role in the success of a program. It is very difficult for the layman to judge design. Results can be measured in a market sense, but only once the hospital is completed. Just the fact that a firm has designed many hospitals is not enough. Creative talent and broad public acceptance of their completed work are essential.

The ideal hospital design combines a very clear, simple traffic configuration with the ability to expand the number of beds and the service base in the future as program growth and change within a hospital structure are continuous. The need for beds does not always grow at the same rate as the need for service programs, but both must have a master plan for direction. The long-range plan must also be flexible enough to allow for technological changes in all areas of health care.

In the design process, the footprint (the land covered by the building) of the hospital must be considered first, though it does not occupy the largest portion of the land. (Parking and multiple entries, discussed below, constitute a larger land use.) There are various approaches to designing the hospital footprint and the patient beds and service base that make it up.

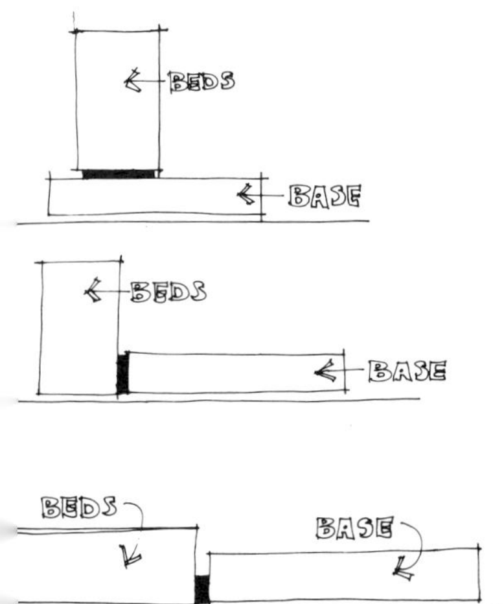

Base. Base services fall into two categories: ancillary services (oriented toward patient care) and service departments (stores, laundry, dietary, housekeeping, and so forth). These elements can be combined into one base structure or they can be housed independently. Different fire ratings for enclosures may determine the approach. The base occupies 500–700 gross square feet per bed and typically requires two to four floors.

Beds. Virtually every possible configuration for bed units has been designed: round, triangular, oval, square, horizontal, vertical, L-shaped, cross-shaped, Y-shaped, H-shaped, T-shaped, and hexagonal. The design chosen should meet the optimum nursing pattern for organization and staffing. Usually twenty to thirty patients are assigned to each nursing team. The mix of private and semiprivate rooms also determines bed floor design, as do minimum federal standards, such as the distance from the end bedroom to the nurses' station and various life safety codes. Specialty units and intensive care units vary in size based upon different programs and levels of care. A long-term or self-care unit may contain more than thirty beds and an intensive care unit should contain a maximum of fourteen to sixteen beds. Since the bed unit is a modular structure, its design may not be compatible with that of the base and different structure and support concepts may be applied to the design of the bed and base units. Interstitial space has recently been incorporated into some hospital designs but the debate over whether the increased building flexibility justifies the higher cost must be settled on an individual basis.

The current ratio of beds to base for a community facility is approximately 400–500 square feet per bed for the nursing units and 500–700 square feet per bed for the base. This average of 1,000 square feet per bed is an overall gross square footage building design. A teaching facility may need up to 1,500 square feet per bed, with university and children's hospitals requiring as many as 2,000 square feet per bed.

The long-range cost implications of fuel also play a key role in design. Solar and reclaimed energy systems may be economically advantageous but they require more building and site space than do conventional systems. Future comfort and space depend upon a great deal of creative engineering now, and this part of the process is of the highest priority.

Long-Range Facility Planning

One of the major problems with many existing hospital facilities is that they lack a long-range plan for expanding or adjusting to new programs. The concept of shared services and levels of care will someday be required, and a good long-range plan will enable the hospital to adjust. Adjustment can require remodeling, expansion, or both, and many older facilities have had to relocate when expansion became necessary due to their total physical obsolescence or the lack of available land. The consultant's program and recommended long-range plan of health needs and delivery systems are important factors in the building scope and future requirements. This is why the facility master plan should be developed before department locations are fixed. The future cost of phasing, relocation, and additions are a critical part of all design, and without a plan or map for the future, the hospital will face delay, cost overrun, and obsolescence.

Structural Elements

Potential vertical or horizontal expansion of the building is one of the most critical issues in the planning stage. Currently, the most popular term in the hospital structural systems market is "interstitial space". The idea is to construct mechanical spaces above occupied areas so that heating, plumbing, and electrical systems can be easily changed when the area below them is reprogrammed. Combined with this, a system of long-span structural elements will allow fewer fixed column locations and, therefore, easier modification of the occupied spaces in the future. Both elements, however, carry a high initial construction cost. Other systems designed to head off high remodeling and maintenance costs in the future have been developed on individual projects. The point is that future remodeling and expansion must be thought out for each new structure in its planning stage, and the long-term cost of the building's operating life must be given high priority. Not everyone will be able to afford the initial costs of advanced systems, even though the operational cost might someday be smaller; but unless these key factors of future change are considered, the long-range plan will lead a short-range life.

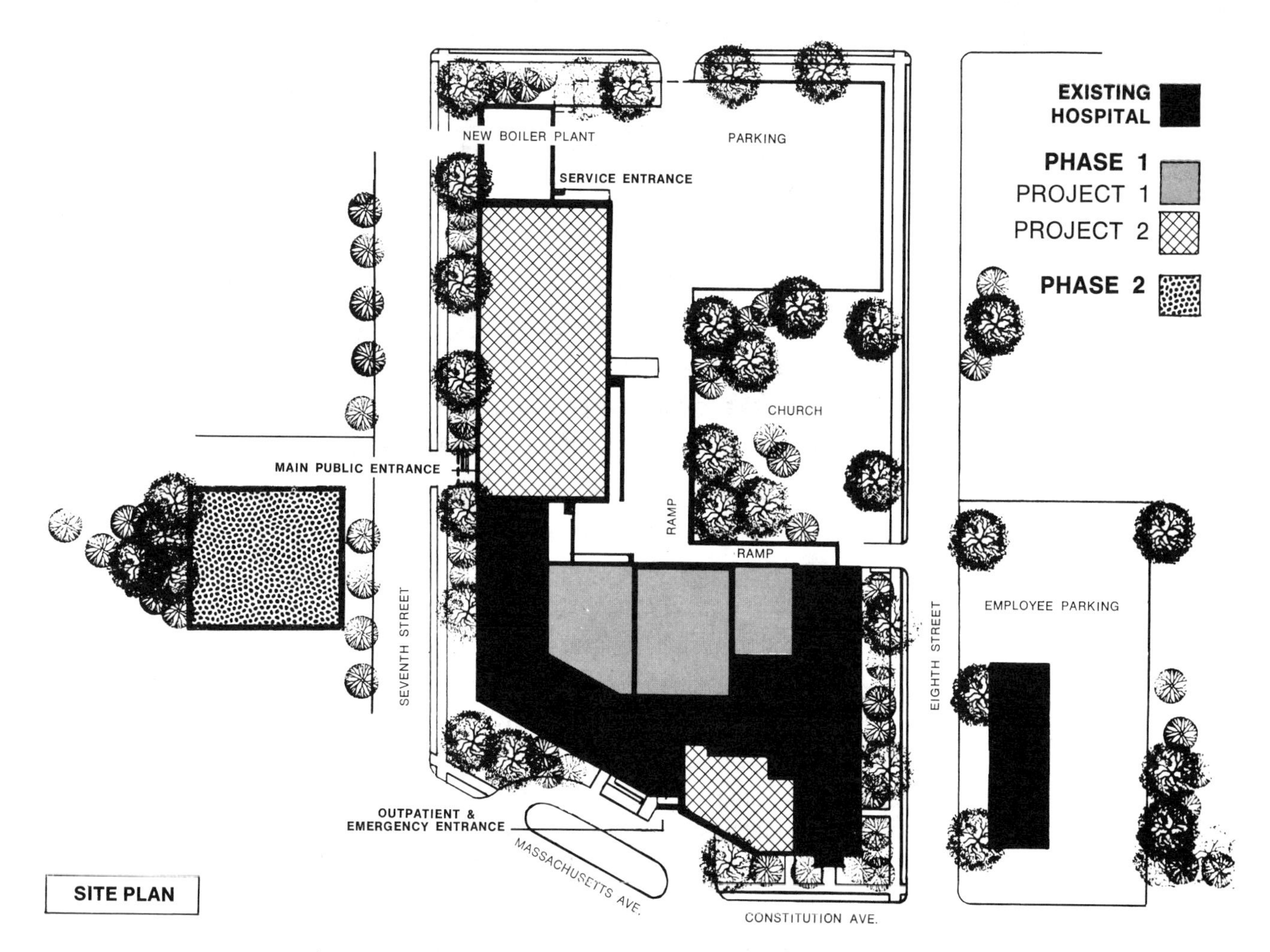

Long-range facility plan. Rogers Memorial Hospital, Washington, D.C.

Interstitial space is an excellent concept, for the hospital service floors and administrators should review the idea before setting department locations, heights, and functions. Interstitial space for nursing floor design, however, is carrying the system too far and cannot be justified. Major changes in the bed areas are not as likely as they are on the service floors, and a much more economical approach, such as flexible vertical mechanical shafts and individual air systems per floor, will allow for reasonable, predictable changes on nursing floors.

Comparisons should also be made in structural system difference, potential, and cost: concrete versus steel versus precast concrete, long-span systems and space frames versus the more conventional spans and erection (these analyses are a part of design and review by the hospital). A full picture of the structural system and its cost should be presented to the hospital by the design team.

Functional Adjacencies

A very important example of functional adjacency is that of the radiology and emergency departments. The radiology department is responsible for the total X-ray needs of a facility. Though the entire radiology staff is not on duty twenty-four hours a day, the emergency room is. It is important, therefore, that a smaller area of radiology can be opened at night for the emergency use. By designing these two areas adjacent to one another both the operational cost and the critical time of travel can be reduced.

Other factors which affect the location of radiology are as follows:

—outpatient X-ray procedures
—admission procedures
—intensive and coronary care procedures
—therapy procedures for extended care patients
—surgery procedures
—special procedures
—inpatient travel and transportation
—outpatient travel and transportation
—operational relationship to nuclear medicine and isotopes
—physical confinement of mass therapy wall design (X-ray shielding, floor loading, and electrical sources)

The final decision on the location of the radiology department will require compromise in some areas, but the major factor must be the cost of operations for staff, travel, and equipment throughout the life of the structure. Secondary factors in deciding department adjacencies are building design, structural economics, future expansion, and site plan.

Traffic, Transportation, and Adjacencies

Subsequent chapters will mention the multiple entrances and exits required in hospital projects, but the arrangement of departments within the structure and their entry requirements must be considered together before ultimate department adjacencies can be designed. Departmental adjacencies are extremely important because they determine the operational costs of staff time and travel throughout the life of the building. One key to a successful functional plan and cost-efficient operation is a simple traffic flow. Maximum separation between public corridors and staff and patient corridors reduces confusion as well as staff and patient transit time. Material supply and trash removal should also have defined routes that do not interfere with the movement of people. It is likewise very important that a hospital be designed so that persons can easily orient themselves within the building; if it is difficult to find departments and not clear where to go, then it follows that staff and supply movement will also be confused and inefficient. Also, the visual impact of travel distance and environment must be pleasant for the public, staff, and patient. Department and individual room adjacencies vary because of the variations in individual hospital programs. General outlines are given in Chapters VIII through XI; the following discussion refers to some specific examples which illustrate the importance of this feature in the operational cost of the hospital.

Site and Parking

The site plan involves all traffic and transportation, parking, entry, exit, material, cost, topography, utilities, future expansion, form, shape, and size. City planning has been a profession since the first caveman occupied a cave, and a hospital contains every possible kind of cave you can name. Every facet of government, industry, and social life is simulated in a hospital. Consequently, site consultants can be hired for landscaping, parking, directional signing, snow melting, truck docking, trash handling, air exhausting, air intaking, fencing, busing, and paving. The master site study by the consulting architect should always be reviewed for any specialty areas that come up. It must be remembered that the physical site size and topography place certain limitations upon potential growth and future expansion. The selection of a site and land acquisition must, therefore, involve long-range planning for 50–100 years.

Three or four major entrances are required for a hospital facility; these entrances are determined by adjacencies and traffic flow inside the facility, and in turn will determine traffic flow outside and location of parking lots. The main hospital entrance is for dropping off visitors and patients; it requires a lot for hourly parking. The ambulatory care entrance is for outpatient, emergency, and ambulance traffic. The service dock is for all supplies' deliveries and trash pickup for the facility. The employee entrance is for current and prospective personnel. All of these entrances require parking lots. The type of parking required and an exact parking count for each entrance are extremely difficult to produce as both are related to the entrances' function. Also, each hospital facility has a different mix of public and private transportation and parking and traffic patterns will vary accordingly: a downtown hospital that serves a walking population may require only one parking space per bed, whereas a suburban hospital may need two parking spaces per bed. In general, one can estimate a need of one and one half to two spaces per bed. The following figures are a guide to design:

—visitors: one space for every three to five patients

—patients: included in visitor's count

—ambulatory care: five spaces per doctor in the outpatient suite, plus emergency parking

—hospital staff: one space for every three employees during the peak daytime shift

—medical staff: one space for each one and a half staff members

The cost of parking lots varies greatly depending on whether the lot is on ground level, above ground, or underground. The overall amount of space allowed per car is 300 square feet, excluding ramps. The cost of a ground level stall is approximately $500 per car, whereas above ground parking varies from $6,000 to $10,000 per car, with an average of about $8,000 per car. Underground lots must be mechanically ventilated and will cost between $8,000 and $12,000 per space. The cost of land plus excavation must also be considered in the parking costs.

Paid parking versus free parking must be worked out by each hospital facility. The initial cost of construction for parking is a major element in the construction budget, and as much review time as required for each department must be given to it.

Material Handling

Material management and handling affect every aspect of hospital organization, operation, and design. Materials-handling systems and electronic aids are fast becoming major cost considerations in the planning budget. The present state of the art relates very unevenly to hospital needs and to the planning process and, furthermore, there does not exist a universally accepted data base or methodology for resolving the issues of whether to have manual or automated transport. Experience has revealed that there is little difference among the functional requirements of hospital material-handling systems, provided the materials are delivered to the user in the desired quantity and quality at the right place and at the right time.

To properly evaluate material-handling systems and other electronic support devices, one must first develop the concept of materials management in the hospital. While there are many definitions of materials management, an organizational and functional concept should provide for efficient planning, coordination, and control of all materials before they are used and for the subsequent disposition of reusables, wastes, and soiled items. To determine the most appropriate system for a particular facility, the materials distribution program should first be planned with respect to specific schedules and user requirements. The job of implementing the handling system is then accomplished through further organization and space planning, equipment selection, engineering design, and training.

Materials management includes planning and anticipating commodity requirements, acquiring needed supplies and materials, introducing and moving them horizontally and vertically, monitoring their status as current assets, accounting for them as charges, and providing them at the right place and at the right time. Materials that fall within the system are medical treatment supplies; nonmedical, general use supplies; pharmaceuticals, biologicals, and drugs; linen (clean and soiled); food; mail and patient gifts; trash; and reprocessibles (trays, bedpans). These commodities usually move within the hospital either as a bulk system (that is, a quantity of supplies loaded aboard a single device going from point A to point B on a programmed basis) or as a small item. Items in the latter category are either nonprogrammable or very small, and they are needed immediately by the user. To meet the transport requirements of both systems, there is a wide choice of modes, from manual to highly sophisticated automation. Essential to the bulk system are carts or modular containers moved either by an employee or by some type of automation. Moving small items falls within a much narrower range, such as pneumatic tubes and box conveyors.

Popular variations of materials-handling hardware and sub-systems include:

—selective vertical conveyor

—tray conveyor and lift

—tow trucks

—box conveyor

—dumbwaiter (cart size)

—elevator (automatic load and off-load)

—elevator (standard for freight)

—overhead monorail conveyor (power and free)

—floor guidance (automatic) systems

—combinations of the above

—pneumatic tube

—chutes

To determine the most efficient system for a facility, management options must first be considered and evaluated, then, all expected movements (on a twenty-four hour, weekly basis) must be simulated on paper. One accurate means of quantifying movement is to base the simulation on a cart-exchange system, even though this method primarily speaks to the bulk delivery requirements. Once this is clear, actual constraints on the most desirable pathways, either horizontal or vertical, become clear. However, engineering or building configurations should not be the deciding factors in achieving the most efficient patterns of movement; building system innovations such as pre-fabricated shaftways and interstitial spaces add great flexibility for the use of automated systems.

Paramount in the selection of any materials-handling system is a life-cycle cost analysis. While life-cycle cost analysis and value engineering have become very popular, there are certain pit-falls to be aware of when making comparisons. Each management method and individual item of equipment should be subjected to thorough cost analysis. To do so, each management principle and piece of equipment should represent solutions to a single problem. It is very easy to slip into comparisons of apples and oranges: be sure that each system is performing the same function under the same conditions.

Each life-cycle evaluation should include initial purchase price of the equipment; periodic overhaul costs; preventive maintenance costs; energy consumption costs; and labor costs. The costs of each of the systems to be evaluated should be derived by using the most appropriate and most recent market data for projections. Numerous methods are used in constructing a life-cycle analysis (I prefer the discount of money concept introduced by the General Accounting Office).

The life-cycle analysis allows a manager to evaluate the method of delivery (for example, manual versus automation) as well as predict initial cost and operational cost to be consumed by the system over a predetermined period of time.

It is important, nonetheless, to develop a broader basis for selecting handling systems before preparing the life-cycle cost analysis. While the cost may be acceptable, other factors such as engineering impracticalities or environmental hazards may render the system unacceptable. Therefore, the basis of selection must be the benefit to patient care, as well as the cost of the system, compatibility with the building, and product reliability.

The field of hospital materials-handling, then, involves industrial engineering, mechanical engineering, production engineering, and architectural and equipment consulting. While it is virtually impossible for hospital administrators to become experts in these fields, their contribution is most important. Operational methods, staffing patterns, and management style must be translated by the materials-handling expert into sensible simulation models reflecting the most efficient system for each facility. Only then can there be a comparison of equipment requirements for manual or automated handling systems.

Electronic Systems

Electronic systems include intercommunications, paper and information flow, monitoring of patients' vital signs, and multiphasic screening. Although these systems do not usually affect the structural or functional layout of the hospital to the extent that the bulk materials system does, they must, nonetheless, be designed before individual departments can be planned.

Modern information systems. Word processing and hard copy electronic record systems are under constant improvement and change. The future use of communications within the hospital and expanded into the home for medical use are around every corner and will dictate the staffing and utilization of hospital design. Even staff communications outside the hospital and two-way ambulance calls are a major design field. The Federal Communications Commission has so many requests for frequency bands that radio systems may face reduction rather than improvement of communications. Communications for a hospital project are as follows:

—intercom (intra- and interdepartmental)

—telephone

—paging (intra- and inter-hospital)

—nurses' call

—computerized visual display terminals

—closed-circuit and cable television

—pneumatic (monitoring systems)

—mechanical life system

—engineering controls and alarm systems

—physiological monitoring

—space satellite hookups

Intercom and nurses call systems have been greatly improved. The cost of advanced manufactured systems, however, is a roadblock for the design team. Evaluations based on manufacturers' literature are dangerous because the life-cycle costs are very difficult to determine. Studies can be done by qualified engineers and equipment can be tested, but very few hospitals can afford to reevaluate these systems for each project. The task of comparing American Telephone and Telegraph's intercom against a privately owned one would be a tremendous effort, and the initial cost of such a study would make it out of the question. It will take a serious effort by the government or private review groups to compare the costs of systems. Also, space technology has affected electronic sensing and communications systems, and innovations hit the market each week. As a consequence, information systems and technology within the hospital will be dramatically improved in the future, and facilities design today should include features such as coaxial cable to every room in order to take advantage of two-way visual systems and multiple display and storage of computerized information.

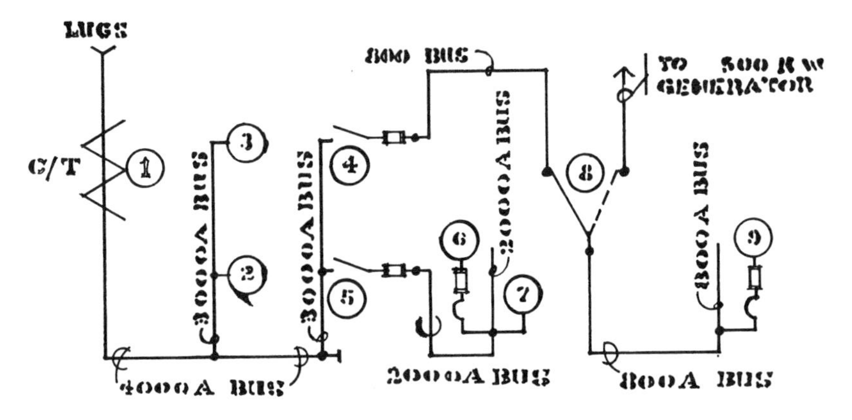

SWITCHBOARD ONE LINE DIAGRAM

Communications requirements and systems are extremely complex and come as close as any area of hospital design to defying solution through the hiring of a technical designer: in this area, experience rather than analytical studies must take precedence. The following list sets out the choices of systems in major categories:

1) Intercommunication systems
   —hospital departments
   —telephone
   —private hospital communications system
   —privately leased systems
   —computer links
   —nursing floors
   —audio intercom (patient to nurse station)
   —visual communicaticn (patient room to nurse station)
   —telephone (patient to nurse station)

2) Medical and administrative departments
   —doctors' page
      –central audio
      –pocket frequency
   —doctors' register
      –visual
      –audio with message storage
   —central dictating
      –telephone
      –private
   —computer systems
      –billing
      –charting and addressing
      –visual display
      –medical records
   —emergency radio bands
   —hospital paging
   —music systems
   —closed-circuit television
   —central clock system
   —television security system
3) Physical monitoring
   —EKG, pulse, respiration, and so on (including remote systems)
   —multi-phasic screening tests
   —visual monitoring
   —biofeedback systems
4) Paper handling
   —pneumatic tube system
   —track
   —lifts
   —electronic sending
   —video
5) Engineering systems
   —remote equipment monitoring (central control)
   —remote heat and lighting control
   —system sensing (heat, cool, light, sound)

—timed switching

—automatic snow melting

—alarm wiring (smoke, emergency power, fire, and so on)

—isolation grounding

Design of electronic systems will greatly affect the total design of the facility. Because life-cycle operational costs can save or cost millions of dollars over the life of a building, the importance of carrying out life-cycle analyses on every possible element of these systems in the initial design phase must be emphasized.

Engineering Systems

Materials handling and electronic systems are dealt with by the engineers on the team who will detail the final systems that are approved by the team. The engineer also takes the lead in the areas of heating, cooling, ventilating, plumbing, and electrical design. These mechanical and electrical systems and their construction account for half the cost of constructing a hospital. The administrator, therefore, must be well advised in this highly technical, but patient-oriented, part of the total design.

The engineering profession has the responsibility for costing out the recommended system. Cost studies thus become a daily part of the engineer's life. Because it is possible to work with known fuel costs and detailed manufactured items, the engineer can justify each system recommended. Still, fuel studies, mechanical system studies, and use of computer analysis are an advanced art in the mechanical and electrical engineering fields and therefore the engineering team members' creative thoughts should be a major effort in the program conception.

Although static-quantity engineering has been described as a straightforward solution, let me warn you that a good engineer is as important to the final success of the building as *any* other member of the team. Comfort control for every individual's thermostat is almost impossible, but it will be that one point that is criticized (never applauded) the most when the building is complete. The wrong decision can make the building shake, sweat, freeze, fry, smoke, leak, dark, dry, loud, and even stop.

Heating, Ventilation, Air Conditioning, and Electrical Systems

The design of the heating, ventilation, and air conditioning systems (HVAC) for a hospital is regulated by state and federal minimum standards; its cost can range from 15–30 percent of the total building cost. A hospital has two main areas of design for HVAC: the exterior walls (typically the patient rooms) and the interior areas (service departments and nursing floors).

Selecting the appropriate air-conditioning system for a hospital is a critical decision facing the architect and engineer. On this decision rests the satisfaction of the entire hospital staff and the patients. Many factors must be analyzed, judged, screened, and coordinated. The desires of the hospital board, the administrator, and the physical plant director, as well as the economic aspects, are all considerations.

The client wants an installation that will provide maximum comfort with minimum operating costs. The engineer must be able to anticipate the behavior of the contemplated air-conditioning system. Complete air-conditioning provides an environment of correct temperature, humidity, air movement, air cleanliness, ventilation, and acoustical level. Anything less is a compromise and is not termed air-conditioning.

The patient rooms of a hospital should be considered like hotel rooms, with the load requirements based on 100 percent occupancy with twenty-four hour, year-round operation. An important factor to remember is that air circulation must be contained within each room. Corridors, nurses' stations, and serving areas must have a separate supply and exhaust system. Each patient room must have an exhaust-creating negative pressure, and there should be no cross-contamination between various areas; individual temperature control must be maintained in patient rooms; and individual temperature, humidity, and ventilation control must be available in special treatment, therapeutic, maternity, surgical, morgue, and other service areas. Absolute cleanliness from duct odors and bacteria is essential; thus, rigid housekeeping procedures are required to ensure that the air-conditioning system will fulfill its basic requirements. The objectives of air-conditioning can be achieved if standard systems and equipment are utilized. They must be simple to operate and maintain, for equipment with extremely complicated control systems in confined spaces soon lacks proper care and attention.

Possibly the best low-maintenance control at the patient room is an all-air system. This is also the most expensive system for total design and cannot always be justified. Two common exterior systems are the fan-coil and the induction unit. With a fan-coil system, outside air and room air are circulated over a heating or cooling coil that is supplied with hot or cold water from a central source. This system can be modified in price and individual room control by having a two-or four-pipe supply. The main objection to the fan coil is the enclosed fan in the unit and the filter, which must be maintained and cleaned. The amount of air that can be recirculated in the room is spelled out in federal construction standards. Induction units are based on air that is warmed or cooled at a central source and that is sent to a room fast enough to cause the air to circulate within the room. This unit does not contain a fan but it does cause a hissing noise that can be objectionable. Also the cost is higher than that of a fan-coil unit. Other variations that have been used for the patient room are radiant heat in the ceiling (hot or cold water run through a grid in the ceiling), electric radiant heat, and package electric units (at each window).

Because humidity control is needed in many of the interior departments, single-or dual-duct air systems are often used. The dual-duct system supplies warm and cool air to a mixing box at the room, and thus individual room temperature control is gained along with humidity control. A single-duct system does not supply individual room control, but rather a zoned area control.

HVAC equipment must be centrally located. Preferably, a boiler room or central plant, separate from the main structure, should be constructed to house the boilers (steam generation), chillers (cold water generation), and all auxiliary equipment needed for their operation. This steam, or hot water and cold water, should be piped through a service tunnel to the main structure. A central mechanical equipment room should be built to house the necessary air-handling units, secondary pumps, converters, and auxiliary equipment for distributing the air and heated and chilled water to meet the system requirements. In addition, a fan room should be located on the roof to house the exhaust fans. The central plant concept includes the use of high-grade commercial equipment with longer life and more economical cost and maintenance.

An important concept in hospital design is that of "total energy". It involves an on-site plant where electric power is generated and the HVAC needs are supplied without using any outside fuel. Initial costs are very high, but if the rate structure for natural gas and oil in a given area is low, the life-cycle of this system could possibly be justified. It cannot usually be justified for the normal-size community hospital.

The mechanical and electrical systems that must be designed in a hospital structure are as follows:

—energy source and solar energy considerations

—boiler

—cooling tower

—gas

—water

—steam

—emergency power generators

—standby fuel

—electrical

—electrical switchgear

—lighting

—lighting protection

—X-ray power transformers

—electrical grounding

—plumbing

—domestic water

—hot and chilled water

—hypothermia system (piped heated or chilled water for a patient blanket system)

—compressed air

—vacuum

—central medical gases

—oxygen

—nitrous oxide

—mechanical

—elevator

—trash disposal

—central monitoring

—exhaust systems (air, boiler, emergency generator, vent)

—site drainage

—storm sewer

—sanitary sewer

—telephone switchgear

Energy considerations for the life of the structure have an enormous effect on operating cost. All possible avenues for recovery of energy, new sources of energy, and energy efficiency should be considered in the design procedure. The design team's duty is to recommend the best possible concept, systems, and lay-outs to the hospital committee and board. The engineering and the details for construction will be worked out by the engineer and coordinated by the architect. It is important that the hospital administrator be well-informed on the systems in order to answer questions.

SPECIFIC FACTORS

Factors that affect design but are specific to the philosophies and objectives of the individual project are found in the following facilities:

—freestanding ambulatory care units

—teaching hospitals

—university hospitals

—hospices

—international facilities

—community mental health facilities

—federal facilities

—osteopathic facilities

—gerontology units

Freestanding Ambulatory Care Units

Programs that give rise to freestanding units for the delivery of health care include:

—physicians' offices

—health maintenance

—primary care centers

—in-out surgery centers

—community health and social centers

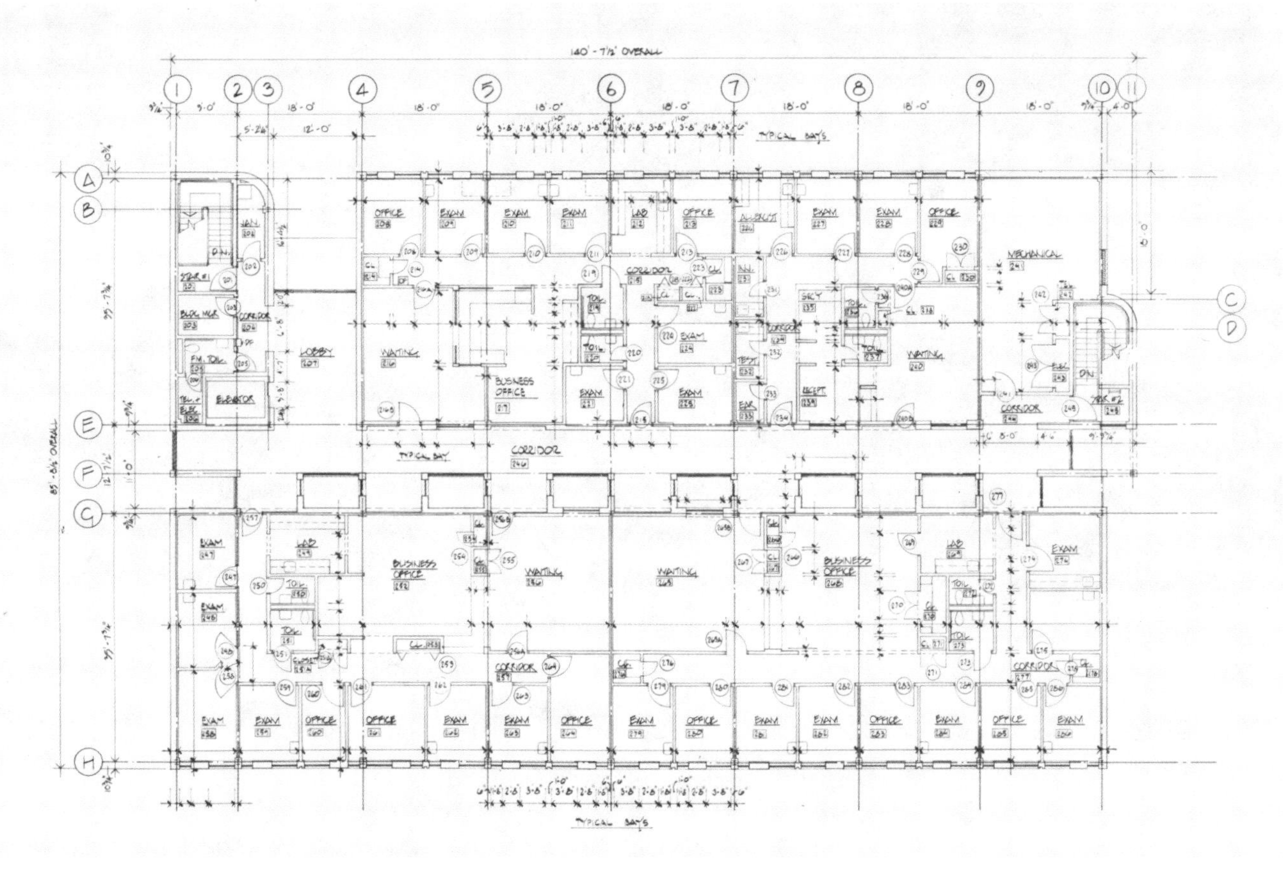

Physicians' office building. Annie M. Warner Hospital, Gettsyburg, Pennsylvania

Ambulatory care includes multiple outpatient services for private and clinic patients. In the search for better preventive care, the independent, freestanding units, programs, and facilities have been tested as to market and effect. Most comprehensive ambulatory care units are attached to hospital facilities in order to share radiology, laboratory, pharmacy, and supply services.

Physician's Office. The physician's office is designed for the individual practitioner or group. If the group is organized to supply comprehensive care, then it resembles an HMO. The typical space requirements run approximately 1,100 gross square feet per physician. This allows the physician to schedule two examinations in separate rooms throughout his day. In addition, this figure provides space for office workers, ten to fifteen waiting people, toilets, equipment, and an office. A building for physician offices contains a common lobby, corridors, service, and mechanical areas. The efficiency factor for the total building is approximately 70–80 percent rentable space for offices and 20–30 percent for common space.

Health Maintenance Organization. The freestanding centers meet many rural needs and act as feeders to the tertiary centers. The Health Maintenance Organization (HMO), as an alternative insurance program, was begun thirty to forty years ago and was aimed at industrial workers. The federal push for HMOs began in the 1970s

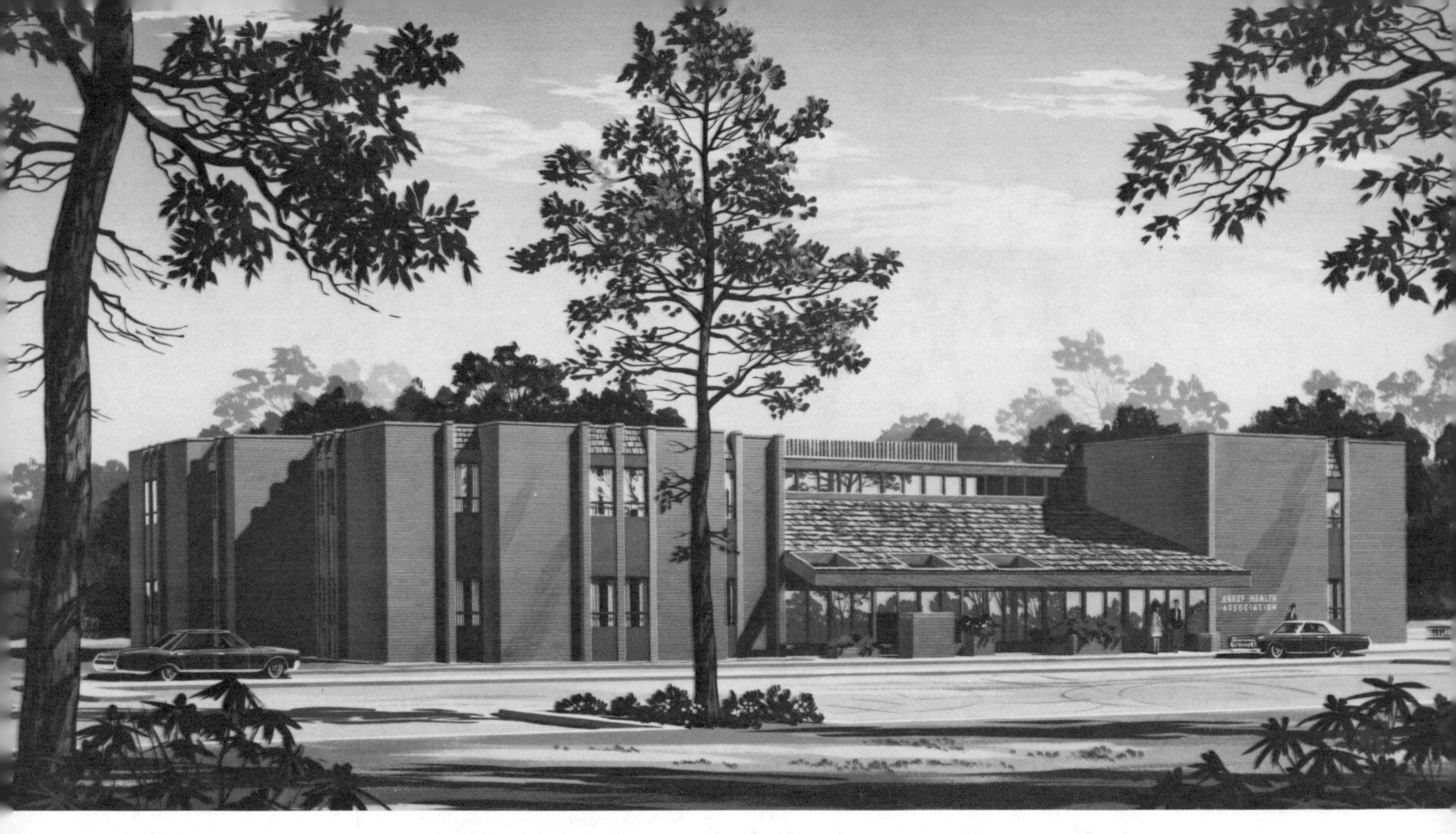

Group Health Association, Rockville, Maryland

as an attempt to reduce the cost of hospital stays. Each HMO begins with a custom program to meet the market needs within a service area. The basic space requirements vary, but they include staff needs and projected load based upon the number of members to be serviced. The space requirement of HMOs vary according to program concept: either a physician's office concept or a nurse practitioner system. Support functions include records, administration, lobby, vending machines and staff lounge, emergency entry, mechanical space, and specialty areas of X-ray, laboratory, EKG, and screening. Space for the examination room, clinic-type waiting areas, and offices depends upon the program offered. Inpatient beds as part of the prepaid insurance plan are located in specific hospital facilities through agreement. A ratio of from one-half to one square foot per enrolled member may be used as a general planning guide.

Primary Care Centers. The primary care center may be aimed at a specific rural population or may serve as a feeder to a larger facility. Design of primary care centers resembles that of an emergency or outpatient unit, with holding beds and doctor's offices attached. Emergency examination and treatment rooms serve for trauma and family outpatient visits. Support areas include records, administration office, conference room, employee lounge and lockers, housekeeping area, storage, and entry waiting area. Full-time primary care physicians and paramedical staff operate these facilities. The space allotment is based upon the characteristics of the service area and predicted number of visits per year. No rule-of-thumb standards yet apply to these facilities, but one can plan on ten visits per gross square foot of space.

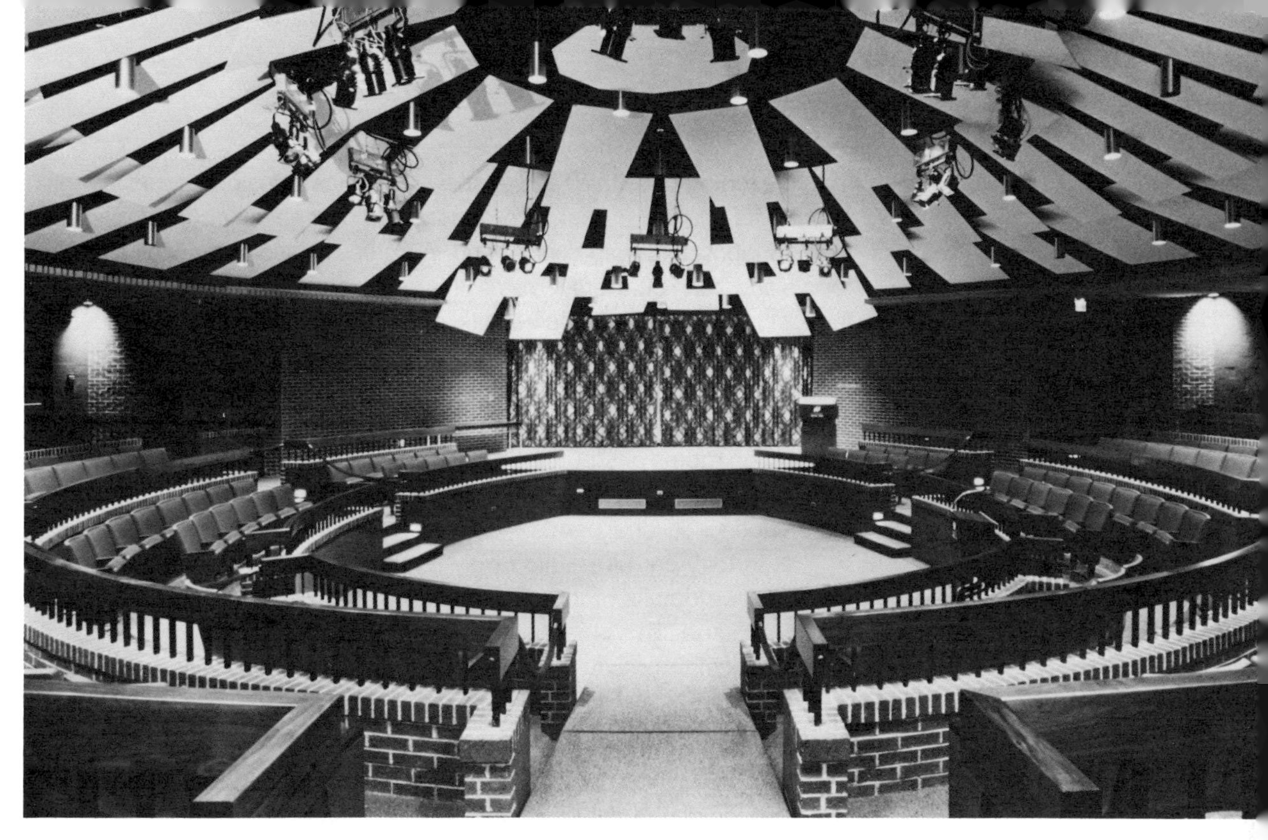

Teaching amphitheatre. Hurley Medical Center, Flint, Michigan

In-Out Surgery Centers. These units are usually connected to a hospital facility or are freestanding close to one. They may be designed to carry up to 50 percent of the hospital's surgical load. The cases involve local anesthesia with the patient's recovering within one to four hours. The utilization projections will determine the number of rooms needed for support services, dressing, examinations, recovery, records, storage, employees, and so on.

Community Health and Social Centers. These units range from an urban free clinic to the community mental health program. Usually funded by local or regional government, these units fulfill varied programs of need. Private buildings for health-related groups are also a key design format.

Teaching Hospitals

The true teaching hospital offers a residency program that involves house staff spaces and medical education but various technical teaching programs exist in many facilities. Some teaching hospitals are affiliated with other facilities so that medical students in specialty programs may be sent to train in the affiliated hospital. For example, a semirural hospital may share a family practice program with a university hospital. Secondary or tertiary private hospitals may also have such affiliations. Most children's hospitals are the teaching arm of university pediatric departments. The teaching hospital with a fulltime residency program may be private or university related.

Teaching hospitals require space to educate residents and interns on the patient floors (clinical areas), in a department of medical education, in research and training laboratories, in clinics, and in nurses' stations, as well as needing classrooms and living quarters. Overall, this space can range from 200–400 gross square feet per bed. The size of the hospital depends on the number of residency programs or technical programs involved. Further, a diploma or graduate nursing school or program also affects the hospital's space needs. Although most diploma programs contain most of the space needed within the school of nursing building, larger medication rooms and nursing stations are required to accommodate the students. An exact calculation of space program and functional areas must be prepared, based upon individual needs.

A tertiary care institution may employ house staff to offset a residency program. These details of larger centers create a need for more staff and additional square footage. This is reflected in the higher cost for delivery of service in tertiary care facilities.

University Hospitals

The university hospital's space needs resemble those of the teaching hospital, with the addition of the medical school's space needs. At some universities, the medical school space is incorporated into the hospital; in others, a separate medical school space is designed. The method of student education determines where student lockers, study carrels, and anatomy laboratories are located. Design concepts can centralize or disperse elements of the medical campus. These elements include the basic science program, allied medicine, student health, reference library, medical school, dental school, nursing school, campus health services, living quarters, and various research institutes.

University medical programming, planning, and design is a specialty that many talented firms practice. It involves special skills such as an understanding of curriculum planning, the state educational system and its goals, and clinic needs for education.

Hospices

The hospice is an inpatient facility or a section of a hospital for dying persons. These patients have special needs in the areas of care, staff training, and programs of service. This type of facility does not come under HSA approval in most states at this time, and reimbursement varies; however, HEW is now conducting pilot cost reimbursement programs.

Very few hospice facilities have been in operation more than a few years in the United States. These programs, within private facilities, have been successfully operated in Europe for the past five years, but within health care systems quite different from that in the United States.

A hospice is designed as a nursing facility with the elements of the long-term care units. The bedrooms are intended to be homelike, with additional space for visitors, privacy, and self-care. The program emphasizes social services, psychological input, and stress management.

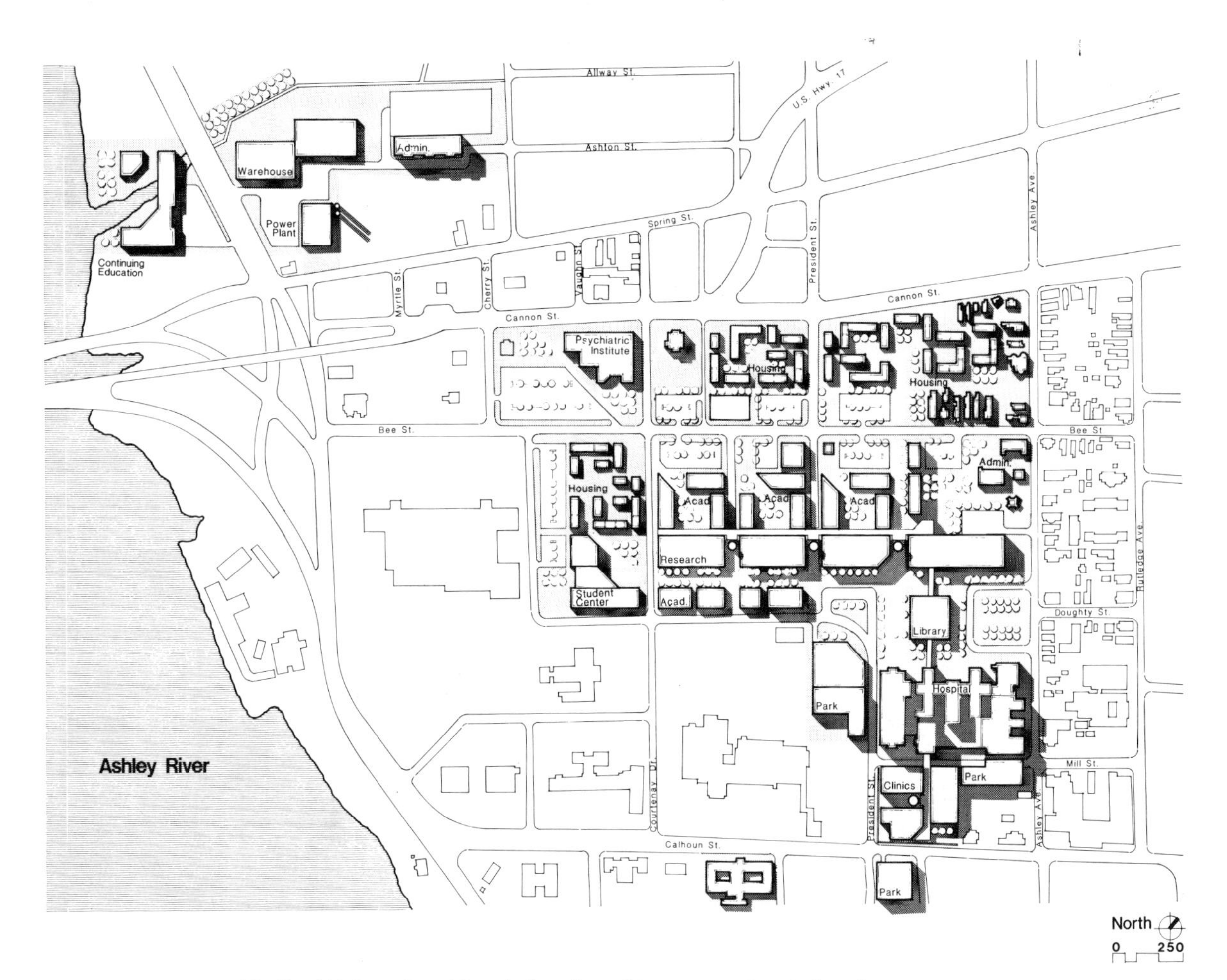

Medical University of South Carolina, Charleston, South Carolina

International Facilities

The late 1970s brought unlimited career opportunities to the health planner, administrator, and nurse overseas: Saudi Arabia alone inundated the newspapers with help-wanted ads. Architectural and engineering commissions soared over night, with many firms making a full commitment to international offices. International work has always existed in design and administration, but the prediction of a recession market in the United States and the flood of new projects abroad tempted many to enter this market. Flights to London and Frankfurt were full of construction workers, managers, dreamers, and designers all ready for adventure.

In the field of health care, planning is underway and some structures have even been completed. The delivery system itself can be built as soon as the populace is ready to use it. Education, training, technology, service, and management must, however, precede use. This will be true in China, Mexico, Saudi Arabia, and anywhere that rapid development occurs.

The single most important feature of international health planning or administration is an understanding of the host country's culture. The emotions, social characteristics, environment, history, and desires of the people must be understood and incorporated into design. For example, a hospital in Saudi Arabia must have sepa-

Charity Hospital, Mecca, Saudi Arabia

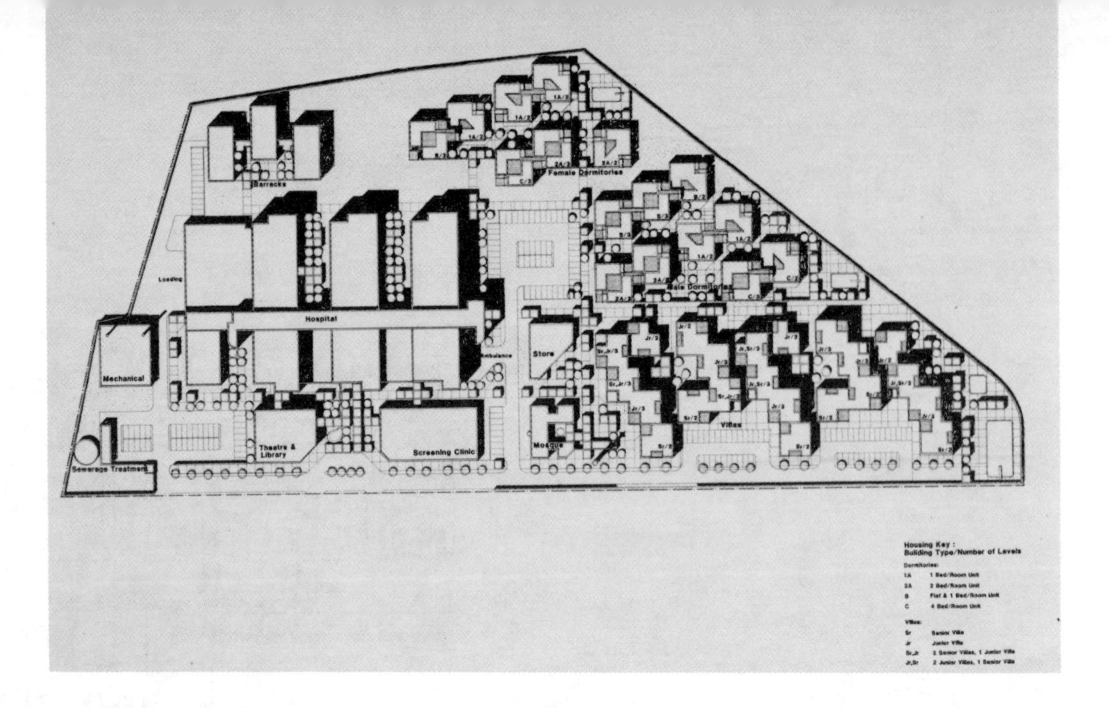

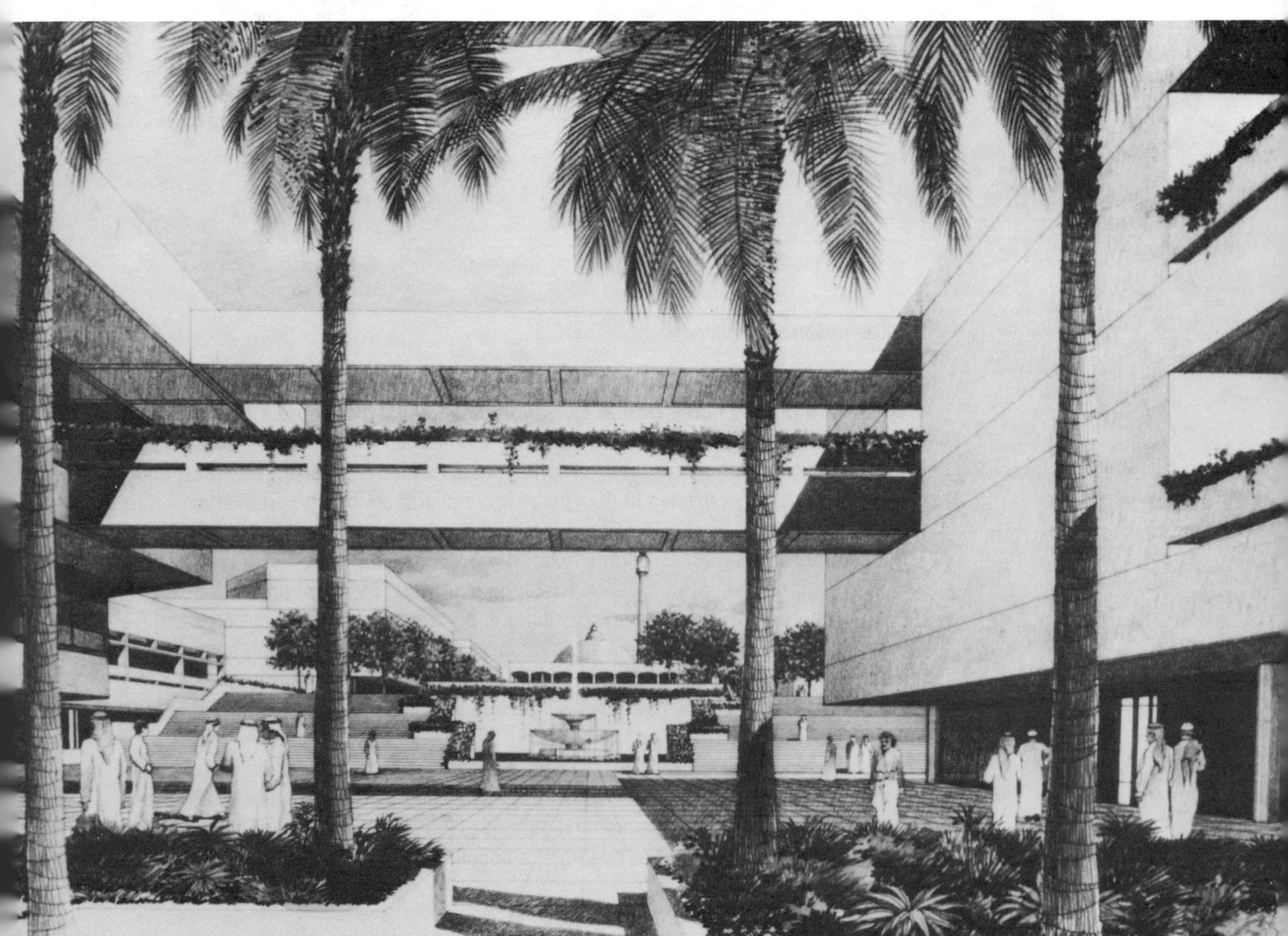

King Abdulaziz University Health Sciences Center, Jeddah, Saudi Arabia

rate areas for men and women, religion is important, water is scarce, maintenance is difficult, more visitors can be expected, and walks must be screened from the sun. In the Virgin Islands and South America, ventilation is necessary and desalinized water must be cooled.

Community Mental Health Facilities

Our nation's mental health needs fall into every age group and have no patterned building program. The National Institutes of Mental Health, with federal funds available in the 1960s and 1970s, produced many community mental health centers. These centers were designed for outpatients in combination with state, local, and private inpatient facilities. With the increase in private insurance and federal payments for mental health needs, this field is still expanding.

Programs range from exclusive private facilities to schools for stress prevention. Social service, nutrition, exercise, medication, group therapy, sex clinics, detoxification units, and headache programs are all interwoven and related to the pressures on, and cracks in, our minds. A physician once explained that sustained pressure will either show up in the physical body or in the mind. Advancements in the understanding of mental health will affect all facility planning and will create new delivery systems for total health.

Federal Facilities

Federal-owned facilities include:

—Veterans Administration (VA) hospitals

—United States Public Health Service(USPHS) hospitals and clinics

—The National Institutes of Health (NIH) facilities

—federal prison health facilities

—military service hospitals and base facilities

Veterans Administration. The VA maintains comprehensive program and design standards, with a full staff in Washington, D.C. and operating staffs at local facilities. Independent national consulting and architectural and engineering firms are retained to complete designs with the VA staff.

VA facilities, located throughout the United States, represent a major health delivery system for veterans and their families. The VA building program in the 1970s produced various "new generation" structures with great experimentation in systems and space concepts. Completely automated materials-handling systems, interstitial space concepts with complete walk-on decks, earthquake-proof structures, design for the handicapped, and layouts resembling shopping malls have been incorporated into the most recent designs.

Facilities include outpatient and ambulatory care centers, long-term care (nursing home) facilities, vast research programs, and complete rehabilitation services. The VA systems maintain affiliations with private hospitals, universities, and state facilities. The VA system is worth studying for its wealth of design and its use of various physical concepts.

Public Health Service. The USPHS system works within a volunteer agreement to meet regional HSA plans. USPHS hospitals serve a mixed population, ranging from merchant marine seamen to residents of our island territories. During the current move towards national health insurance and ambulatory services, these facilities may have an increased role. The procedures issued for the development of facility master plans for all federal-owned facilities parallel the standards of the private health industry and are an excellent guide.

National Institutes of Health. The NIH reaches out into many educational communities with funded research programs and facilities, and its standards are the industry's standards for outpatient- and inpatient-related research in medical schools. The main NIH campus in Bethesda, Maryland, contains a clinical center of approximately 2 million square feet, comprising a vast complex of research laboratories, administration offices, and the National Library of Medicine. This complex of institutes is devoted to research, understanding, and prevention of disease. The ambulatory care research facility addition to the clinical center was programmed and designed for research on clinical, preventive medicine. The advanced technology used and the design studies performed by NIH should be studied as a state-of-the-art in the health care field.

Federal Prison Health Facilities. These are specialty programs designed by each state system and by federal institutions.

Military Facilities. Two structures are prime examples of innovation in this field: the Walter Reed Medical Center and the National Naval Medical Center, both in suburban Washington, D.C. Military health care facilities are located throughout the world and are used by servicemen and their dependents. Staff planning expertise is provided to private design firms by the Surgeon General's office and military service departments. A closer tie between military and private hospitals may come about as world tension and the threat of war increase.

Osteopathic Facilities

Most regions have an osteopathic hospital, and the D.O. (Doctor of Osteopathy) and M.D. (Medical Doctor, or allopathic physician) are equal staff members at many hospital facilities. Various osteopathic medical schools exist throughout the United States and a large number of this country's registered beds are in osteopathic hospitals. These facilities are approved by the HSA process and most meet federal design standards and life safety codes. There is essentially no difference in the design and space programs of the osteopathic and the allopathic facility.

Gerontology Facilities

The social and housing needs of the aged are a design field in themselves. Because increasing numbers of persons are reaching their senior years, sufficient facilities are not available. Consequently, this design field is one that will see continuous growth in the 1980s and 1990s.

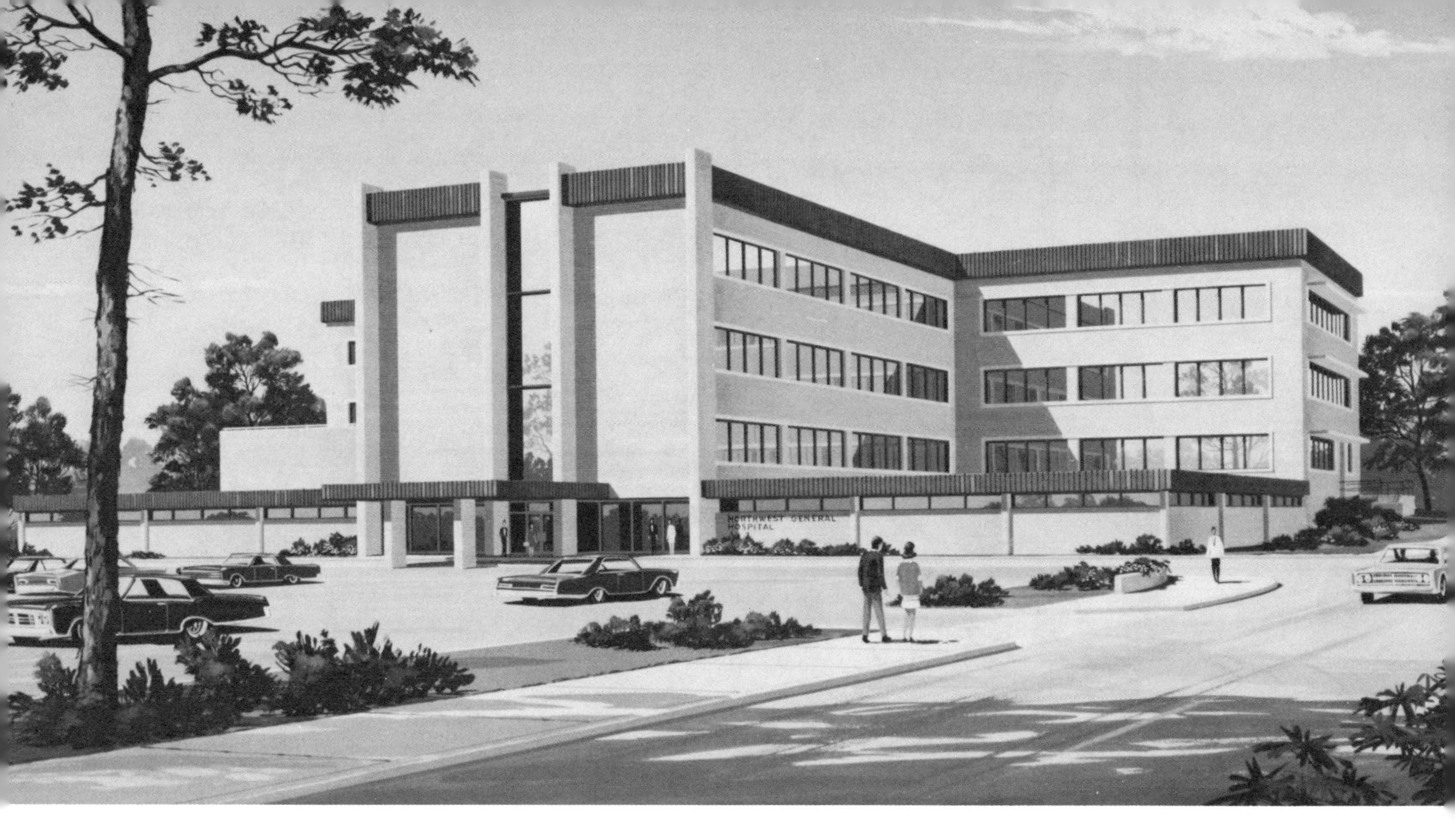

Northwest General Osteopathic Hospital, Milwaukee, Wisconsin

PRODUCTION OF DESIGN DOCUMENTS

Taste is indefinable. A building that is functional and pleasing to those who use it follows no set of rules or procedures in its conception. The site, landscaping, building facade, and interior spaces are a variable mixture of materials designed to satisfy human emotions.

Concept

The concept of a building is the interpretation of the programs, education, operation, and identity it will embody into functional form. Block department plans, traffic and transportation layouts, structural concepts, energy directions, material form, and siting concepts are developed to meet cost ideas and massing direction.

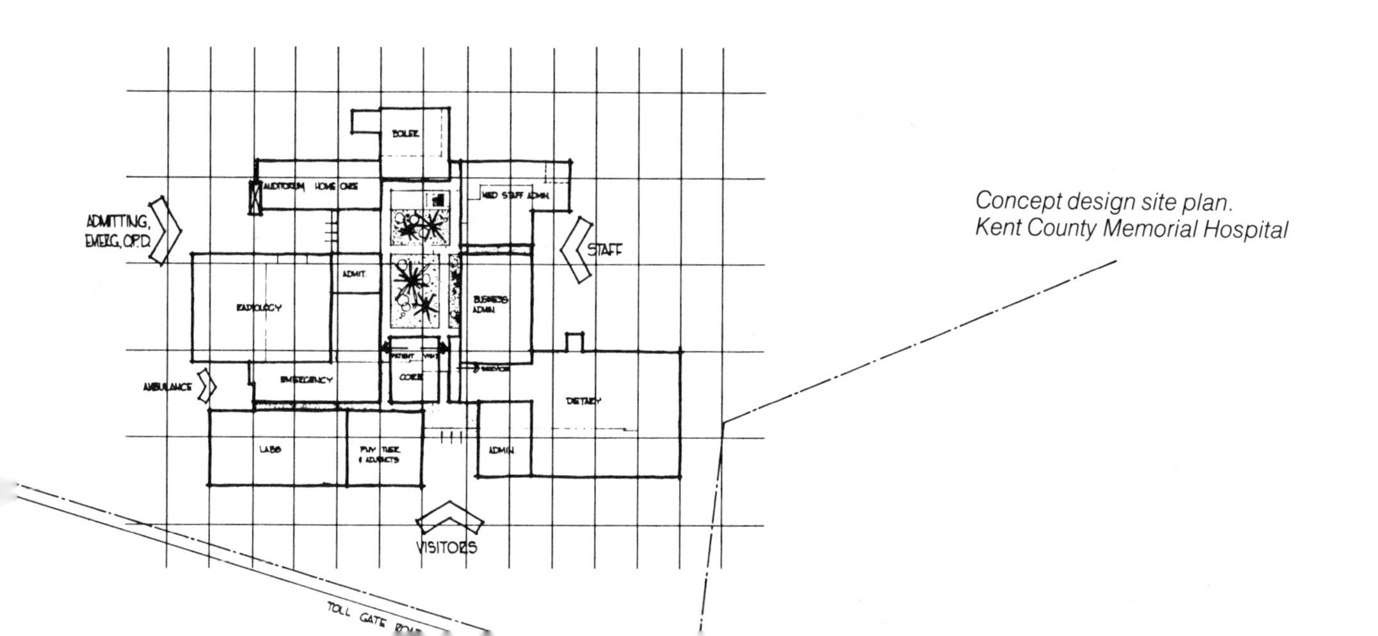

Concept design site plan.
Kent County Memorial Hospital

This page:
Heart House,
American College of Cardiology,
Bethesda, Maryland

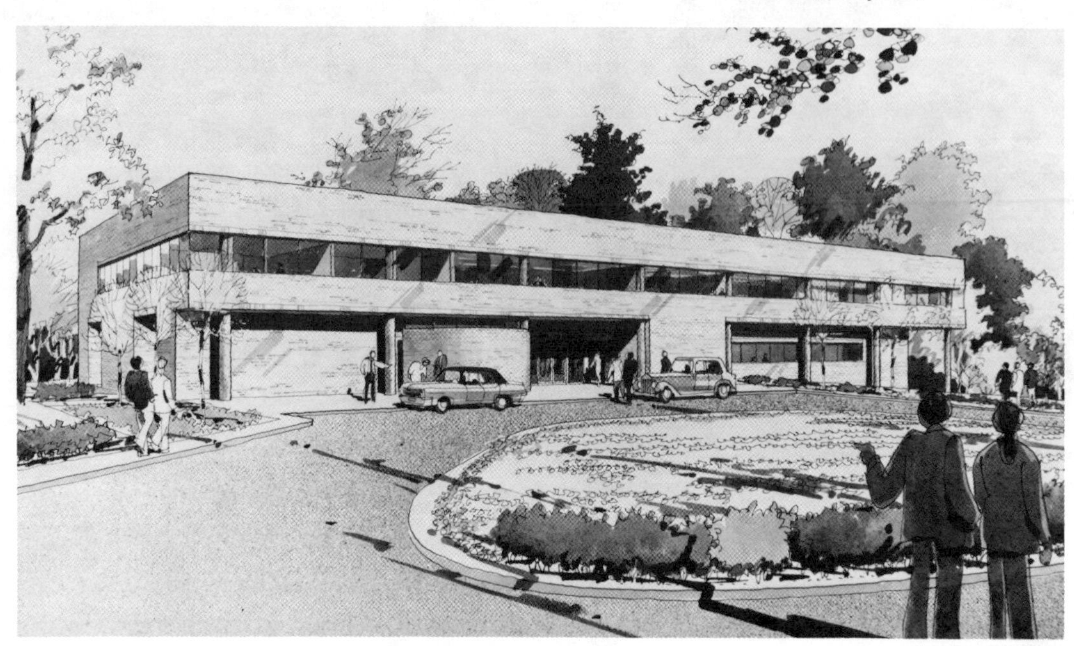

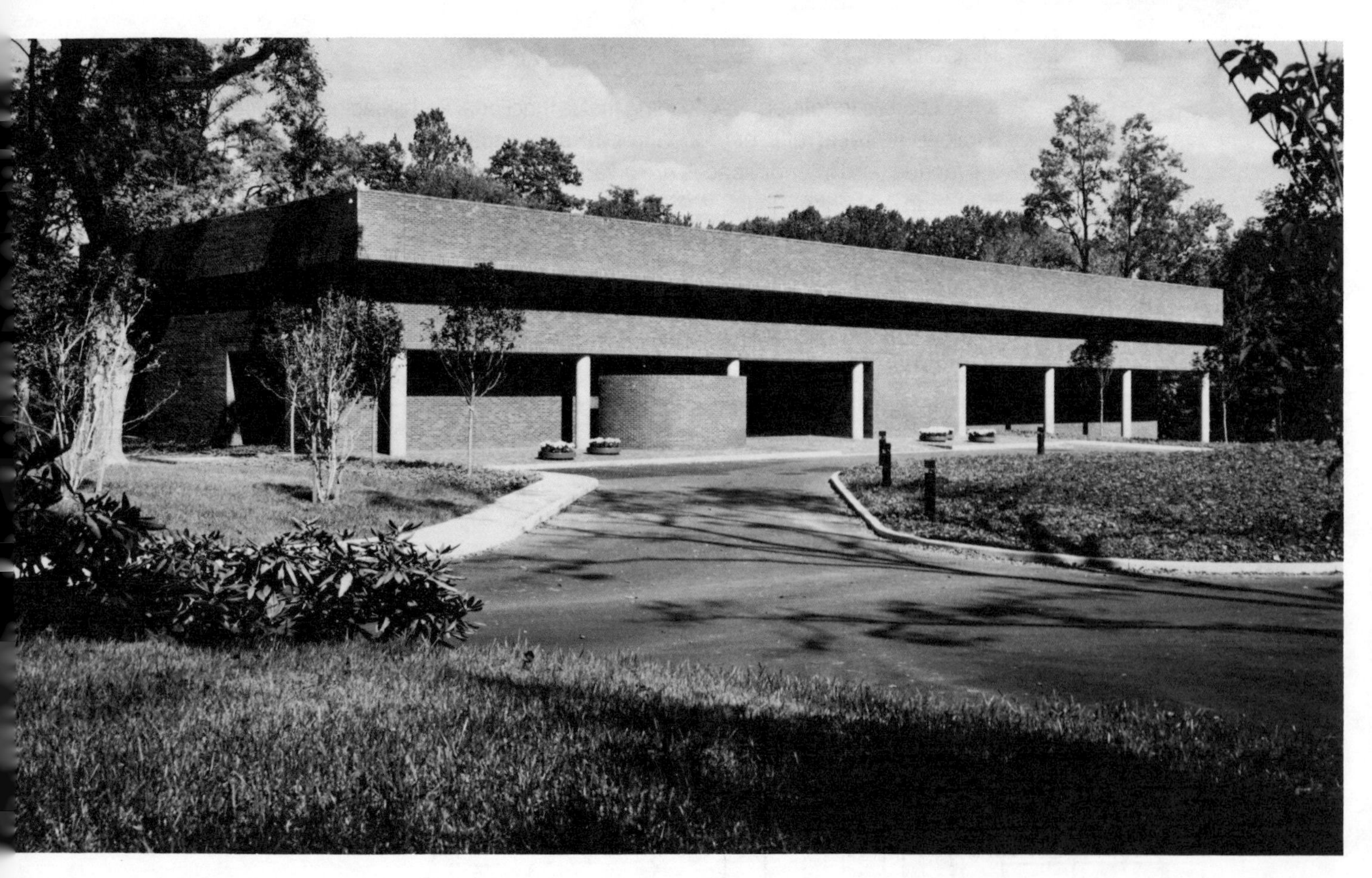

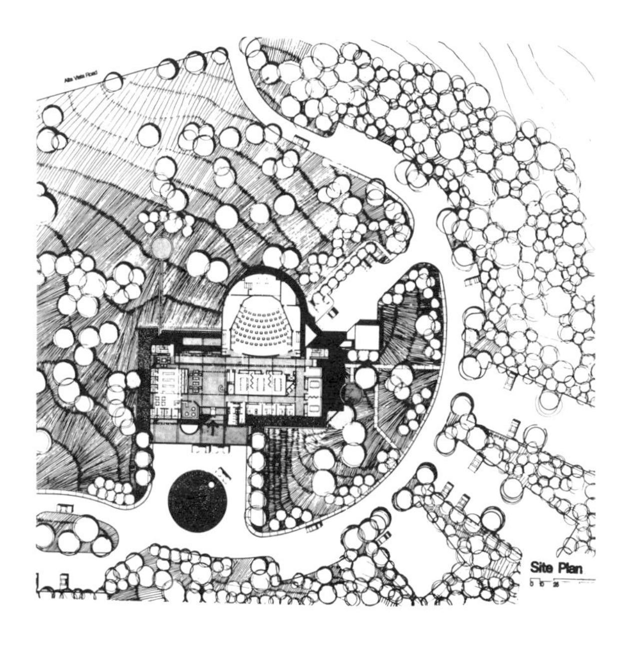

This page:

Heart House,
American College of Cardiology,
Bethesda, Maryland

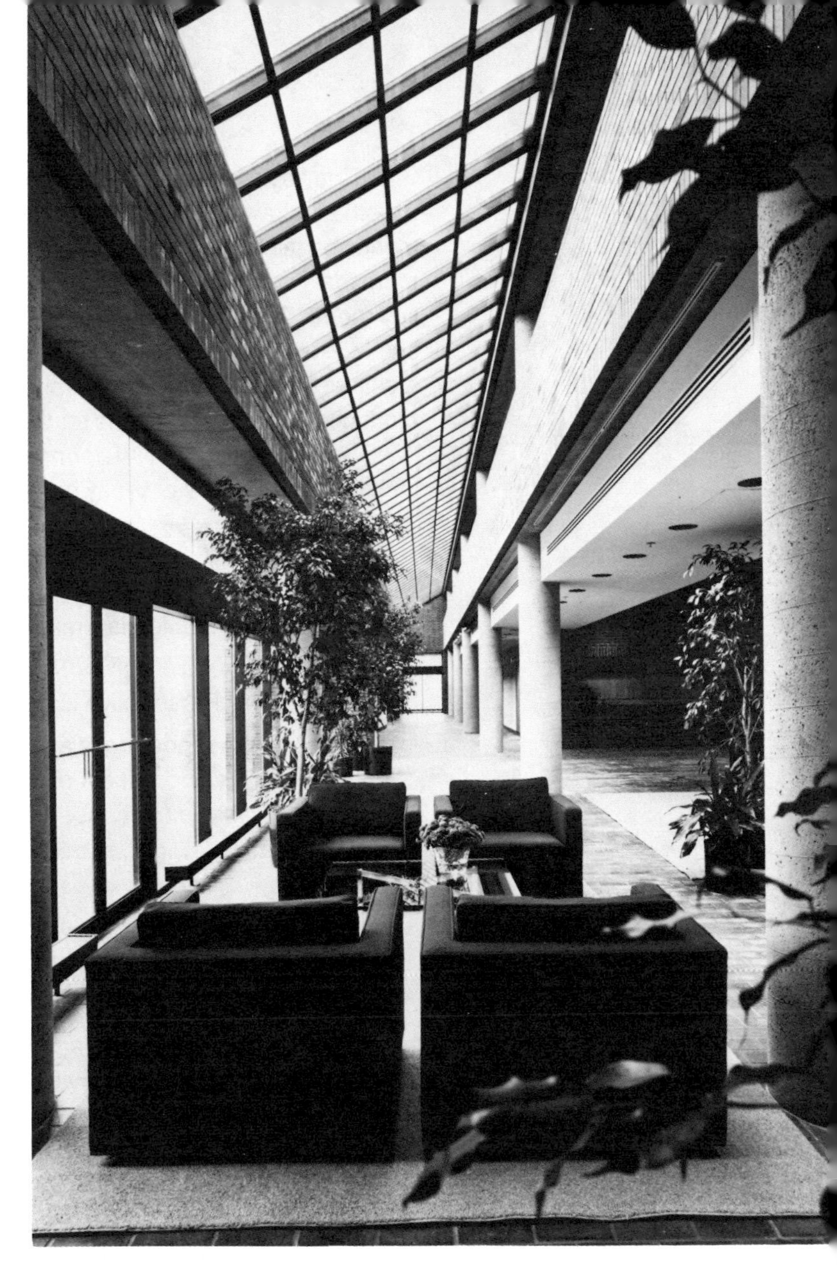

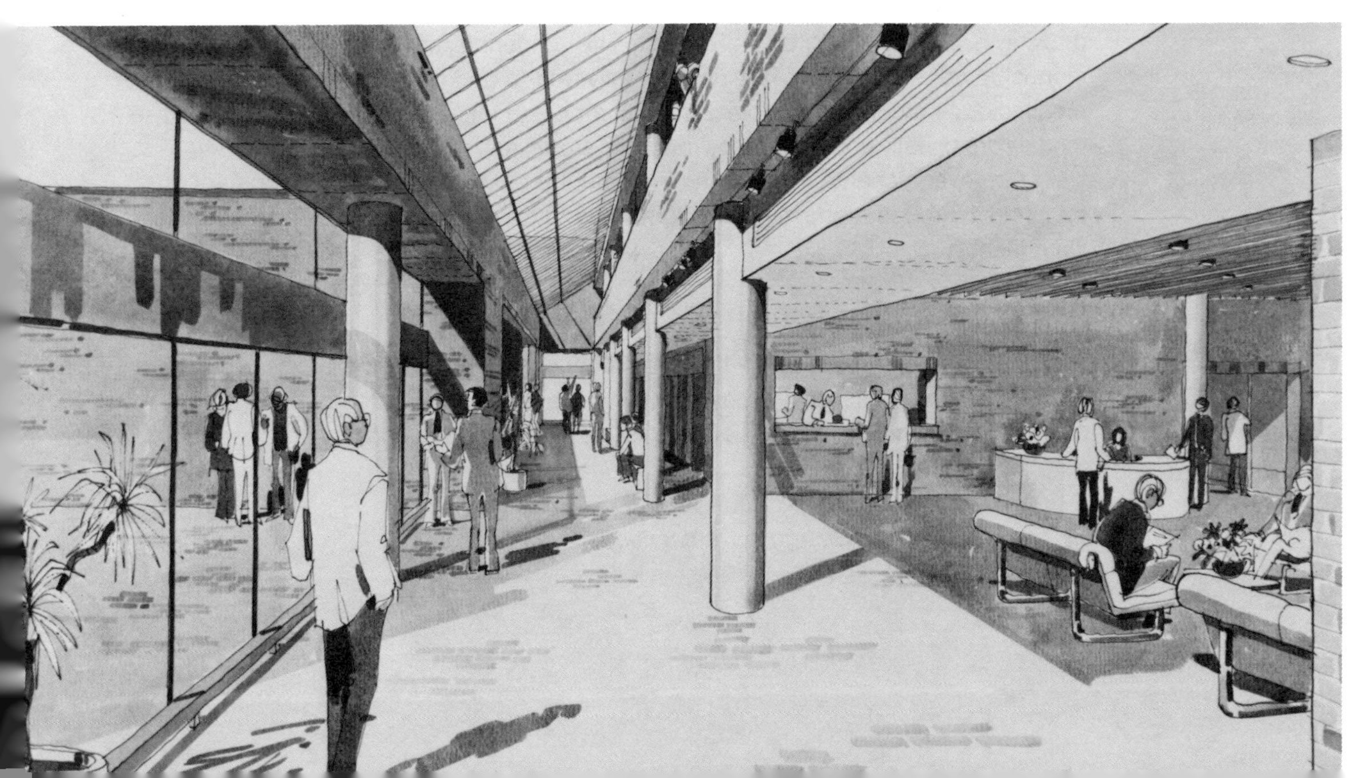

The key to a successful project may be the ability of the hospital staff to read schematic drawings and project the volume represented in them. One of the best means of gaining an understanding of schematic drawings is to study drawings of a room the same size as an existing room. Another means is using full size models of key rooms. The design architect has many ways of presenting the physical layouts and is extensively trained in such presentation. The administrator must rely on the architect's advice in this phase and give him the freedom to design space that will produce improved conditions for the patients.

Some explanation of terminology common to drawings developed during architectural design work may be helpful at this point.

PLAN. The plan is the top view.

ELEVATION. The elevation is the side view.

SECTION. The section is similar to an elevation, but it shows what remains after an imaginary slice (section) has been cut through the object.

PERSPECTIVE. Perspective is a three-dimensional drawing of an object.

RENDERING. A rendering is a finished architectural perspective drawing indicating materials and effects of light, shade, and shadow to help explain form or shape. Plans, elevations, and sections are also referred to as "rendered" when materials, light, shade, and shadow are shown.

PLAN SECTION. The term "plan" is used interchangeably to refer to a top view and to what is actually a plan section. A plan section is a horizontal (rather than vertical) section of a building. It shows the top view of what remains after everything above the slice has been removed.

PLAN * = top view.

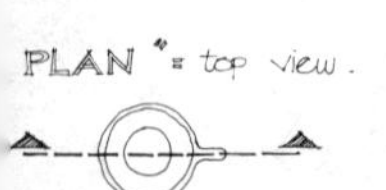

ELEVATION * = side view.

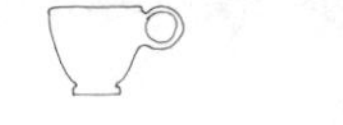

SECTION * = Indicates a view similar to elevation, but showing what remains after an imaginary slice or "section" has been cut through the object.

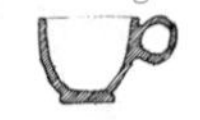

Plan, section, elevation, and perspective drawings are used to communicate architectural development in reviews with administrative staff and departmental personnel throughout the course of the project. Once functional relationships among the departments, traffic, material, site, and utilities have been established, schematic drawings of the design solution are presented for review and approval. Such drawings are the basis for fixing the scope of the project and for making the survey estimate of cost required to insure that project scope and budget are compatible.

When schematic drawings have been approved, a rendered perspective drawing is usually made of the project. The rendering may be black and white, monochrome, or full color. It is usually delivered to and paid for by the client. An architectural model of the project may also be commissioned. Finished, detailed models are usually constructed by specialty stores and paid for by the client.

Approved schematic drawings become the basis for further development of the project through a phase of the work referred to as preliminaries, or design development.

Schematics

At this stage of planning, the overall concept, or block drawings, have produced general traffic and transportation adjacencies and department design criteria. It is now time to gather all the thoughts of the program and develop them into

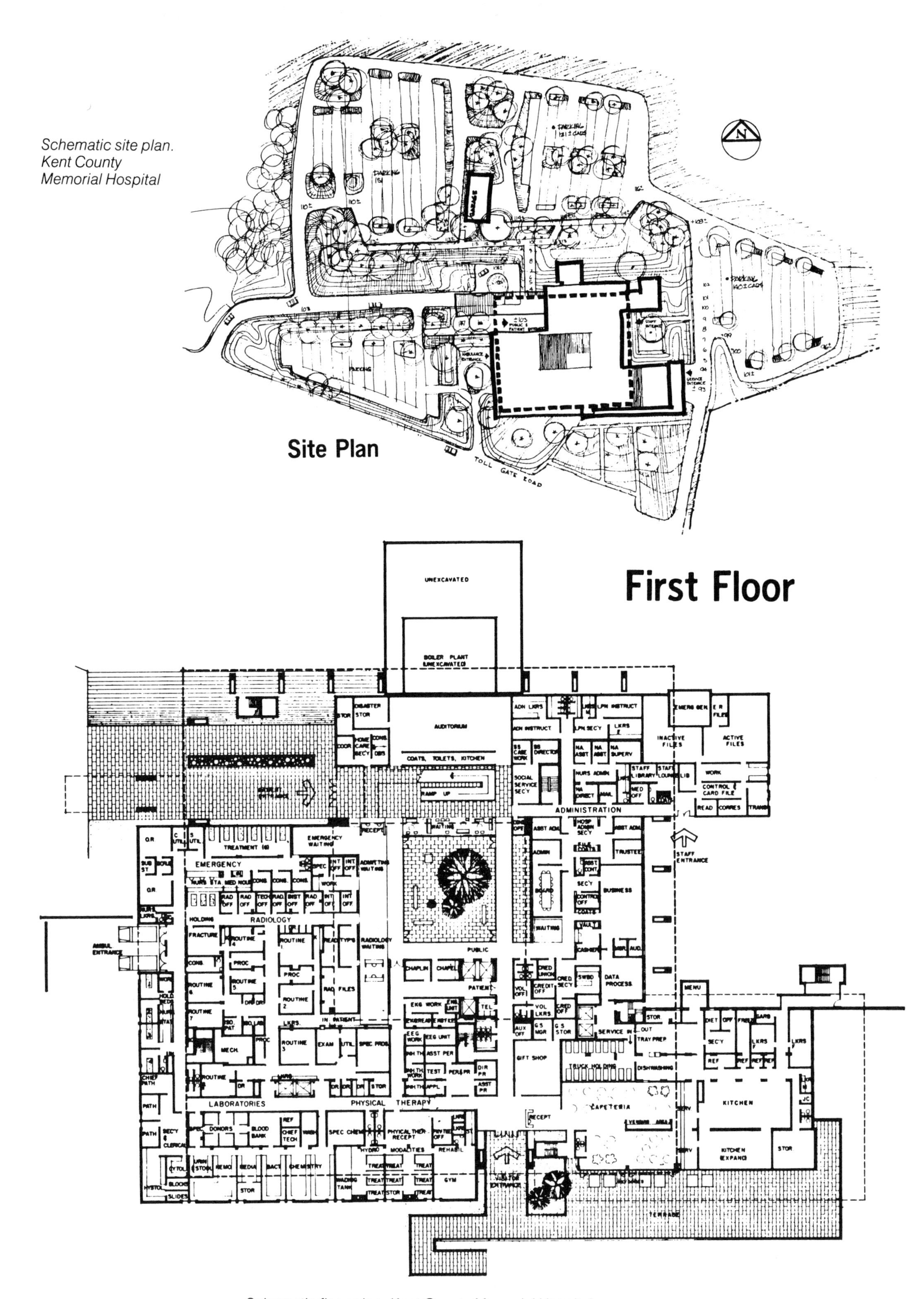

Schematic site plan. Kent County Memorial Hospital

Schematic floor plan. Kent County Memorial Hospital

single-line schematic drawings. At this stage the hospital administrator must rely heavily on the architect who will draw up a single-line design showing the program scope and the budget in one concept.

The architect takes into account all of the elements that have stimulated the concept and produces the innovations and basic building that will meet the stated needs. The hospital administrator should be totally involved in the results of schematics, for he will be asked to approve, support, and present the final recommendations; he must become familiar with the tools of the architect and with the drawings of what will someday be his physical plant.

At this stage of project development, detailed review and confirmation of the functional, operational, and architectural program is required in order for physical plan development to represent consensus and current hospital needs. Medical staff and departmental input in program review is important, since plan development and subsequent reviews will be based on approved programs.

Careful attention must also be paid to the budget and how it is related to the scope of the program. The budget can be checked by projecting the amount of space required to "house" the program (with appropriate allowances for equipment, site work, and so on) and applying a cost per square foot to the resulting area. In order to be realistic, these costs must be projected to the anticipated midpoint of construction. As a result of such a check, the direction to be taken in the development of schematic plans is established, and project scope, at the completion of schematics, should be on budget. In some situations, the hospital may elect to design according to a program that is not adequately covered by the budget; this presents no problem as long as resources are available for increasing the budget.

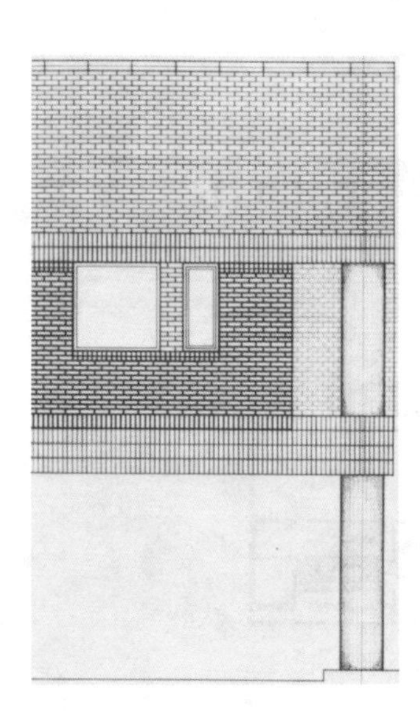

Early schematic architectural development is normally diagrammatic in nature, with plan areas, or blocks, representing program elements being organized and reorganized in search of the best functional relationships, given necessary adjacencies. Drawings at this point are single line, often freehand so that changes can be easily made.

Elevations

Exterior elevations, or drawings of how each face of the building will look, is the beginning of combining the function and the form. The building materials, windows, columns, roof lines, shadows, and color are all like notes in a beautiful symphony. Environmental factors of sun, shading, passive solar energy, insulation, cost, and beauty are elements of this creative effort.

There are several stages in the design of a building elevation. Elevations combine into three-dimensional form with the functions inside the structure, the topography of the land, and the land forms of trees, shrubs, flowers, parking lots, and human scale. Structural elements of the building are often exposed converting function into form. The smallest details of shade and shadows, dark and light, and form and volume are studied and reflected in the design. Design carries through the entire building process, as each wall, ceiling, light, and floor is melded into the structure. The results are for everyone—those who use it, those who spend their lives working in it, and the society it reflects.

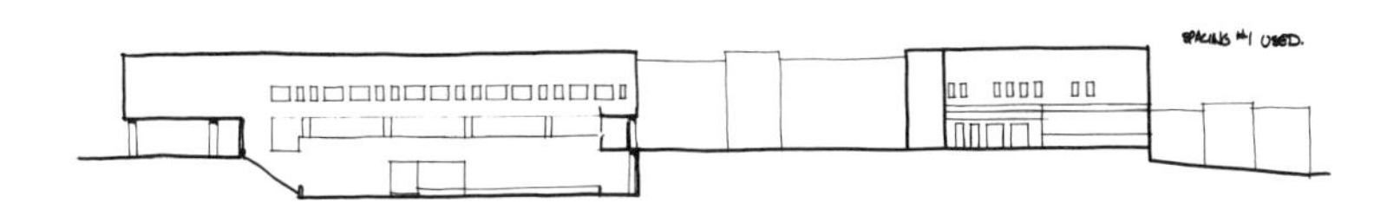

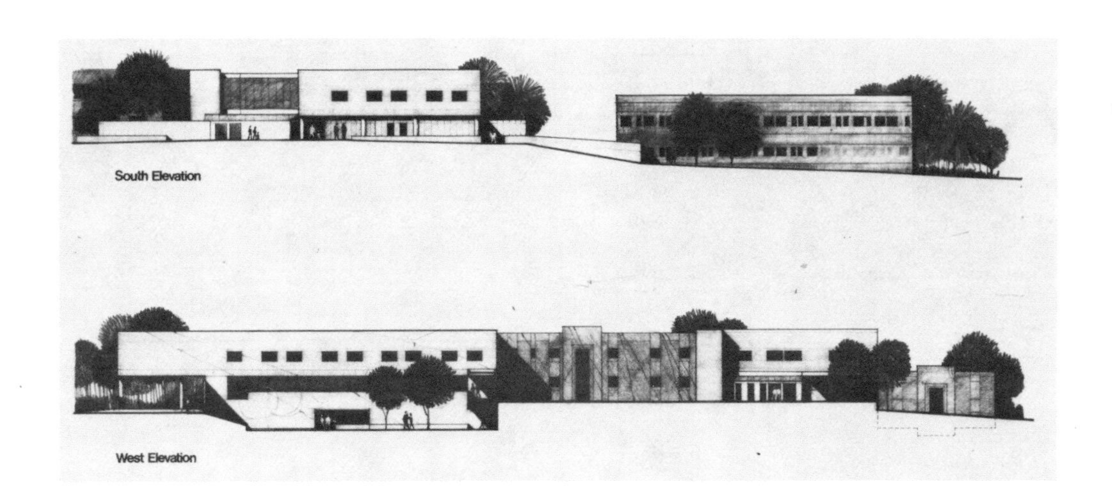

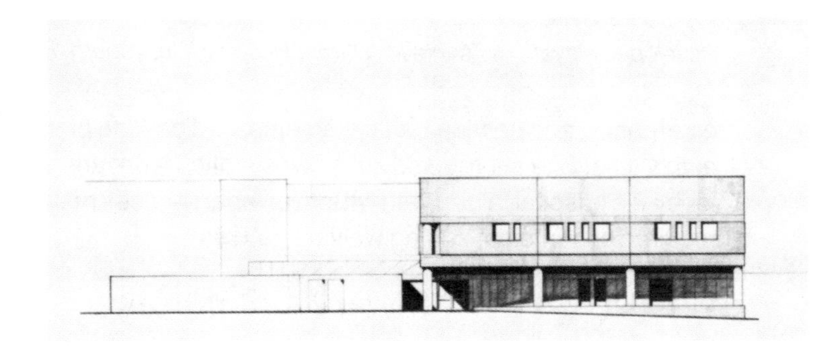

Illustrations, pages 100-101: Concept and schematic elevations. Annie M. Warner Hospital, Gettysburg, Pennsylvania

DESIGN DEVELOPMENT

After schematics have been approved, architectural development becomes more technical and detailed. Virtually all work done during design development is an elaboration on concepts developed in the programming and schematics phases.

Site

If survey, soils investigation, and utility information are still incomplete at this point, the necessary work must be completed and information collected to support development of initial studies in foundation and structural framing, sanitary and storm sewer systems, site development and grading, and electrical power and energy services. Access of traffic to the building entrances, separation of public,

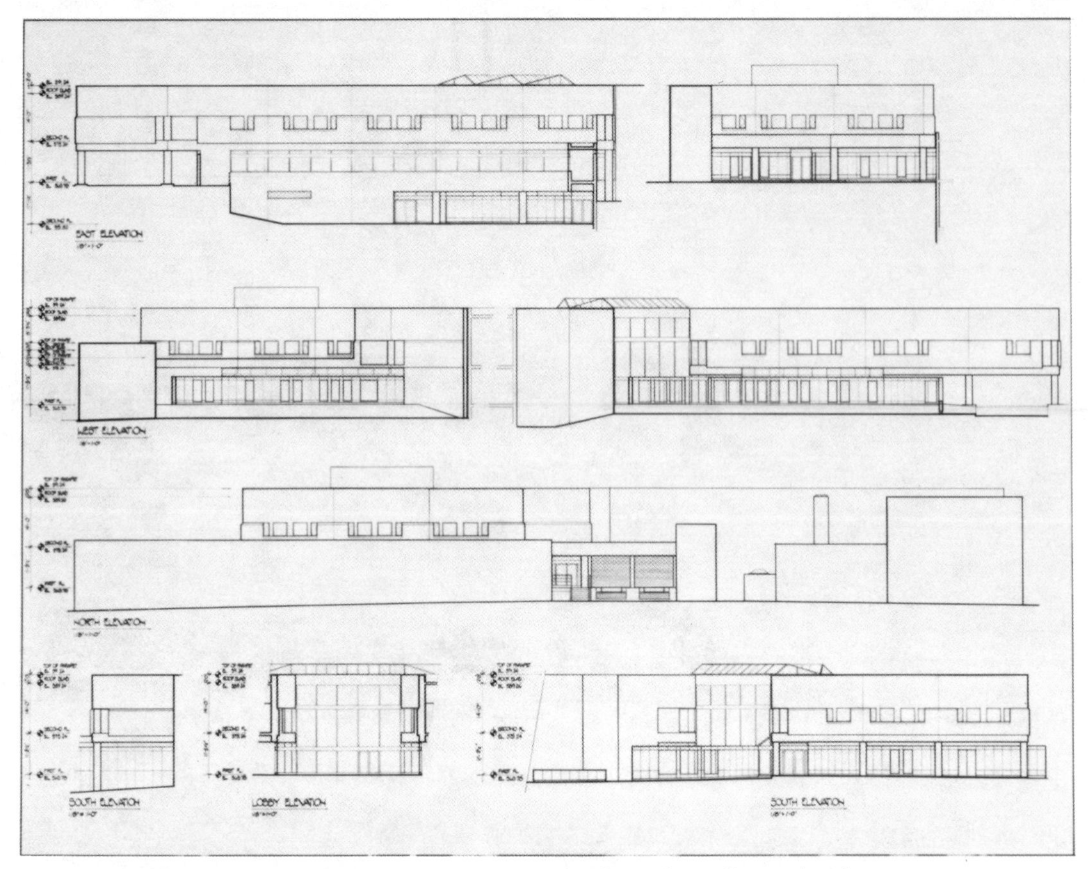

Developed elevations. Annie M. Warner Hospital, Gettysburg, Pennsylvania

emergency, and service traffic elements, and parking provisions are further studied at this time. Site survey and soils investigation work are normally ordered and paid for by the hospital, along with whatever legal services may be necessary in securing required easements, zoning waivers, and so on.

Building

Architectural development includes further study and decisions regarding materials, windows, exterior finishes, architectural treatment and detail; refinement of space layout within the facility, selection of finishes and materials in keeping with maintenance and durability requirements; and comparative cost studies of methods and materials for partition systems and exterior walls, ceiling, and windows.

Engineering

Further development is also required on concepts of air handling, air conditioning, electrical distribution-lighting-communications systems, and medical gas, plumbing, and piping systems. During design development these systems are worked out sufficiently to allow cost studies and basic interfacing decisions to be made. Drawings are normally single-line indications of piping or duct work. Total service requirements for electrical power, natural gas or fuel oil, sanitary and storm sewers, water, and solid waste disposal are now established.

ROOFING 6

1. Flat Roofs	Positive 1/8" to 1/4" pitch to drains. Insulated with tapered insulation board. Roofing to be 4 ply built-up of 20 year bond construction with gravel cover. "U" Factor .08 or better.
2. Courtyard	4" x 8" brick pavers in bituminous setting bed over waterproofing.

EXTERIOR WALL 7

1. Walls	Concrete walls - 8" reinforced architectural concrete, light sand blasted. Brick walls - 4" reinforced face brick, 1" cavity to the building interior, back-up of 6" structural steel studs with 6" fiberglass batt insulation.
2. Skylights	Anodized aluminum tube system with 1/4" pinstriped wire glass on inside and 1/4" tempered solar glass on the exterior.
3. Exterior Windows and Door Frames	Anodized Aluminum Frames. Glass types to be 1" insulating, 1/2" butt jointed glass at exterior, 1/4" clear tempered glass interior. Entrance doors to be anodized aluminum with 1/4" tempered glass.
4. Architectural Louvers	Anodized aluminum. Storm proof type with insect screens.

PARTITIONS 8

1. Masonry	4" ground faced concrete block, laid in running bond with a 4" starter base course and a "switch course" starting 3'-0" above finished floor. 16" concrete block units, laid in running bond. 6" semi-solid 2 hr. fire rated block with furring, and 1/2" layer gypsum board.

2. Gypsum Board	Remaining partitions shall be 3-5/8" metal studs with 5/8" layer of gypsum board each side and 2-1/2" metal studs with (2)1/2" layers of gypsum board each side, STC rating of 50.
3. Interior Borrowed Lights	Frames to be oak with 1/4" clear tempered glass.
STAIRS 9	
Concrete Stairs	Reinforced architectural concrete, with painted 1-1/2" pipe handrail.
FINISHES 10	
1. Concrete	Light sandblasted; cement to be Type 1 Buff.
2. Masonry	4" face brick to be laid in running bond, color range and colored mortar to match existing brick. ground faced concrete block with clear silicone sealer.
3. Gypsum Board	Painted, semi-gloss enamel special wall coating. In Toilets, Labs and Utility areas.
4. Ceramic Tile Walls & Floor	2" x 2" full height in all toilets, bathrooms, showers, and janitors closets.
5. Ceilings	Exterior Soffits: 1" cement plaster on galvanized metal lath. Toilet Rooms: Painted gypsum board. Shower Room: Keenes cement plaster on galvanized metal lath. General: 2 x 4 acoustical panels with exposed spline.
6. Flooring	Sheet Vinyl: Heavy gauge, nondirectional pattern. Carpet-Construction. Brick paver - 4" x 8" x 1-1/2" running bond. Ceramic tile - 2" x 2" unglazed - pantry, public toilets, shower and locker areas.

Equipment

Hospital planning requires careful attention to the fixed and movable equipment that will be needed to implement the operational program. Early in design development, equipment and room detail interviews are held with medical and staff personnel. In these sessions, equipment requirements are documented. The information is used in coordinating room sizes, utility services, lighting, and work flow. Documentation usually takes the form of room-by-room equipment lists, or room data sheets, and are submitted for administrative, medical staff, and departmental review after compilation.

Systems

Complex systems of various types are often incorporated, in concept form, in the schematic design. Functionally, these include communications, information transmission, storage and retrieval, materials handling, security, food preparation, and others. Each system that is to be incorporated must be studied in detail and interfaced with equipment common to other building systems; space and structural requirements are often extensive. Justification of systems is critical, since initial and maintenance costs are usually high.

Design development drawings normally show considerably greater detail than do schematic drawings. Major equipment and furniture are shown in the plans in order to facilitate engineering coordination of utilities and lighting. Plans show wall thickness, door and window function, and more detail regarding vertical circulation and materials. Sections and elevations at larger scale depict relationships between materials. Outline specifications, to supplement the drawings, are compiled for each material, system, and element of work. A room-by-room equipment list, or room data book, is included to record equipment requirements.

A design development is desirable to provide summary discussion of operational concepts, materials, special equipment, and environmental systems. When design development documents are completed, a cost estimate is prepared and presented with the drawings, outline specifications, equipment information, and narrative for hospital review. The estimate provides a current check on project scope related to budget.

After approval, design development documents provide the basis for the working drawing or contract document phase of the project. The design development phase sets the detailed operation of each room and leads to approval of all systems, fixed equipment, material types, and building construction. This is the most important part of the administrator's role on the team, as it sets all of the ideas, programs, needs, and designs into the final building plan. All anticipation of future needs are now fixed, as the following phases only detail and construct what is now the final design product.

V

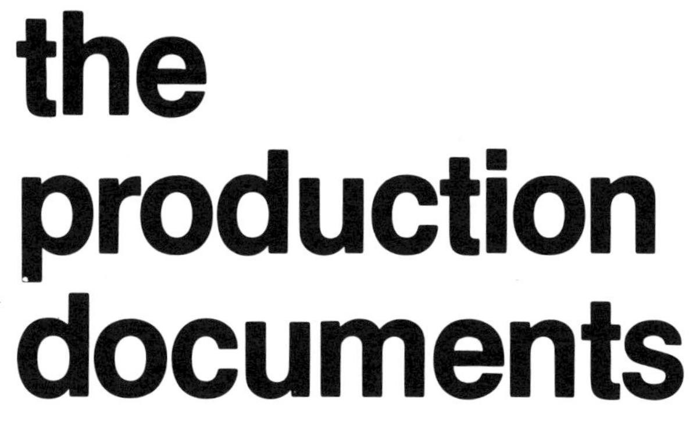

the production documents

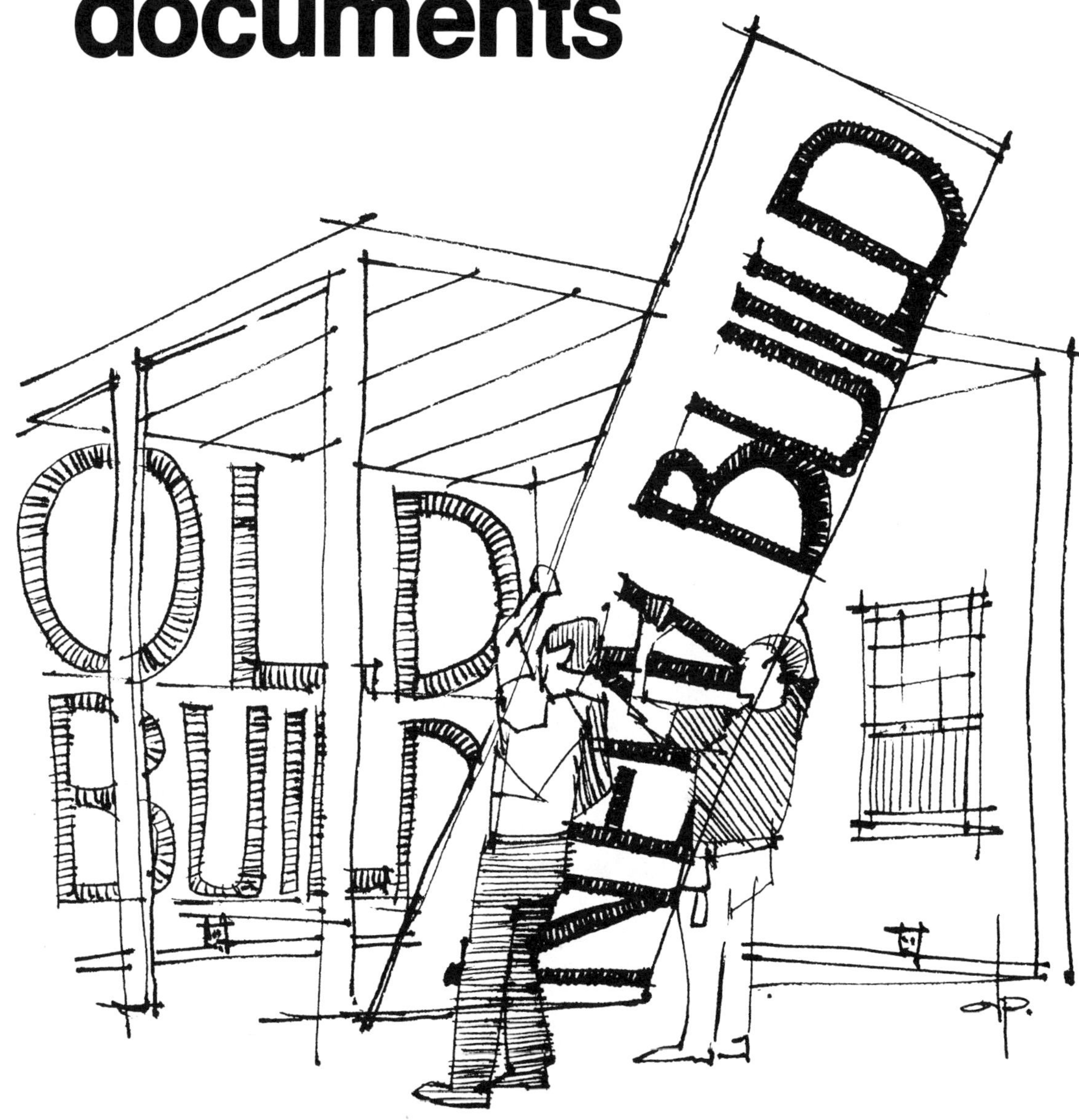

The "production phase" of a health care facility is much more than just the construction of the physical plant; in fact, it begins and ends with the execution of legal activities. From the production and execution of the owner–contractor agreement, to the final inspections and acceptance of the completed structure, the hospital administrator and board will find themselves involved with complex and critical legal documents and activities. In addition to these clearly legal activities, a new kind of architectural drawing must now be produced: the working drawings. The working drawings, along with written specifications, are in themselves a form of legal document as they describe in pictures and in words what the contractors have legally agreed to build and the purchaser has legally agreed to pay for.

Given these considerations, it is as important that the hospital administrator and the board members understand these documents and activities as it was that they understood the earlier design documents and activities. What follows in this chapter is a brief discussion of what these documents are composed of, what they mean, and how to read them.

The contract documents consist of the owner–contractor agreement, general and supplementary conditions, drawings, specifications, and all addenda issued before the execution of the agreement. The owner–contractor agreement is considered the basic contract because it is the only one that requires the signature of both the owner (client) and the contractor and it incorporates all other documents referred to in it. The agreement provides a statement of the contract sum, identifies the nature of the project, establishes the time of commencement and completion, and describes the manner wherein the contractor will be reimbursed for work performed.

The general conditions set forth the legal and regulatory requirements of the contract, and are usually included as part of the contract through a standard form from the American Institute of Architects "General Conditions of the Contract for Construction," which is accepted by the construction industry as a standard. The supplementary conditions extend and modify the general conditions, defining the specific requirements of a particular project. The drawings are graphic representations of the work to be performed and contain information about design, location, and dimensions of the elements of the project. The specifications are a statement of particulars. Construction specifications are written instructions, distinguishing or limiting and describing in detail the construction work to be undertaken which provide technical information about the materials indicated on the drawings.

The publication of a standard form that would reflect the studied approach of the architectural, construction, and legal professions was first undertaken by the American Institute of Architects in 1888. Since then, the form has been revised twelve times. These modifications of format and content have resulted from thorough reviews of contract procedures and the desire for contract stipulations that are equally fair to, and protective of, the interests of the owner and the contractor. In order for the form to be useful nationwide, some of its provisions had to be written in general, rather than specific, language. Provisions reflecting local or regional requirements were not included. The standard provisions also allow for modifications to meet special circumstances. Although the standardized format has kept pace with the changes in construction practice, there developed the need for a supplement that would translate general provisions into specific project requirements. This led to two separate but related documents: the general and the supplementary conditions.

GENERAL CONDITIONS

The "General Conditions of the Contract for Construction" is now the basis for a further review to determine whether supplementary conditions should be part of the contract. Provisions are grouped into fourteen logically developed sequential articles.

—*Article 1: Contract Documents.* This article includes discussions of the following: contract documents, contract, work, execution, correlation, intent and interpretations, and copies furnished and their ownership. Also the components of the contract documents, the scope of the work to be included, and what constitutes the project are defined. The contractor is obligated by this article to familiarize himself with the site, local conditions affecting the work, and the requirements of the contract documents. The number of contract documents to be issued to the contractor is stated, together with the contingency that all such documents be returned to the architect.

—*Article 2: Architect.* This article has two sections: a definition and an explanation of the administration of the contract. The architect is defined as the

ABBREVIATIONS

Term	Abbreviation
ACOUSTICAL TILE	AT
ADDITION	ADD
ADJUSTABLE	ADJ
AIR CONDITIONING	A/C
AIR HANDLING UNIT	AHU
ALTERNATE	ALT
ANGLE	∠
APPROXIMATE	APPROX
ARCHITECTURAL	ARCH
ASBESTOS	ASB
ASPHALT TILE	AT
AUTOMATIC	AUTO
ALUMINUM	AL
AVERAGE	AVG
BASEMENT	BSMT
BEAM	BM
BEARING	BRG
BEVELED	BEV
BENCH MARK	BM
BLOCK	BLK
BLOCKING	BLKG.
BOARD	BD
BOTTOM	BOT
BORROWED LIGHT	B LT.
BRACKET	BRKT.
BRITISH THERMAL UNITS	BTU
BUILDING	BLDG.
BULLETIN	BUL.
CABINET	CAB.
CALKING	CLKG.

Term	Abbreviation
CAPACITY	CAP.
CASEMENT	CSMT
CAST IRON	CI
CEILING	CLG
CEMENT	CEM
CENTER	CTR.
CENTER LINE	CL OR ℄
CENTER TO CENTER	C/C OR C-C
CERAMIC TILE	CER. T.
CHANNEL	[
CLEANOUT	CO
CLEAR	CL
COLD WATER	CW
COLD ROLLED	CR
COLUMN	COL
COMPOSITION FLOORING	CF
COMPRESSIBLE	COMPR
CONCRETE	CONC
CONCRETE MASONRY UNIT	CMU
CONNECTION	CONN.
CONSTRUCTION JOINT	CONST. JT
CONTINUOUS	CONT.
CONTRACTOR	CONTR
CONTROL JOINT	CJ
CORNER GUARD	CG.
CORRIDOR	CORR.
CORRUGATED	CORR.
COUNTER SUNK	CSK
COURSE	C
COMMON	COM
COVERED	COV
CUBIC YARD	CY
CYLINDER-CYLINDRICAL	CYL
CLOSET	CLO
COMBINATION	COMB.

person or firm licensed by the state to practice architecture and identified as such in the agreement. Notice is also provided that there exists no contractual obligation between the architect and the contractor for though the architect provides general administration of the construction contract he is not responsible for directing the work. His authority to function as the owner's representative is outlined in the contract.

—*Article 3: Owner.* This article includes the following areas: definition, information and services required by the owner, owner's right to stop the work, and owner's right to carry out the work. The owner is defined as the person or firm executing the agreement with the contractor. The owner is obligated by this article to furnish all surveys, site investigation studies, easements, and legal access to the site. The right of the owner to stop the work or to have deficiencies resulting from the contractor's defaults or neglect corrected by others at the contractor's expense is spelled out.

—*Article 4: Contractor.* This article covers the following: definition, review of contract documents, supervision and construction procedures, labor and materials, warranty, taxes, permits, fees and notices, cash allowances, superintendent, responsibility for those performing the work, cleaning up, progress schedule, drawings and specifications at the site, shop drawings and samples, use of site, cutting and patching the work, communications, and indemnification. The contractor, defined as the person or firm executing the agreement with the owner, is obligated to review all contract documents carefully and report any deficiencies noted to the architect. He is to supervise the work and be responsible for construction methods, coordination, and procedures, using materials and workmanship that accord with contract requirements. By his execution of the contract, he warrants that all work will be in conformance with the contract documents. The contractor is obliged to pay all taxes and to pay for all permits, fees, and licenses applicable at the time bids are received. The primary representative of the contractor during construction is the superintendent, who is responsible for daily progress of the work and the conduct of all those performing on the site. A schedule of anticipated progress leading to completion of the work is prepared by the contractor for distribution to everyone involved in the project. A set of drawings is provided to the contractor for recording all changes made during construction which will be surrendered to the owner to function as an "as-built" record. Shop drawings, which include drawings, diagrams, brochures, and other data sufficient to illustrate individual portions of the work, are prepared by the contractor and submitted to the architect for approval. Samples, where they serve the same purpose, are also submitted. All communications between owner and contractor go through the architect. The indemnification provision requires that the contractor hold harmless the owner and architect in casualty situations where personal injury involves a contractor's employee or other member of the public, where property damage results from construction operations, and where either casualty is caused in whole or in part by negligent act or omission of the contractor or his forces.

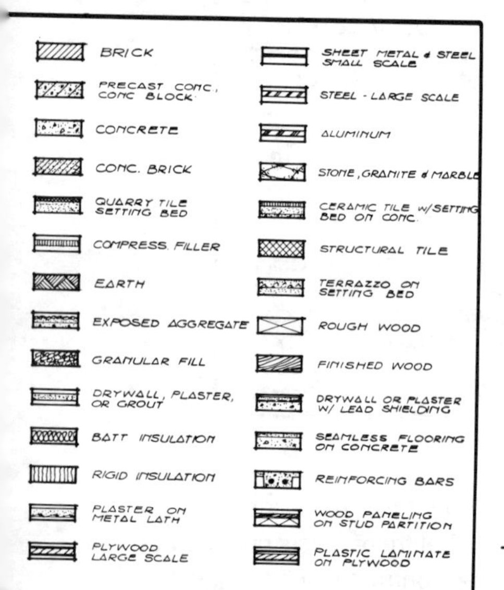

—*Article 5: Subcontractors.* Subcontractors may be needed on the site to carry out work required by the contract. This article confirms that no contractual relationship exists between the owner and any subcontractor but that the identity of all subcontractors is to be made known to the owner so that he or she may express any reasonable cause for rejecting a subcontractor. While neither architect nor owner has any legal obligation with respect to payments to subcontractors, the procedures relative to such payments are spelled out in this article so that the contractor must assume them as part of his contract obligation.

—*Article 6: Additional Contracts.* Article 6 reserves the right to award additional contracts to others who will pursue certain portions of the work simultaneously with the original contractor. It then becomes necessary to define mutual areas of responsibilities as they will apply to the separate contractors performing simultaneous work on the project.

—*Article 7: Miscellaneous Legal Provisions.* Included here are: restrictions against the assignment of the contract procedures related to processing claims for damages, testing requirements to satisfy the orders of a public authority, the arbitration process that will be instituted in the event of an alleged breach of contract.

—*Article 8: Time.* Article 8 is concerned with the definition of time as the term will be employed in other contract provisions. The sections that apply to all construction projects are those concerned with the commencement date and the date of substantial completion. The latter is significant because it signals the inauguration of the one-year guaranty period. The remaining sections, which deal with delays and extensions of time, become particularly meaningful when the contract contains clauses entitling the owner to penalize the contractor for delays in completing the project within an allocated period of time.

—*Article 9: Periodic Payments Procedures.* This article elaborates the processes to be employed in confirming the basis on which payments are made to the contractor as the work progresses. On projects in which large sums of money and an extended period of construction are involved, progress payments are normally made on a monthly basis to reflect work performed during the preceding month. The amount paid is usually 90 or 95 percent of the monies earned with the remainder being retained by the owner to ensure faithful completion of the project. Requests for payment are forwarded by the contractor to the architect, who certifies their correctness and transmits them to the owner with his endorsement that they be honored.

ABBREVIATIONS - CONT

Term	Abbreviation
DEGREE	° OR DEG
DEPARTMENT	DEPT.
DETAIL	DET
DEPRESSION OR DEPRESSED	DEPR.
DIAGONAL	DIAG.
DIAMETER	⌀ OR DIA.
DIMENSION	DIM.
DOOR	DR
DOUBLE ACTING	DA
DOUBLE HUNG	DH
DOWN	DN
DOWN SPOUT	DS
DRAIN	DR.
DRAWING	DWG
DRINKING FOUNTAIN	DF
EAST	E
EACH	EA
ELECTRIC/ELECTRICAL	ELEC
ELECTRIC WATER COOLER	EWC
ELEVATION - GRADE OR BLDG. OR INTERIOR	EL.
ELEVATOR	ELEV.
EXPANSION JOINT	EJ
ENTRANCE	ENT.
EQUIPMENT	EQUIP
ESTIMATE	EST
EXCAVATE	EXC
EXHAUST	EXH
EXISTING	EXIST
EXPOSED	EXPD.
EXPANSION OR EXPANDED	EXP
EXTERIOR	EXT

Term	Abbreviation
FHARENHEIT	F
FEET	FT
FIELD CHECK	FC
FIGURE	FIG
FINISH	FIN.
FIRE EXTINGUISHER	FE
FIRE EXTINGUISHER CABINET	FEC.
FIRE HOSE CABINET	FHC
FIXTURE	FIX.
FLOOR	FL.
FLOORING	FLG
FLOOR DRAIN	FD
FOOTING	FTG.
FOUNDATION	FDT.
FLUORESCENT	FLUOR.
FURNISHED	FURN.
FINISHED OPENING	F.O.
GAGE OR GAUGE	GA
GALLON	GAL
GALLON PER MINUTE	GPM
GALVANIZED	GALV.
GALVANIZED IRON	G.I
GENERAL	GEN
GLASS	GL
GLAZED STRUCTURAL UNITS	GSU
GRADE	GR
GRATING	GRTG
GROUND	GRD.
GYPSUM	GYP.

—*Article 10: Safety.* Article 10 delineates the responsibilities imposed on the contractor to ensure protection of persons and property. Project safety is the exclusive responsibility of the contractor, who must take all reasonable safety precautions necessary to protect the work, the people affected by the work, the site, and the property adjacent to the site. Damage to the work or property resulting from inadequate protection are to be remedied by the contractor, except where damage can be attributed to faulty drawings or specifications or to acts of the owner or architect not attributable to faults or negligence of the contractor.

—*Article 11: Insurance.* This article identifies the type of insurance coverage to be provided by each of the parties to the contract. The contractor must secure worker's compensation coverage and bodily and property liability insurance. The owner must purchase and maintain property insurance that protects him and the contractor and his forces against fire, extended coverage, vandalism, and malicious mischief. The owner may also obtain liability insurance.

—*Article 12: Changes.* This article contains the details involved in formulating changes in the work defined in the original contract documents. Such changes, which normally will affect the contract sum, are formalized through a change order. Normally, the architect describes the intended change in writing or drawings and transmits the description to the contractor along with a request for the price of the work described. The contractor submits his proposal of the cost for such work to the architect, who recommends acceptance, rejection, or negotiation of the proposal to the owner. If the owner and contractor agree on the proposal, the architect prepares the change order for execution by all three parties.

—*Article 13: Uncovering and Correcting.* Article 13 is concerned with the uncovering and correcting of work performed by the contractor. If work is covered by the contract contrary to the request of the architect, the contractor must bear the expense of uncovering and recovering, even when the work is found to be in accordance with contract requirements. If the architect does not specifically request that the work be kept uncovered, then the contractor is liable only if the uncovered work is not in accordance with the contract documents. The cost of removing and correcting all work rejected by the architect as being defective is borne by the contractor, whether it occurs before substantial completion or within a year after substantial completion.

—*Article 14: Termination.* This article defines the circumstances under which the owner or contractor may legally terminate the contract before the project is completed.

SUPPLEMENTARY CONDITIONS

The supplementary conditions contain amendments to the general conditions and are usually attached to them. Common modifications include the following:

ABBREVIATIONS · CONT.

Term	Abbreviation
HANDRAIL	HR
HARDWARE	HDW
HEAD	HD
HEADER	HDR
HEATER	HTR
HEATING	HTG
HEIGHT	HT
HIGH PRESSURE	HP
HOLLOW METAL	HM
HORIZONTAL	HORIZ
HORSE POWER	HP
HOSE BIB	HB
HOT WATER	HW
HOUR	HR
HYDRAULIC OR HYDRANT	HYD
HIGH POINT	H.P.
INCH	IN
INCLUDE	INCL
INFORMATION	INFO
INSIDE DIAMETER	ID
INSULATION	INSUL
INTERIOR	INT
JANITOR'S CLOSET	JC
JOINT	JT
JOIST	JST
JUNCTION	JCT
KEENES' CEMENT PLASTER	KCP
KICK PLATE	KP
KITCHEN	KIT
LABORATORY	LAB
LAMINATE	LAM
LANDING	LDG
LAVATORY	LAV
LIGHT / LIGHTING	LT/LTG
LINEAR FEET	LF
LINEN CLOSET	LIN CLO
LINTEL	L
LINOLEUM	LINO
LIVING ROOM	LR
LOAD	LD
LOADING	LDG
LOCKER	LKR
LONG	LG
LOW POINT	LP
LOW PRESSURE	LP
LUMBER	LBR
LENGTH	LGTH
MACHINE	MACH
MANHOLE	MH
MANUFACTURER	MFR
MANUFACTURING	MFG
MARBLE	MAR
MASONRY	MAS
MASONRY OPENING	MO
MASONRY UNIT	MU
MATERIAL	MATL
MAXIMUM	MAX
MECHANICAL	MECH
MEDICINE CABINET	MC
MEMBRANE	MEMB
METAL	MET
METAL LATH	ML

—alteration of Article 1 by giving the number of sets of drawings and specifications the contractor will be furnished free of charge

—alteration of Article 7 to require that the contractor furnish performance and labor and material bonds in the amount of 100 percent of the contract sum

—alteration of Article 11 to establish the limit of liability in dollar amounts that must be covered in the insurance taken out by the contractor

Where federal funds are involved in the project, the government requires the inclusion of supplementary conditions concerning the right of federal access to and inspection of the work, compliance with equal opportunity requirements, adherence to a schedule of prevailing wages, and extra compensation for overtime, and submission by the contractor of weekly affidavits certifying compliance with federal regulations.

SPECIFICATIONS

Specifications are written instructions describing in detail the construction work to be undertaken. Specifications and drawings serve complementary functions. The drawings represent, in graphic form, the size, shape, and location of the various building elements and the manner in which they relate to each other, thus defining the quantity and type of each building component. The specifications express the quality, performance standards, and end result expected from the assembly of the materials and equipment items identified on the drawings. Notes on the drawings are usually stated in general terms, with the more detailed information being incorporated in the specifications.

The preparation of specifications is an essential feature of the design process and proceeds most effectively when it is done concurrently with the drawings. During the evolution of the specifications, it is often necessary to confer with manufacturer's representatives and for contracting personnel to become fully conversant with materials and methods applicable to the project. The selection of materials and equipment is essentially the responsibility of the architect, and before being included in the specifications, products must be appraised by the architect as to their suitability for the use intended.

A working knowledge of the materials used in the building includes their basic composition, the manner of their fabrication and installation, and their suitability for the use intended. Such knowledge is vital to the development of the specifications. Because the specifications are written, they are more readily comprehensible to persons not affiliated with the construction industry than are the drawings; thus, the owner and his legal and financial counselors are better able to understand the nature of the building elements and their relative significance through reading the specifications.

Once the most suitable product is determined, the architect must specify it in such a manner as to allow competitive bidding. Four of the most common practices employed for this purpose can be briefly described as follows:

—*Contractor's Option.* This type of specification lists every acceptable trade name for each product. After execution of the contract, the contractor may use any product listed, but only products listed.

—*Product Approval.* This type of specification lists one or more trade names for each product; it includes a statement that any request for substitutions by a bidder must be made a given number of days before the opening of bids and that all approvals will be issued in the form of an addendum.

—*Approved Equal.* This type of specification lists one or more trade names for each product required and adds the phrase "or approved equal." After execution of the contract, the contractor may use any of the listed products or may request permission from the architect to substitute an unlisted one he considers equal. It is to be understood by the contractor that the phrase allowing substitution requires written approval of the architect and that no substitutions may be made without such written approval.

—*Product Description.* This type of specification describes completely all details, qualities, functions, and sizes of a product without mentioning a trade or a brand name. Any product that meets all of the detailed specifications will be approved.

It is sometimes advantageous to include within the specifications a request for alternative prices for a single element or for certain areas of the total project. There are two basic reasons why alternative prices are requested: (1) to reach a final decision between two different materials or methods on the basis of their comparative value; (2) to adjust the bids received so that the contract sum can be made to fit within the budget established for the project. Alternatives should be held to a minimum, since an overabundance of them tends only to complicate the bidding process. Where alternative prices are requested, the form of proposal submitted by each bidder should identify alternative prices separately from the lump sum proposal.

The specifications will be indexed and bound in book form, by trade activities, that have been accepted by the construction industry. In the final specifications, the technical sections will be preceded by documents that involve various aspects of project involvement, but that do not amplify or describe the work illustrated on the drawings. In addition to the title page and the table of contents, these sections will include bidding requirements, contract documents, and general requirements.

The bidding requirements section of the specification is concerned with inviting firms to submit proposals and delineates a set of bidding requirements on the

ABBREVIATIONS - CONT.

Term	Abbreviation
METAL THRESHOLD	MT
MINIMUM	MIN
MOULDING	MLDG
MOUNTING	MTG
MOVABLE PARTITION-MOV	PART.
METAL TOILET PARTITION	MTP
NORTH	N
NOT IN CONTRACT	NIC
NUMBER	# OR NO
NOMINAL	NOM
NOT TO SCALE	NTS
OBSCURE	OBSC
OFFICE	OFF
ON CENTER	OC
OPENING	OPG
OPPOSITE	OPP
OUT TO OUT	O/O OR O TO O
OUTSIDE DIAMETER	OD
OVERALL	OA
OVERHEAD	OVHD
PAINTED	PTD
PAIR	PR
PANEL	PNL
PARTITION	PTN.
PASSAGE	PASS
PENNEY (AS NAIL 10d)	d
PERFORATED	PERF
PIECE	PC
PLASTER	PLAS
PLASTIC	PLAST

Term	Abbreviation
PLATE	⅊ OR PL
PLUMBING	PLBG.
PLYWOOD	PLY WD.
POINT	PT
POLISHED	POL
PORTABLE	PORT
PORTLAND CEMENT	PC
POUNDS	LBS
PRECAST	PRCST
PREFABRICATED	PREFAB
PROJECTION	PROJ
PUBLIC ADDRESS	PA
QUARRY TILE	QT
QUART	QT
RADIUS	R
RECEPTACLE	RECP
REFERENCE	REF
REFRIGERATOR	REFR
REINFORCEMENT	REINF.
REMOVABLE	REMOV
REQUIRED	REQD.
RESILIENT	RESIL
REVISION	REV
RISER	R
ROOF DRAIN	RD
ROOFING	RFG
ROOM	RM
ROUND	Φ OR RD
RUBBER	RB

procedures for the preparation and submission of those proposals. The invitation identifies the project, owner, and architect, establishes the time and location for the receipt of bids, and tells where bidding documents may be obtained. The instructions define the format in which bids are to be tendered, for what period bids are to remain binding, how questions related to interpretation or bidding documents are to be formulated, what bonds are to be executed, and what actions are to be expected of the owner following his review of the bids.

The contract documents section of the specification contains a sample form of the agreement to be executed by the owner and the winning contractor, general conditions of the contract, and supplementary conditions.

The general requirements section of the specification includes general references to the contractor's work and resemble in content the supplementary conditions of the contract. However, since they are concerned with activities on the site once construction has begun, they are traditionally isolated from the contract itself. A listing of typical general requirements would include:

—temporary power

—temporary water

—temporary heat

—temporary ventilation

—temporary field offices

—temporary toilet facilities

—commencement and completion dates

—job meetings

—construction sign

—sequence of construction

—measurements where existing buildings are included

—access to existing buildings

It is customary to arrange the sections of the specifications in the order in which the respective trades normally begin their principal work at the site. In addition to the sequential evolution of the trade activity, current specification writing also dictates that no single section cover the work of more than one subcontractor or material supplier. Adherence to this principle will tend to minimize the chance of duplication, omission, or confusion. It is understood, however, that while the architect organizes the specification sections, he cannot assume responsibility for allotting portions of the work to specific subcontractors.

Specifications are currently subdivided by anticipated trade involvement on the site into sixteen headings:

—Division 1, general requirements

—Division 2, site work

—Division 3, concrete work

ABBREVIATIONS - CONT.

SCHEDULE	SCHED
SHEET	SHT
SECRETARY	SECY
SECTION	SECT
SHEET METAL	SH. MET
SHOWER	SH
SLOP SINK OR SERVICE SINK	SS
SOUTH	S
SPECIFICATION	SPEC
SQUARE	□ OR SQ
STAGGERED	STAG
STAINLESS STEEL	SS
STANDARD	STD
STATION	STA
STEEL	STL
STERILIZER	STER
STORAGE	STOR
STRUCTURAL	STRUCT
STRUCTURAL FACING UNIT	SFU
SUPERINTENDENT	SUPT.
SUSPENDED	SUSP
SYMMETRICAL	SYM
TELEPHONE	TEL
TEMPERATURE	TEMP
TERRAZZO	TERR
THICK	THK
THRESHOLD	THRESH
TOILET	TOIL
TONGUE & GROOVE	T&G
TREAD	T
TELEVISION	TV
TYPICAL	TYP
UNEXCAVATED	UNEXC
UNFINISHED	UNFIN
UNIT HEATER	UH
URINAL	UR
UTILITY	UTIL
VENTILATION	VENT
VENTILATOR	VENT
VERTICAL	VERT
VESTIBULE	VEST
VINYL ASBESTOS TILE	VAT
VINYL TILE	VT
VOLUME	VOL
VENT THRU ROOF	VTR
WAINSCOT	WSCT
WATER CLOSET	WC
WATER HEATER	WH
WATERPROOF OR WATERPROOFING	WP
WEATHER STRIPPING	WS
WEIGHT	WT
WELDED WIRE MESH	WWM
WEEP HOLE	WH
WEST	W
WIDE FLANGE	WF
WINDOW DIMENSION	WD

—Division 4, masonry work

—Division 5, metals

—Division 6, carpentry

—Division 7, moisture protection

—Division 8, doors, windows, and glass

—Division 9, finishes

—Division 10, specialties

—Division 11, equipment

—Division 12, furnishings

—Division 13, special construction

—Division 14, conveying equipment

—Division 15, mechanical

—Division 16, electrical

Each of these is further subdivided into a number of individual sections that progress from the general to the particular. An instance could be found where the heading for Division 9 is "finishes" and typical section headings would read "vinyl wall covering," "resilient flooring," "acoustical ceilings," "painting," and so on.

In summary, a set of project specifications is the written material that accompanies the drawings for a construction project. This material has as its objectives the following:

—to describe what is shown on the drawings and to portray information and establish requirements that can be done best in writing rather than in graphic form

—to include all of the legal requirements that are to apply to the owner and contractor upon finalization of the contract

—to provide the necessary accompaniment to the drawings in establishing a firm base for the preparation of competitive bids and the execution of the work required by the contract

—to assist the contractor in organizing his bidding, purchasing, and construction procedures by classifying the various trade activities into the sixteen divisions identified above

—to function as a guide for owner, contractor, and architect during construction and inspection of the work

—to regulate payments and to provide the basis for legal interpretations

ABBREVIATIONS

WIRE GLASS	W. GL.
WINDOW DIMENSION	WD.
WITH	W/
WITHOUT	W/O
WOOD	WD
WOOD THRESHOLD	WT
WROUGHT IRON	WI
YARD	YD.

PHASING AND REMODELING

One of the key words in hospital construction is "phasing." When a project involves existing facilities or renovated facilities, a phasing plan for construction and operation must be worked out. The common notion that "we can just relocate our existing equipment in the new building to save cost" is one of the most difficult problems in construction. During hospital remodeling, the existing facility must be kept operational at all times. If an entire department is to be replaced, the new department must be ready before the existing one can move. This makes it almost impossible to relocate fixed equipment without shutting down the operation. Some fixed items, such as millwork, can only be reused in a department that will be phased out later. By the time wood or metal cabinets are torn out, moved, refinished, and installed again, the cost of the old equipment will be very close to that of new items.

Phasing of operations and work flow involve the entire hospital staff. Once a plan is coordinated with the contractor, the staff must be notified, equipment and utilities must be put in place, and traffic and time elements must be worked out. It is necessary at many phases for the contractor to work at night or on weekends so that utilities can be disconnected and replaced. Time is critical on an hourly basis and takes a maximum effort by the administrator, architect, and contractor. The hospital administrator must attempt to anticipate all of the problems that can occur. A phasing program connected with remodeling must be accomplished before the final plans are given to various contractors for bidding, and the time frames and temporary construction conditions must be clearly defined. Once a contractor is chosen, he should be made aware of the key areas of hospital operation concerned with the departments he will remodel.

Costs for major renovation can be as high as those for new construction and hidden pipes and undocumented structures can cause disputes. The expertise of a remodeling contractor is as important, if not more so, than that of a new building contractor. Renovation design and operation is very difficult and only experienced professionals should be employed to attempt it.

ALTERNATIVES AND COSTS

By this stage of the project development, the major decisions of the design team have been carried out and are very costly to change. The hospital consultant completed his job before working drawings were started, and the architect is now 70 percent finished. The department heads' input plus all fixed equipment and functional design have been set for months. The documents are by now supposed to contain every approval, thought, mood, change, and quality of all the various people involved over the design period. Construction prices, however, have been only estimates, and a final price can only be obtained with the complete scope of drawings, specifications, and conditions of the contract. It is at this point, before bidding, that *deductive, add-on* alternatives, or both, should be included. Though most alternatives were conceived early in the design, because of the budget, the formal proposal is only now drawn up.

What is an alternative and why is it necessary? An alternative is designed to meet the taste of the client on the day final prices are received. Anyone who has shopped for a major appliance for his home has faced the same situation: an estimated price is established on the basis of experience and advertisements; then the extras to be added on or the features that may have to be taken off are considered.

Typical deductive alternatives for a hospital may be a price for eliminating the material-handling system, the laundry, or a complete bed floor. Add-on alternatives may include vinyl wall covering, wood paneling, parking structures, or extra landscaping. Furthermore, an anticipated labor problem, economy change, code enforcement, or even the weather can vary the final price drastically. Therefore, the hospital should be prepared to face a situation in which its extra wants can be either deducted or added on. Deductible alternative estimates do not usually reflect a fair market price of the work items and construction; therefore, add-on alternatives must cover the real costs and are the preferred format.

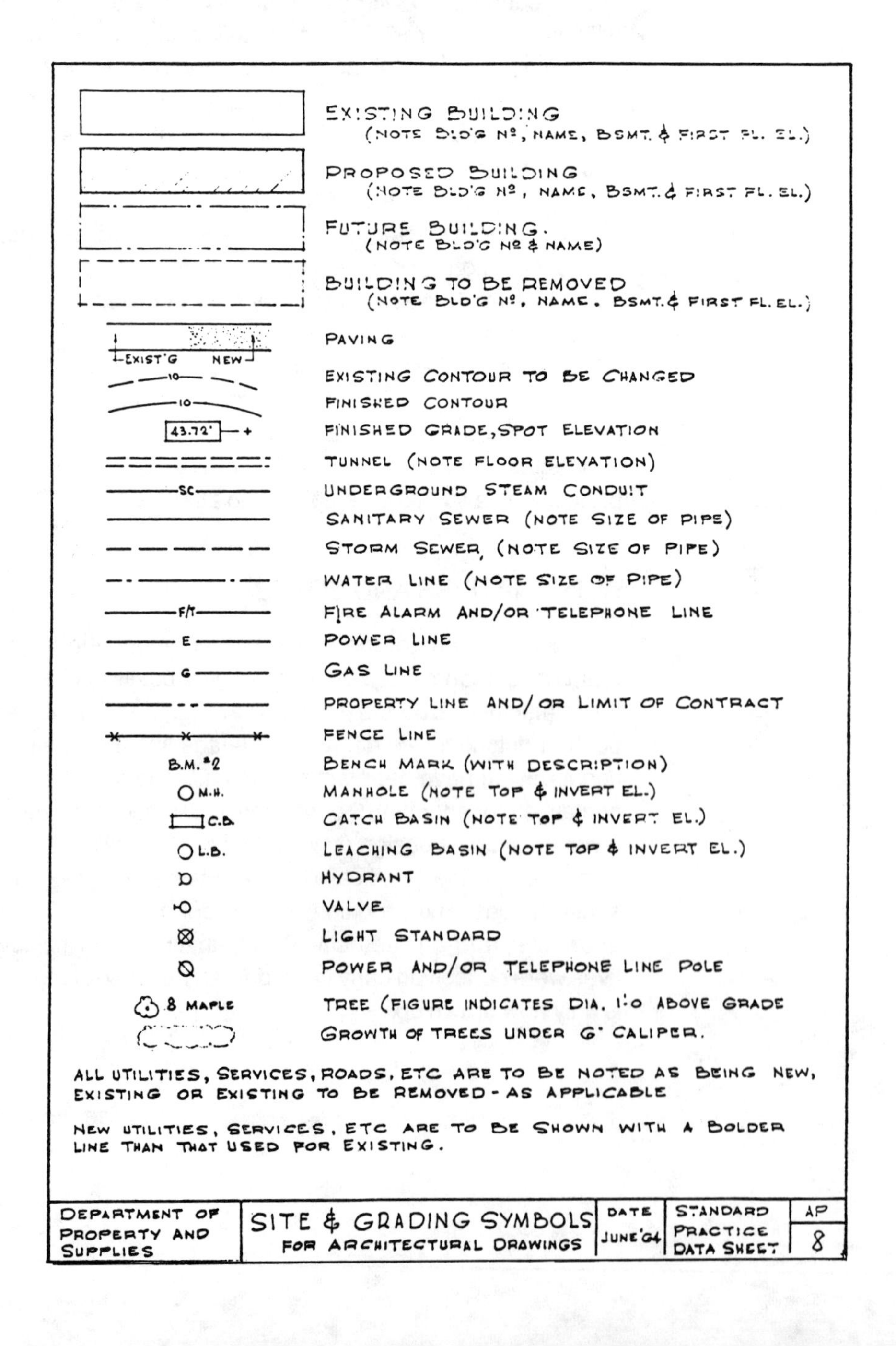

In a system of scope set, pricing design, and guaranteed prices, alternatives are negotiated in or out of a project as the final prices are being put together. Quality control is absolutely necessary during the entire program and design stages, but a final decision on what items can be deducted or added must be made by the administrator.

WORKING DRAWINGS

Working drawings represent the culmination of the architect's efforts in interpreting the client's program requirements. They are intended to explain fully and in detail the volume of the building to be erected. This detail is necessary in bidding to determine total building cost; following receipt of bids and selection of the contractor, it is needed to erect the building.

Working drawings and specifications together are called the construction documents. The drawings graphically portray the design, while the specifications supply complementary verbal descriptions. As such, they are mutually extensive, and what is required by one is required by the other. In the event of conflict between the two documents, the architect is the interpreter. Another, older definition states that the drawings tell the builders what to do, while the specifications tell him how to do it. Whereas this definition may once have been valid, it may be more accurate now to say, in laymen's terms, that the drawings tell the builder where, what, and how to erect the building, and the specifications establish quality control.

The purpose of working drawings is to depict graphically the characteristics and extent of the project. Properly prepared drawings describe, locate, give dimensions, and give physical properties of, or specifically detail the assembly of, various materials. When issued, all working drawings, regardless of building type, must represent a coordinated effort of the general construction trades, and of structural, mechanical, and electrical designers and trades. Throughout the project's development, the architect has headed the efforts of all consulting engineers. Coordinating their design and project requirement implementation, as well as interpreting and complying with applicable codes, is the architect's responsibility. Specifications evolve concurrently with the development of working drawings. Ideally, the specifications define physical properties and performance criteria of each item to be incorporated into the structure. In addition, they identify acceptable materials, manufacturers, and materials and application standards. Regardless of the size of a project, the sequence of working drawings should be as follows.

The title sheet identifies the building or project. Supplemental sheets may enumerate the working drawings to follow, normally defined as to trade and further trade-related by specific drawing enumeration such as A–1, 2, 3 for architectural (general construction) drawings; S–1, 2, 3 for structural drawings; P–1, 2, 3 for plumbing; M–1, 2, 3 for mechanical; and E–1, 2, 3 for electrical.

The site plan and detailed drawings illustrate how the building is situated on a real piece of ground; advise through an area location map as to community location and relationship; and delineate new and existing utilities, new and existing grade, roads, improvements, retaining walls, outbuildings, and landscaping. In short, it would delineate the scope of the project and the limits of the contract.

ORGANIZATION OF DRAWINGS

COVER	Project Title Index	
CIVIL	Drawings in this category shall be arranged in the order indicated. The first plan shall be numbered C1-1 and additional plans shall be numbered consecutively C1-1, C1-2, C1-3, etc.	
	C1-1	Location Plans
	C1-2	Site Plan
	C1-3	Demolition
	C1-4	Grading
	C1-5	Paving & Drainage
	C1-6	Sitework Details
	C1-7	Landscaping (if involved)

ARCHITECTURAL

A1-1, A1-2, etc.	Plans
A2-1, A2-2, etc.	Elevations and General Sections
A3-1, A3-2, etc.	Finish Schedule Door Schedule & Details Equipment Schedules (Millwork, Material, etc.)
A4-1, A4-2, etc.	Wall Sections & Exterior Details
A5-1, A5-2, etc.	Interior Details
A6-1, A6-2, etc.	Reflected Ceiling Plans

STRUCTURAL

S1-1, S1-2, etc.	Plans
S2-1, S2-2, etc.	Schedules
S3-1, S3-2, etc.	Details
S4-1, S4-2, etc.	Elevations & General Sections

MECHANICAL

M1-1, M1-2, etc.	Plans - Heating and A.C.
M2-1, M2-2, etc.	Plans - Plumbing and Special Systems
M3-1, M3-2, etc.	Schedules
M4-1, M4-2, etc.	Details & Schematics

ELECTRICAL

E1-1, E1-2, etc.	Plans - Lighting
E2-1, E2-2, etc.	Plans - Power and Special Systems
E3-1, E3-2, etc.	Schedule
E4-1, E4-2, etc.	Details and Diagrams

Architectural drawings follow. These typically include consecutive floor plans, the roof plan, elevations of the building, sections, details, and room finish and door schedule drawings.

Structural drawings generally consist of foundation plans, floor and roof forming plans, structural sections and details, column schedules, miscellaneous structural element schedules, fireproofing requirements, and structural requirements for the specific project.

Mechanical drawings usually begin with a site utilities drawing delineating incoming water supply service, fire hydrant and underground fire protection water piping system, and storm water and sewer line networks. This drawing very closely follows the site plan. After this come the plumbing drawings, consisting of plans for normal plumbing fixtures, piping to and from them, medical gas systems, pneumatic tube systems, roof drainage systems, and sprinkler systems. Mechanical drawings also include plans illustrating heating, ventilating, and air conditioning systems (especially equipment definitions, duct systems, and hot and cold water piping systems). Equipment schedules and details complete this section, along with system and fixture schedules and stack diagrams.

Electrical drawings begin with a site plan that illustrates incoming power, its point of entry into the building, and site and exterior building lighting. Electrical plans are normally separate efforts designed to show interior lighting fixture arrangement; to define interior power (equipment and receptacle requirements); and to define other systems such as nurses' call and intercommunications, telephones, electrostatic shielding, special grounding, and fire alarms. Plan drawings would be supplemented by fixture schedules, various system riser diagrams, and details.

In addition to the above drawings the architect makes topographic survey drawings and test boring records available to the contractor. These are not usually included with the contract drawings, since they were not prepared by the architect or under his supervision or authority (they are provided directly to the owner by independent professionals).

READING THE WORKING DRAWINGS

At first glance, working drawings are formidable, especially those of a typical hospital project. Yet, if it is remembered that these documents tell the contractor exactly how the building is to be built, they become like a foreign language; the more one learns about them, the less mysterious they become. Taking part in the development of these drawings, from schematics to working drawings, for a single hospital project would provide a complete education, but it would take from two to four years on the average.

Another approach is to analyze a small portion of the total drawing effort. This limited approach can still be confusing because all the "trades" drawings rely heavily on standard material and equipment representations, on symbols, and on industry-accepted abbreviations.

Essentially, each trades drawing is meant to complement the others. The architect is responsible for coordinating the trades drawings, while the general contractor is charged with coordinating the work of subcontractors. In addition, the specifications require that all contractors study the work of other contractors as defined

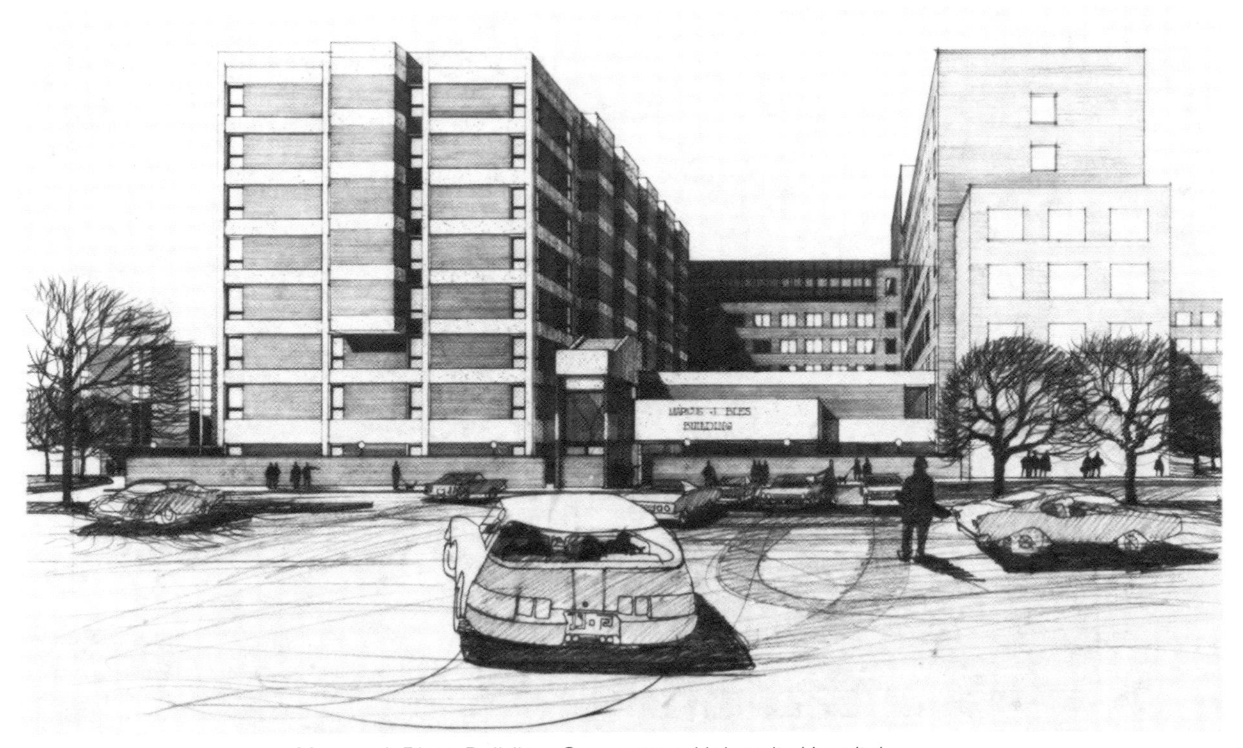

Marcus J. Bless Building, Georgetown University Hospital

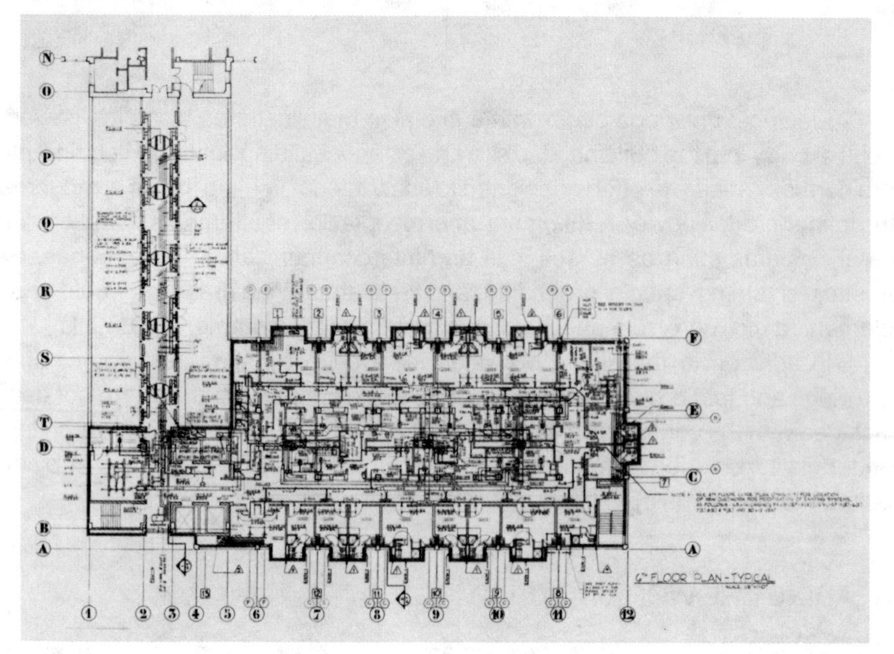

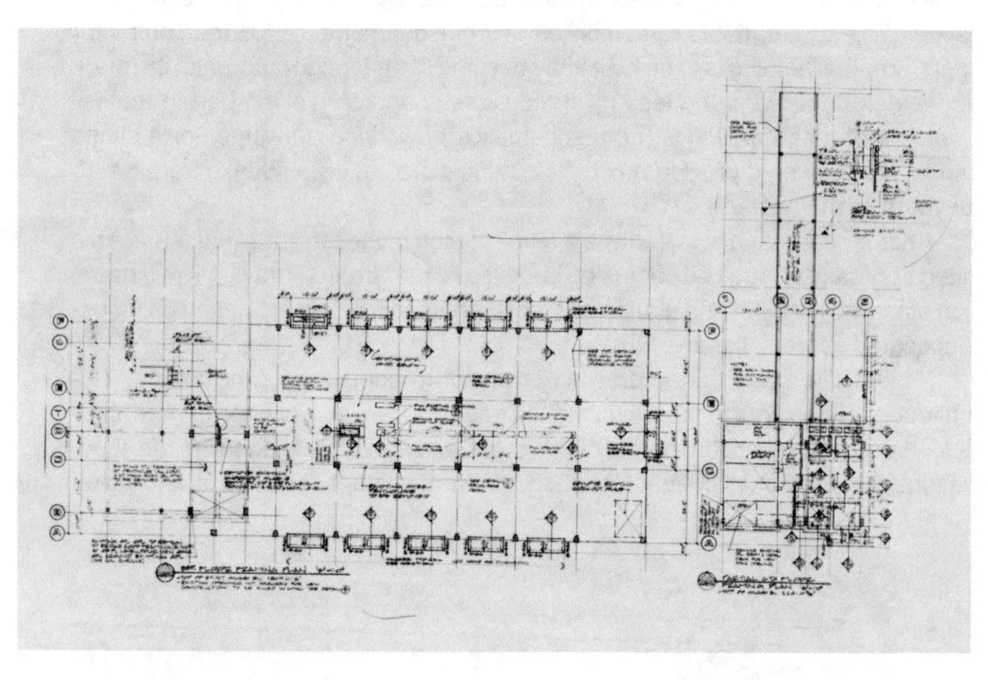

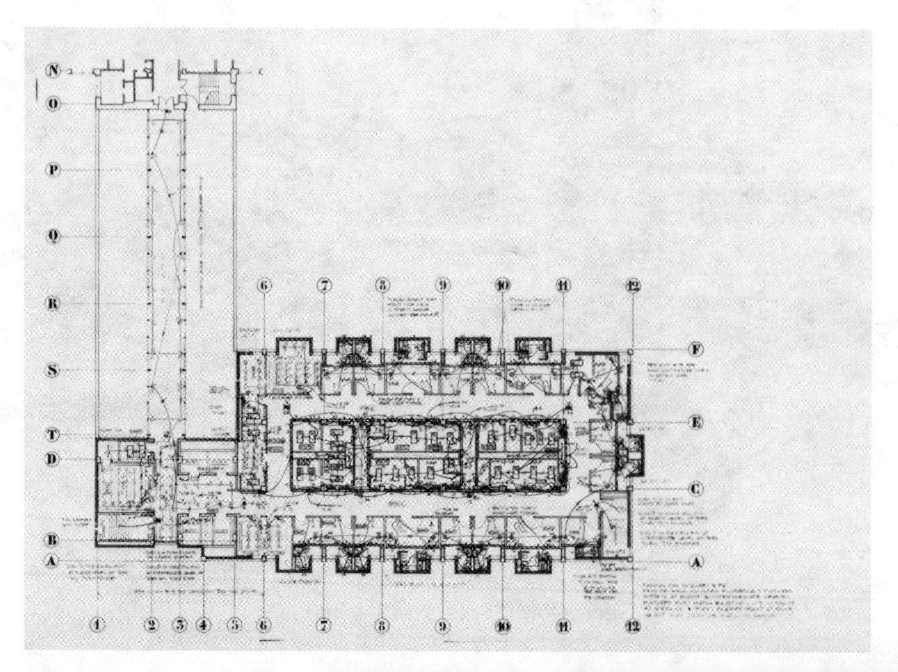

This page:
Working drawings.
Marcus J. Bless Building,
Georgetown University Hospital

by the working drawings and specifications. Some architectural firms require composite drawings that laid out, on a large scale, the major elements of the plumbing, mechanical, and electrical systems. Such drawings not only forced the engineers to coordinate their work in the field, but dictated the order in which system components were actually installed. Following completion of the work, the drawings were turned over to the client and became a valuable part of the as-built record of construction, enabling the in-house engineering personnel to more easily repair and control the systems. Should future alterations or additions be needed, these as-built records would be extremely useful.

CONSTRUCTION

Bidding Requirements and Procedures

As explained in the previous chapters, the system of construction management and guaranteed prices has become very popular in the hospital field. Tradi-

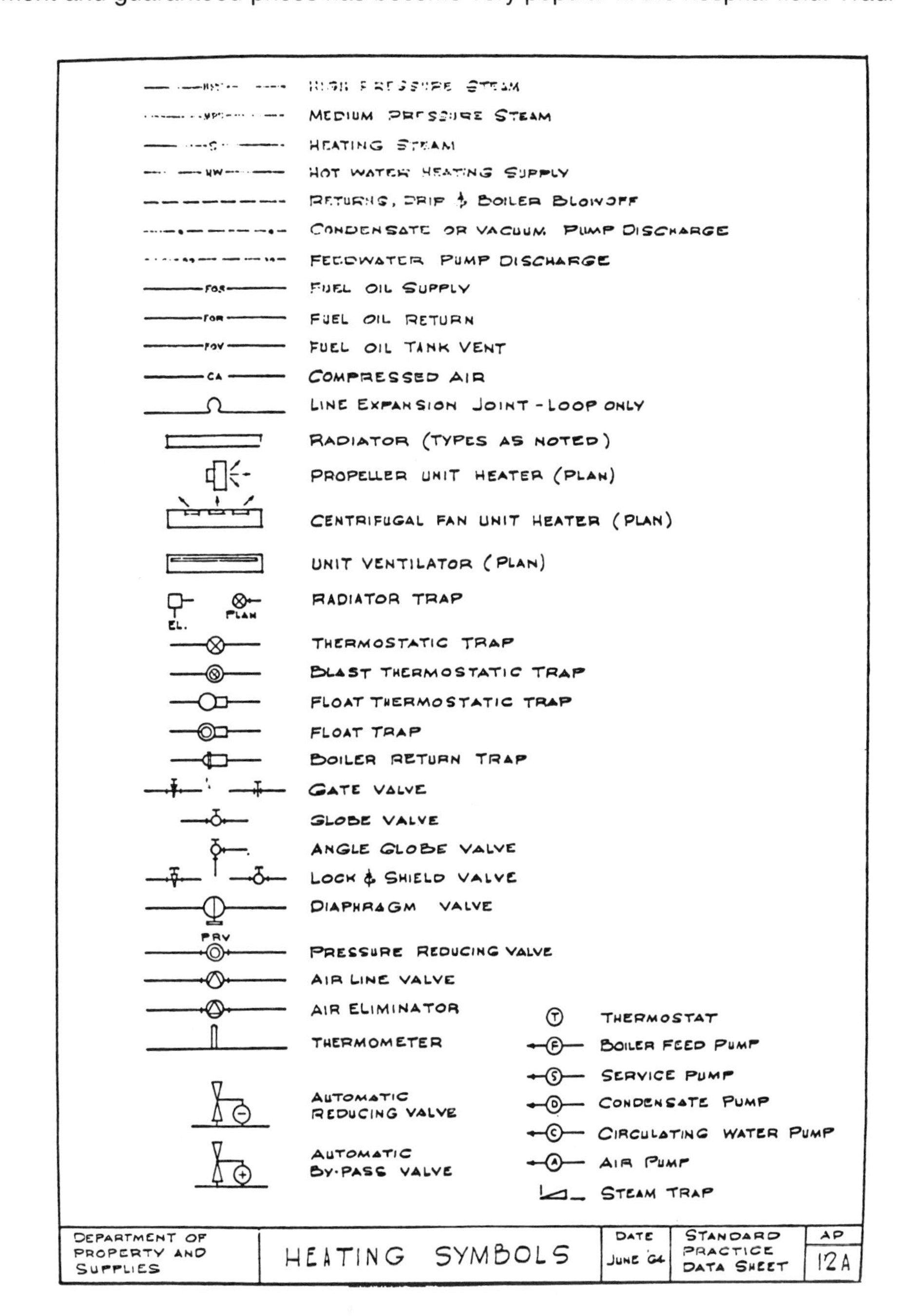

tionally, a series of building contractors would submit sealed prices in competition for the total building project and competitive bidding will remain one of the most widely used methods of obtaining construction prices.

The discussion on general conditions outlined the responsibilities and conditions that a contractor must assume to complete a building project. The sections on specifications and working drawings defined the materials produced by the architect. This phase of a building program now commits the hospital client to sign a separate contract with the construction contractor, with the architect acting as the client's representative. When using competitive bidding, it is wise to pre-qualify the contractors who will be involved. That is, the architect designs a form that asks each interested contractor to submit references and data on experience, financial condition, and ability to be bonded.

An invitation to bid, as described above, outlines the time, place, scope, and location of the final plans and actual bid. The sets of plans and specifications are usually very large rolls, and specification books must be distributed to the general contractors and kept at trade locations for the information of the subcontractors. The architect will supply a minimum number of bid sets; it is the hospital's responsibility to pay for additional sets (this responsibility should be verified by the administrator in the original architect–engineer contract, as the cost can annoy the hospital board if they are not aware of it.) Deposits can be collected to assure that contractors who do not win the bid will return the sets.

The bidding contractors should be allowed approximately four weeks to come up with their final price. During this time, a conference may be held to make sure each bidder realizes the scope of the project; when so many people are looking at a set of plans and specifications there are bound to be questions. Clarifications and item changes should be worked up by the architect, and addendums issued showing each bidder the exact change. When bids are received, all addenda and alternatives are acknowledged. The final price submittals must be evaluated by the architect, who will advise the client as to technical accuracy. The contract can then be awarded. The lowest qualified bidder should receive the project. At this time, the architect and the hospital's legal counsel must draft a contract that is agreeable to the hospital and to the contractor.

In many states, as a financing mechanism, it is required that the general, mechanical, and electrical contracts be bid separately. The mechanical and electrical engineering contracts are then assigned to the successful general contractor so that one company is responsible for the project.

Once the bids are received and the contracts signed, the client has very little control over the selection of subcontractors. The bid documents may require that a list of subcontractors be submitted, but this does not always come about. Whatever prices the general contractor used to formulate his total, he can now negotiate each item: any savings that result will not be available to the hospital. The contractor must, however, meet the quality and quantity as described in the drawings and specifications. Changes at this point will be very expensive.

DESCRIPTION	SYMBOL	DESCRIPTION	SYMBOL
FAN AND MOTOR WITH BELT GUARD AND FLEXIBLE CONNECTIONS		VOLUME DAMPER	V.D.
VENTILATING UNIT (TYPE AS SPECIFIED)		GOOSENECK HOOD (COWL)	
UNIT HEATER (DOWNBLAST)		BACK DRAFT DAMPER	BDD
UNIT HEATER (HORIZONTAL)		AUTOMATIC AIR DAMPERS (MOTOR OPERATED)	SECT. AAD EL
UNIT HEATER - PLAN (CENTRIFUGAL FAN)		ACCESS DOOR (A.D.) ACCESS PANEL (A.P.)	A.D.
THERMOSTAT	T	DAMPER AS SPECIFIED	
POWER OR GRAVITY ROOF VENTILATOR - EXHAUST (ERV)		ACOUSTICAL LINING	
POWER OR GRAVITY ROOF VENTILATOR - INTAKE (SRV)		SOUND TRAP	ST
POWER OR GRAVITY ROOF VENTILATOR - LOUVERED		FIRE DAMPER & SLEEVE	F.D.
MIXING PLENUM	H C MB	FLEXIBLE DUCT	
LOUVERS AND SCREEN		EXHAUST OR RETURN AIR INLET CEILING (INDICATE TYPE)	12"x20" GR. 700 CFM
DIRECTION OF FLOW		SUPPLY OUTLET, CEILING, ROUND. (TYPE AS SPECIFIED) INDICATE DIRECTION OF FLOW	20"Φ 700 CFM
SPLITTER DAMPER		SUPPLY OUTLET, CEILING, SQUARE (TYPE AS SPECIFIED) INDICATE DIRECTION OF FLOW	12"x12" 700 CFM
DUCT SECTION (EXHAUST OR RETURN)	E OR R 12"x20"	SUPPLY OUTLET WALL	12"x20" GR 700 CFM
DUCT SECTION (SUPPLY)	S 12"x20"	SUPPLY GRILLE (SG)	12"x20" SG 700 CFM
DUCT (1ST FIGURE = SIDE SHOWN 2ND FIGURE = SIDE NOT SHOWN)	12"x20"	RETURN GRILLE - NOTE AT CEILING OR FLOOR	12"x20 RG 700 CFM
INCLINED DROP IN RESPECT TO AIR FLOW	D	EXHAUST GRILLE (EG)	12"x20" EG 700 CFM
INCLINED RISE IN RESPECT TO AIR FLOW	R	EXHAUST OR RETURN INLET-WALL (EG OR RG)	12"x20" G 700 CFM
TURNING VANES		DOOR GRILLE	DG 12"x6"
		NOTE: GRILLES W/ VOLUME CONTROL DESIGNATE AS - SR, RR or ER	

DEPARTMENT OF PROPERTY AND SUPPLIES	VENTILATION-AIR CONDITIONING SYMBOLS	DATE JUNE '64	STANDARD PRACTICE DATA SHEET	AP 12 B

Permits

The contractor must obtain the proper building permits from all local building and environmental authorities. Utility permits, site permits, and building permits have previously been approved according to the plan layouts but they must be paid for before construction begins. These costs are usually in the contract, but the client can pay for them independently to avoid the contractor's markup.

Symbol	Description
RD	REFRIGERANT DISCHARGE
RS	REFRIGERANT SUCTION
C	CONDENSER WATER SUPPLY
CR	CONDENSER WATER RETURN
CH	CIRCULATING CHILLED OR HOT WATER SUPPLY
CHR	CIRCULATING CHILLED OR HOT WATER RETURN
	MAKE-UP WATER
H	HUMIDIFICATION LINE
	DRAIN PIPING
B	BRINE SUPPLY
BR	BRINE RETURN
T	THERMOSTAT - SELF CONTAINED
T	THERMOSTAT - REMOTE BULB
P	PRESSURESTAT
P	PRESSURESTAT W/ HIGH PRESSURE CUT-OUT
	HAND EXPANSION VALVE
	AUTOMATIC EXPANSION VALVE
	THERMOSTATIC EXPANSION VALVE
	HAND SHUT-OFF VALVE
M	MAGNETIC STOP VALVE
S	SOLENOID VALVE
	SNAP ACTION VALVE
	CHECK VALVE - LIQUID OR SUCTION
	SUCTION VAPOR REGULATING VALVE
	CONSTANT PRESSURE VALVE - SUCTION
	THERMO SUCTION VALVE
	THERMAL BULB
	SCALE TRAP
	DRYER
	STRAINER
	VIBRATION ABSORBER - LINE
	FILTER - LINE
	FILTER & STRAINER - LINE

DEPARTMENT OF PROPERTY AND SUPPLIES	REFRIGERATION SYMBOLS	DATE JUNE '64	STANDARD PRACTICE DATA SHEET	AP 12C

General Contractor

The general conditions defined the liabilities and role of all general contractors and subcontractors. The contractor must also understand hospital operations in order to disrupt hospital routine as little as possible.

Construction touches special nerves of the administrator and hospital staff. The administrator will be blamed for the noise, site confusion, distractions, and labor

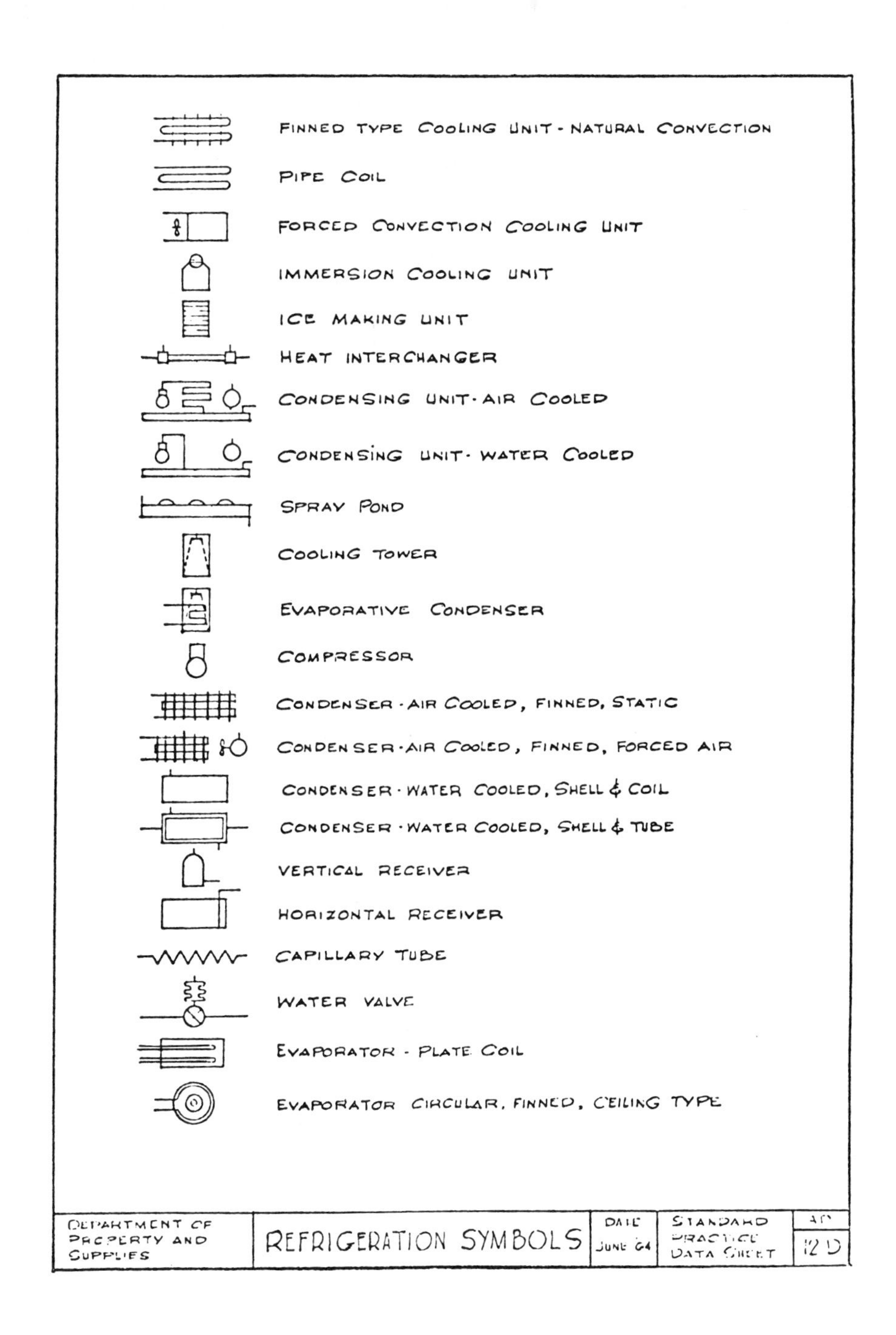

strikes. These things are part of normal construction, but they place an unfamiliar burden on the hospital's normal operation. The best advice that can be given to an administrator is to leave on vacation during construction and come back when the project is finished! Of course, this is impossible. The administrator should, however, leave construction problems up to the experienced professionals who have been hired to deal with them. Day-by-day construction seems like endless delay and problems to the layman; it is a way of life for the architect and the contractor.

The administrator must rely on the contractor and realize that the contractor's aim is to build an excellent facility that will carry his reputation in the community. The building contractor must be experienced, in order to handle problem situations that occur every day. The contractor must, at one and the same time, coordinate thirty to forty different trades (all with experience and advice), solve all labor problems, and build a complicated hospital without creating noise, dust, delay, error, or sparks.

Inspection

One way to save the client some of the headaches mentioned above is to employ a clerk-of-the-works. This person represents the client; he is experienced in construction and is hired by the hospital to check daily progress. Although the architect acts as the client's representative during construction, he only performs inspection as it is required; he will not be on the site every day and, in fact, may negotiate extra fees for inspection services. The architect's duty here is to check shop drawings (detail of each item specified and submitted by the manufacturer for approval), verify the contractor's invoices to the owner, and see that quality and design are met. The architect does not tell the contractor how to build the building: he defines the size, shape, and quality of the building.

R — REFRIGERATOR · ABOVE 32°F.

F — FREEZER ROOM

HIGH SIDE FLOAT

LOW SIDE FLOAT

GAGE

A.C. D.C. — MOTORS

CS — COMPRESSOR SUCTION PRESSURE LIMITING VALVE, THROTTLING TYPE

ES — EVAPORATOR PRESSURE REGULATING VALVE, THROTTLING TYPE

EVAPORATOR PRESSURE REGULATING VALVE, THERMOSTATIC THROTTLING TYPE

S — EVAPORATOR PRESSURE REGULATING VALVE, SNAP ACTION TYPE

DEPARTMENT OF PROPERTY AND SUPPLIES	REFRIGERATION SYMBOLS	DATE JUNE '64	STANDARD PRACTICE DATA SHEET	AP 12 E

Symbol	Description
o	WASTE, CONDUCTOR OR VENT RISERS
o	WATER SUPPLY RISERS
———	SANITARY SEWER
— — —	STORM WATER AND DRAINAGE
—·—	COLD WATER (MAIN)
—F—	FIRE LINE (MAIN)
—G—	GAS (MAIN)
- - - -	VENT LINE
—·—	COLD WATER SUPPLY
—··—	HOT WATER SUPPLY
—···—	HOT WATER RETURN
—DW—	DRINKING WATER SUPPLY
—DWR—	DRINKING WATER RETURN
—D—	DISTILLED WATER
—S—	SPRINKLER (MAIN SUPPLY)
—o—o—	SPRINKLER BRANCH AND HEADS
—F—	FIRE LINE
—G—	GAS LINE
—V—	VACUUM LINE
—CA—	COMPRESSED AIR
ACID	ACID WASTE
O.S.H.	SHOWER HEAD
	VACUUM OUTLET
F.D.	FLOOR DRAIN
A.D.	AREA DRAIN
oOo	MIXING VALVE
	FLUSHING VALVE
	BACK WATER VALVE
	CHECK VALVES
	LOCK & SHIELD VALVES
	ANGLE GLOBE VALVE
	GLOBE VALVE
	GATE VALVE
HW T	HOT WATER TANK
WT	WATER HEATER
GT	GREASE TRAP
C.O.	CLEANOUT
H.B. / S.C.	HOSE BIBB & SILL COCK

DEPARTMENT OF PROPERTY AND SUPPLIES	PLUMBING SYMBOLS	DATE JUNE '64	STANDARD PRACTICE DATA SHEET	AP 12 G

WALL	CEILING	Description
	A 300W	INCANDESCENT OUTLET LETTER DENOTES FIXTURE TYPE, Nº DENOTES WATTAGE.
E	E	EMERGENCY ONLY
N	N	INCANDESCENT OUTLET - NORMAL & EMERGENCY
		EXIT LIGHT OUTLET - DIRECTION ARROWS AS INDICATED
P.C.	P.C.	INCANDESCENT OUTLET W/ PULL CHAIN
J	J	JUNCTION BOX
C	C	CLOCK OUTLET
B	B	BLANKED OUTLET
		FLUORESCENT OUTLET
S	S	SPEAKER OUTLET
		DUPLEX CONVENIENCE OUTLET
1,3		CONVENIENCE OUTLET OTHER THAN DUPLEX 1 = SINGLE, 3 = TRIPLEX, ETC.
WP		WEATHERPROOF CONVENIENCE OUTLET
R		RANGE OUTLET
S		SWITCH AND CONVENIENCE OUTLET
		SPECIAL PURPOSE OUTLET DESCRIBE IN SPECS OR SYMBOL LIST
F		FAN OUTLET
		FLOOR OUTLET
TV		TELEVISION OUTLET
T		ELECTRIC THERMOSTAT
S		SINGLE POLE SWITCH
S_3		THREE WAY SWITCH
S_4		FOUR WAY SWITCH
S_D		AUTOMATIC DOOR SWITCH
S_K		KEY-OPERATED SWITCH
S_P		SWITCH AND PILOT LIGHT
S_{MC}		MOMENTARY CONTACT SWITCH
S_{RC}		REMOTE CONTROL SWITCH
S_{WP}		WEATHERPROOF SWITCH

Symbol	Description
	PUSHBUTTON
	BUZZER
	BELL
	ANNUNCIATOR
	OUTSIDE TELEPHONE
	INTERCONNECTING TELEPHONE
T	BELL RINGING TRANSFORMER
F	FIRE ALARM STATION
F	FIRE ALARM BELL
W	WATCHMAN'S STATION
W	WATCHMAN'S CENTRAL STATION
	HORN
N	NURSES SIGNAL PLUG
M	MAIDS SIGNAL PLUG
R	RADIO OUTLET.
M	MICROPHONE OUTLET
	BATTERY OPERATED EMERGENCY LIGHTING UNIT - Nº OF TRIANGLES DENOTES Nº OF HEADS.
	REMOTE EMERGENCY HEAD
	LIGHTING PANEL
	POWER PANEL
———	BRANCH CIRCUIT CONCEALED IN CEILING OR WALL CONSTRUCTION
- - - -	BRANCH CIRCUIT CONCEALED IN FLOOR CONSTRUCTION
	CIRCUIT TO PANEL BOARD - INDICATE Nº OF CIRCUITS BY Nº OF ARROWS NOTE: ANY CIRCUIT WITHOUT FURTHER DESIGNATION INDICATES A TWO WIRE CIRCUIT. FOR A GREATER Nº OF WIRES INDICATE AS FOLLOWS: (3 WIRES), (4 WIRES), ETC.
G	GENERATOR
	MOTOR
	MAGNETIC STARTER W/ THERMAL OVERLOAD SWITCH
	MANUAL STARTER W/ THERMAL OVERLOAD SWITCH
	DISCONNECT SWITCH - HORSEPOWER RATED AND NON-FUSED UNLESS OTHERWISE NOTED.

DEPARTMENT OF PROPERTY AND SUPPLIES	ELECTRICAL SYMBOLS	DATE JUNE '64	STANDARD PRACTICE DATA SHEET	AP 13 B

VI

public affairs

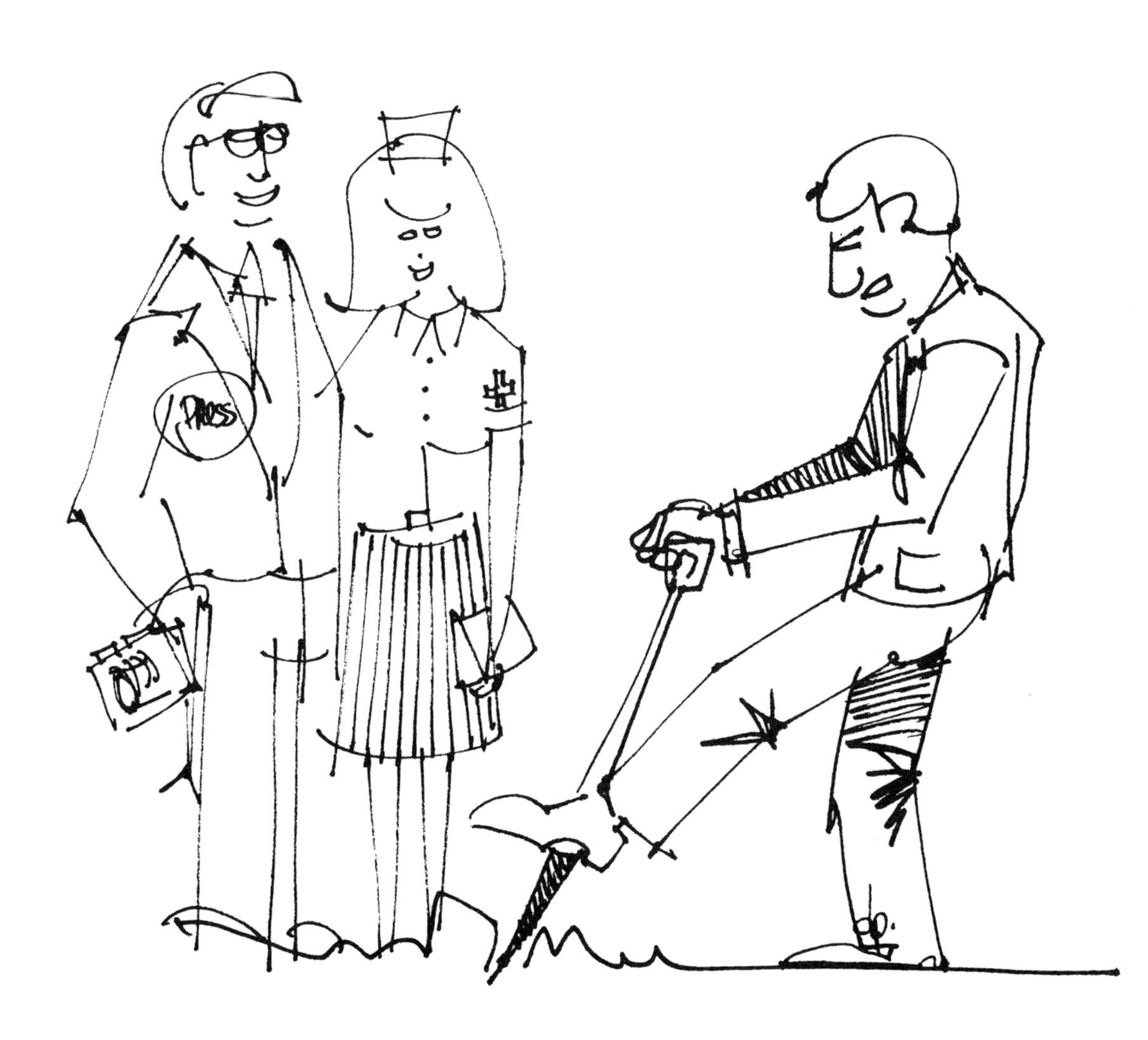

Public affairs, or health design communications, is assuming important new roles in the billion-dollar health industry. No longer the mere conveyor of publicity messages, the public relations person is involved with the administrator in policy making. Becoming, lately, the consumer advocate weighing the impact of new programs on the community, the public relations professional has become an important part of the health care delivery team, particularly in the vital area of health design and administration.

The new concept of health design communications goes beyond communicating with the conventional audiences within the hospital—trustees, medical staff, paramedics, and employees—and the power structure in the area: it reaches out into the community. The advantages and services of the new hospital wing or medical center should be presented to everyone who lives in the area. People should know how to get help before a condition becomes acute, what transportation to the new outpatient department is available, who is eligible for care, how to apply for Medicare and Medicaid, and so on. A sound, concerned hospital communication program will educate all the people in the community through various media, including newspaper, radio, television, and a speaker's bureau. Health construction offers unique opportunities for the hospital and medical center involved in a new building or an expansion program to achieve excellent public and community relations. The administrator must be sensitive to, and knowledgeable about, the events that afford exceptional vehicles for communicating the philosophy, goals, and services of the center.

COMMUNICATIONS: INTERNAL

Internal communications have several audiences: the board of directors, medical staff, professionals and paramedics, volunteers, employees, patients, and visitors. Health design communicators should use all available hospital health care literature as information media. News stories and features should be included in:

—hospital newsletters

—annual reports

—hospital trade magazines

—patient news bulletins

—employee guides and magazines

—information kits

—visitors' pamphlets

—doctors' and medical staff's bulletins

—special events brochures

—board meetings

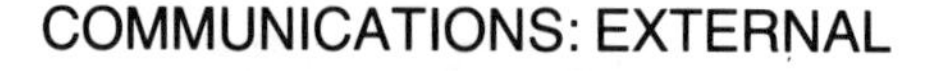

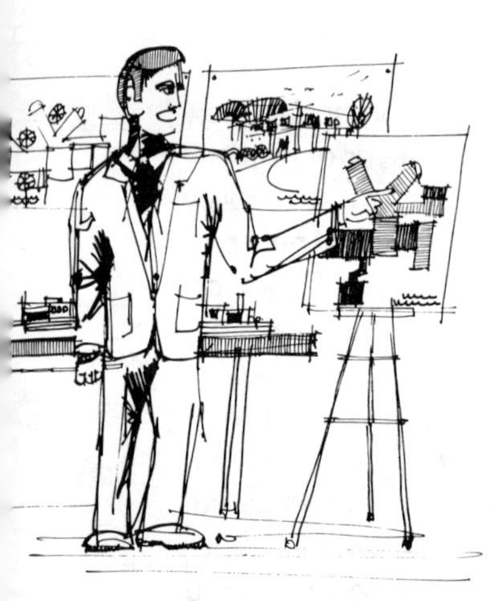

COMMUNICATIONS: EXTERNAL

External communications are aimed at the entire community and the wider public—legislators, government officials, opinion makers, social service and health organizations, and community groups. The media available for such communications include:

—daily newspapers

—wire services (Associated Press and United Press International)

—the local press

—television stations

—radio stations

—national and regional magazines

—Chamber of Commerce and community bulletins

—health and social service organization newsletters

—annual reports

—films, videotapes, closed circuit television

—audiovisual slide presentations

A speakers' bureau should be available for scheduled talks to luncheon and service clubs, the Chamber of Commerce, and community service, educational, and child care organizations. Other means of external communications include:

—open-house tours

—press tours

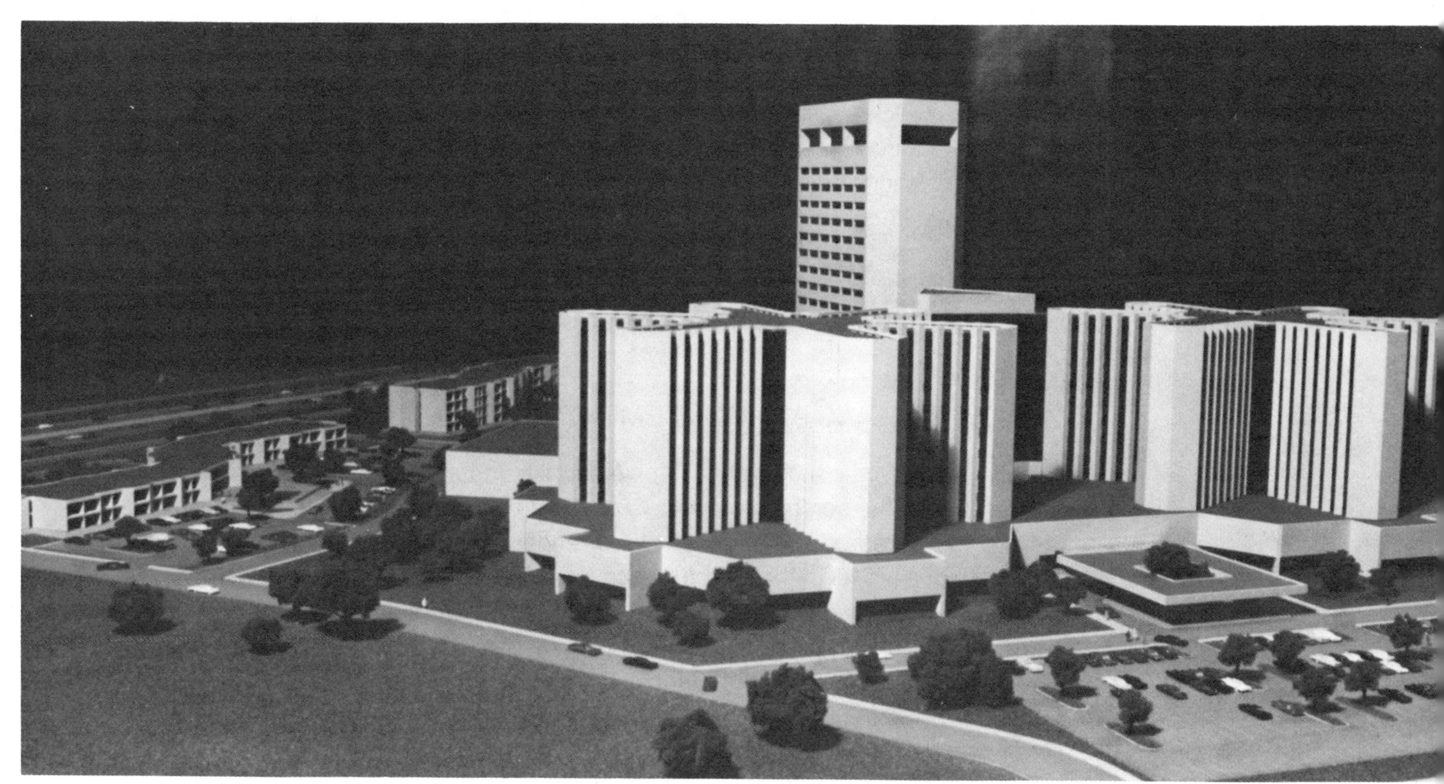

Houston Memorial Baptist Hospital

—announcement of plans and programs

—booklets and newsletters

—anniversaries and birthdays

—the volunteers and auxiliary

—the candy stripers

—county and school publications

The following, in chronological order, are major building design events:

—long-range plan and program development

—announcement of architect's building plans

—groundbreaking ceremonies

—openings and dedications

Additional opportunities present themselves at various stages of building and in expansion programs. It is at these important occasions in the life of a medical center that the administrator should consult his health design professional. In health design, the public relations professional's role is considerably more complex than planning a program to maximize the public relations potential of events. He or she must also be concerned with and involve many internal and external elements, including the staff and the community.

Knowledgeable administrators and health design communicators should be familiar with the public relations program and goals of the American Hospital Association, which aims to make the hospital the coordinator in providing health care to all Americans: the educational roles of the hospital are defined and encouraged; the public relations function is changed and encouraged to become a planning and educational aid to management. In addition to defining the jobs of communicating to particular audiences and groups within and without the hospital, public relations must ask such questions as, "How will we get cooperation and approval of the community, top opinion leaders, and the press?"

NEW BUILDING ANNOUNCEMENTS

When announcing expansion plans, it is important to contact the architect. The architect is the person most able to articulate and interpret the structure. He should provide a "reproducible" photo of the rendering of the building. (When possible, a photo of a model of the structure can be very effective.) A visit to news editors and television and radio news directors can be most rewarding. The resulting scrapbook of press clippings can be valuable to the hospital. The administrator should delegate the responsibility to an experienced public relations practitioner for best results.

GROUNDBREAKING CEREMONIES

Groundbreaking is almost a magic word—it means you have finally made it! It is the real beginning. After the presentations, proposals, conferences, and approvals, groundbreaking calls for a kind of celebration. It is an ideal time to educate and communicate. Everything should be geared to making the groundbreaking ceremony a successful event, one that has a positive impact on the community and its leaders, as well as on the hospital staff.

When planning groundbreaking ceremonies, one should:

—create a theme; express the meaning of the new building and the medical services it can contribute

—select the date: make it a convenient one for guests, the community, and the press

—invite the speakers: choose leaders who have something important to say and who can say it interestingly

There are many details in setting up groundbreaking ceremonies, all of them important. One has to consider and evaluate the place, atmosphere, placement of speaker tables, audience, microphone, and podium. Arrangements have to be made for simple refreshments and for music, if desired. A warm and friendly, but professional, atmosphere has to be created. If the speeches are to be taped, preparations must be made in advance. If the weather is inclement, ceremonies will have to be held indoors; guests can gather at the site afterwards for digging and bulldozer cere-

Tucson Medical Center, Tucson, Arizona

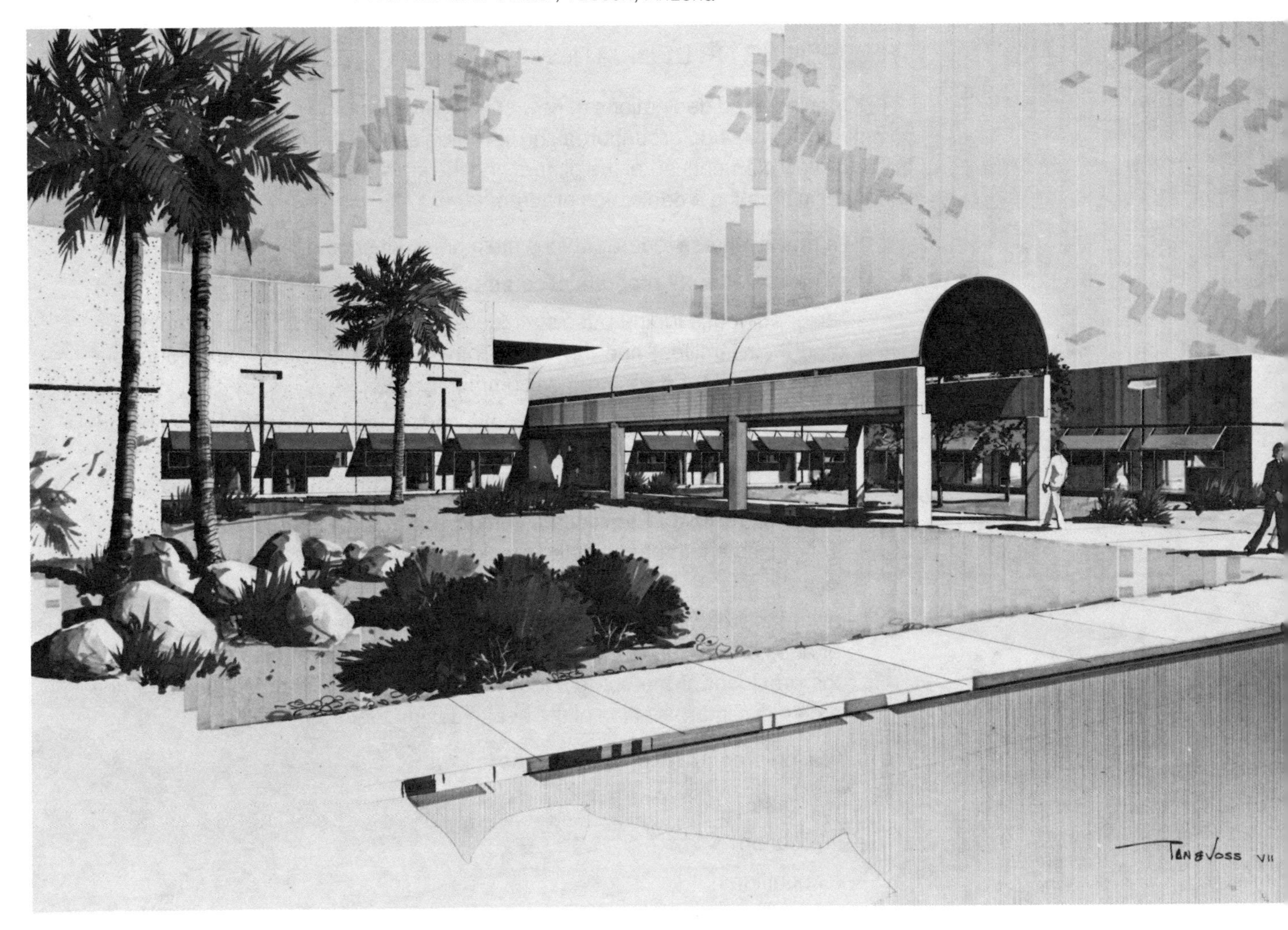

monies and photos. It is a good idea for the hospital to have its own photographer, not only to document the event, but to have immediate photos for press coverage.

Imagination is needed in invitation design and in the making up of the invitation list in order to reach the government leaders in the community and the VIP guests. To accomplish this, the program brochure should be attractive. Also useful is an exhibit of plans, renderings, models, and possibly interior designs mounted on easels or wall boards. As in every health design event, the public relations communicator should plan the program far ahead of time. Renderings, models, photographs, speakers, logistics of the site, all have to be planned well in advance. The guest list takes time to select, call, and refine. An interested assistant or executive secretary should be selected to coordinate details: this person's follow-through work is vital in assuring that all the important people are invited and in making numerous day-before telephone calls reminding VIP guests, officials, and press to be present.

THE OPENING OR DEDICATION

Openings and dedications of new buildings require the same intensive use of communications as do groundbreaking ceremonies, but they take place in the new building. New elements enter the picture and the logistics change. The following are important in creating a dedication program:

—a preview press tour (at which time a press kit should be distributed)

—a more elaborate program of ceremonies

—an open house for in-house staff (doctors, nurses, paramedics, employees, and their families) and the community (opinion leaders, government officials, and a broad spectrum of community groups)

—television news coverage, if possible, and taping of the speeches for broadcast by a local radio station

—a more comprehensive speaker program, featuring leaders in the community or in the field of health care, the governor, the mayor, U.S. senators and congressmen, the head of the medical staff, or the president of the hospital board

—an attractively designed brochure (including the meaning of the new building or addition, its relation to existing structures, photographs, renderings, and the president of the board's message; a page should be set aside for the architect's interpretation of the health design features)

The dedication program might proceed as follows:

—welcome

—invocation

—recognitions

—dedication remarks

—introduction of honored guests

—introduction of speakers

—principal speaker

—music

—refreshments

The techniques for making up a VIP guest list are similar to those used for the groundbreaking ceremonies. A coordinator can help make the event a greater success. Friendly telephone calls are needed to remind important guests and members of the press corps to attend.

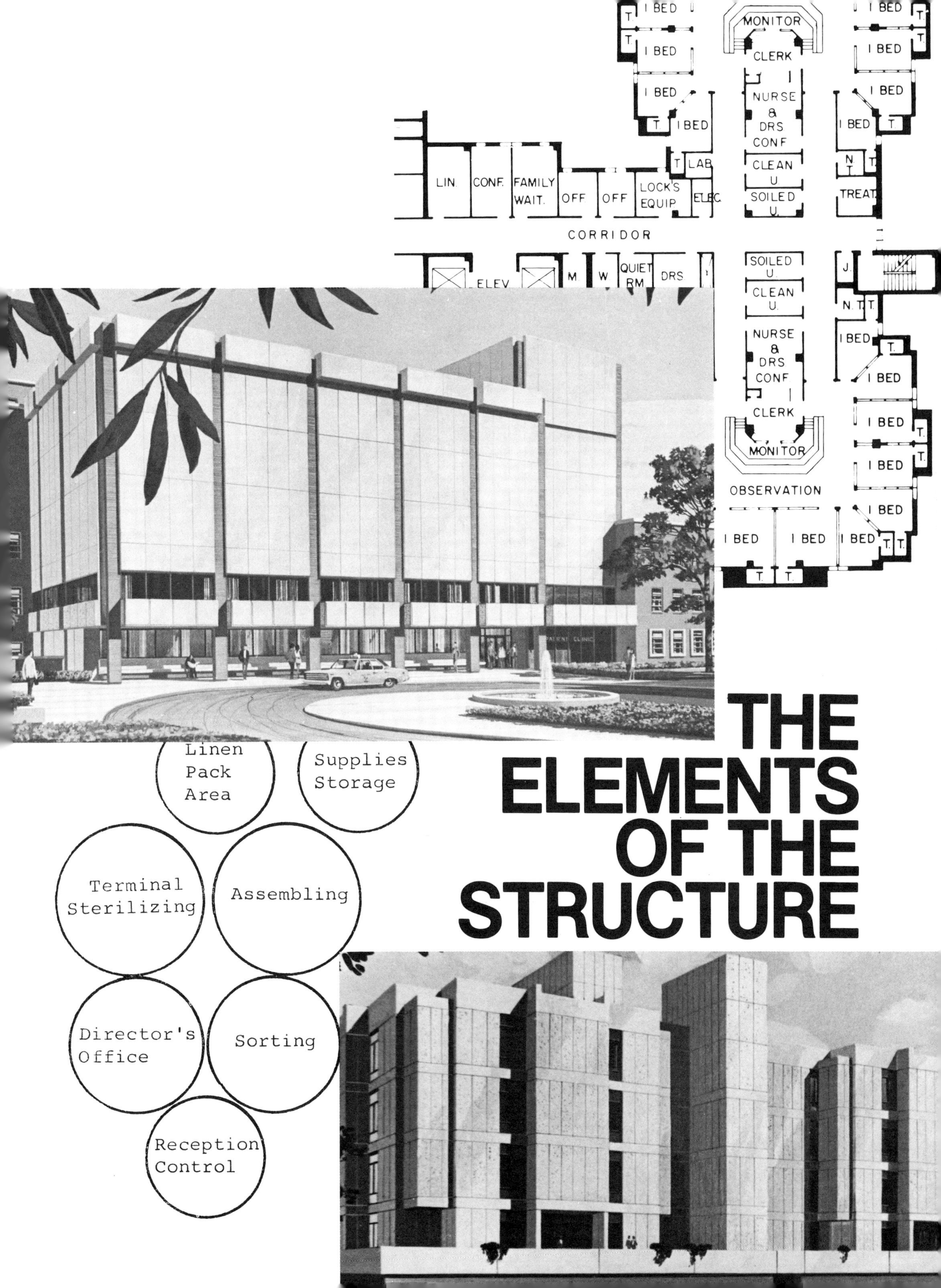

THE ELEMENTS OF THE STRUCTURE

VII

patient environment

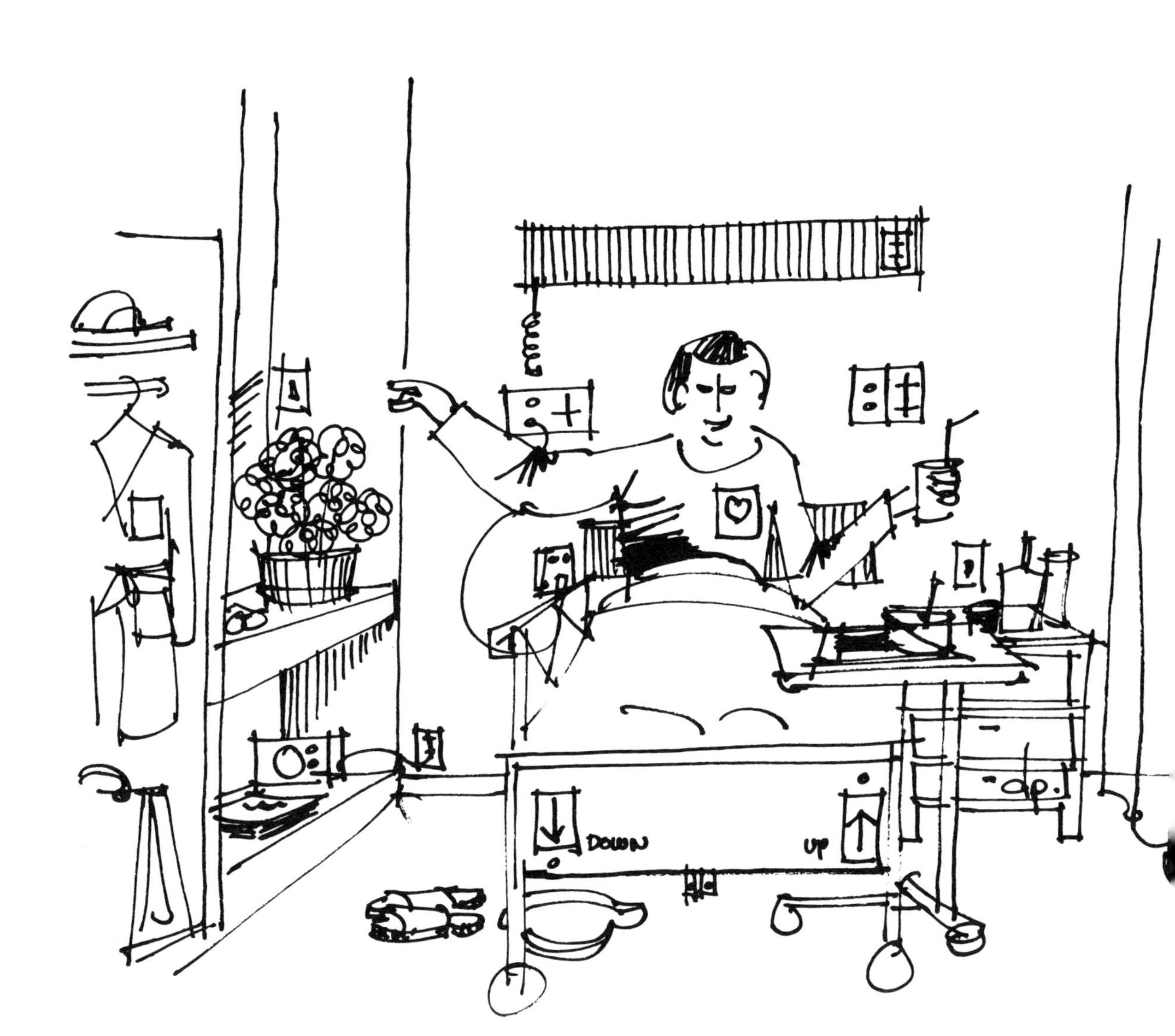

After working on the planning and design of 160 health care facilities over the past twenty years, I still cannot say that a patient has ever attended a design meeting. I have always felt responsibility for representing the patients and, even more so, their families. The time spent in the hospital, clinic, or doctor's office can be traumatic. The planning team must ensure that patient and family needs are understood and that all possible comforts are offered.

Along with the facility master plans and cost reimbursement formulas, a patient needs study should be undertaken. Each community has an ethnic, religious, social, and economic profile. The hospital administrator must understand this profile and plan for it.

THE PATIENT

The patient is admitted to a facility at his doctor's choice, but the patient is the most important customer in the entire system. A patient profile reflecting current preferences, tastes, and specific needs is a valuable tool in planning and daily performance. Such intangibles as a neat appearance and friendliness on the part of the staff, unwavering respect for the dignity of the patient, and tender loving care are at the top of the list for the patient's overall comfort.

Fear of pain, separation from family, death, and unknown changes in life-style directly affect the patient's adjustment and recovery. In addition, the patient will experience an increased awareness of his physical environment. Noise, color, lighting, odors, and air temperature are amplified; combined with the lack of privacy, delays, and attitudes of the staff, these stimuli can seem alien to the patient. The architect must be aware of these anxieties and environmental factors in order to design a medical facility that will promote the patient's recovery.

Most patients undergo a set sequence of events during their hospitalization. Because of the complexity of diagnostic and therapeutic services a patient may receive, it is vital that the departments providing these services be physically close to each other; speed, comfort, and efficiency must be at a maximum. The following is a typical sequence of events, written by Jody Taylor, a specialist in health care architecture. Although the patient does not physically go to the majority of the departments, staff and supplies from these departments are utilized in his care and are usually brought to him.

—The patient is transported to the hospital by private vehicle, public transportation, or ambulance (emergency).

—He enters (emergency, public spaces, outpatient department) by wheelchair, on stretcher (equipment storage), or on foot.

—He is assisted (auxiliary) to his room on the ward (nursing administration, medical, surgical, and gynecological bed unit, obstetrical bed unit, pediatric bed unit, psychiatric bed unit, intensive care, long-term care).

—He changes into hospital gown (laundry). His clothes are placed in his individual wardrobe or locker. He is given a receipt for any valuables (nursing administration), and they are taken (nursing administration, auxiliary) to be securely stored (business office).

—He is examined (central sterile supply, central storage and distribution) by a physician (medical staff facilities).

—He undergoes diagnostic tests (laboratories, radiology, nuclear medicine, physical medicine, EEG, EKG, cardiopulmonary function).

—The patient is wheeled on a stretcher (equipment storage) to surgery (operating suite, delivery suite), where he may be anesthetized (nursing, administration, anesthesiology). Medical staff (physicians, nursing administration) perform surgery with the aid of sterile supplies (central sterile supply, central storage and distribution). While in surgery, a section (laboratories) or X-ray may be taken (radiology).

—The patient goes to the recovery room (operating suite or delivery suite) for observation or is moved to an intensive care unit (central storage and distribution, pharmacy, dietary, radiology, inhalation therapy, laboratories).

—He is wheeled on a stretcher (equipment storage) back to the nursing unit for additional care (nursing administration, dietary, pharmacy), physical comfort (laundry, housekeeping), psychological comfort (telephone, solarium, gift shop, mail room, meditation area, library, and reading room), therapy, and recovery.

—He leaves the nursing unit (auxiliary) and is discharged from the hospital (admit-credit-insurance, business office, medical records).

OR

—He dies. An autopsy may be performed (laboratories, morgue). His body is removed to a private funeral home. His family is comforted (meditation area). His records are cleared (admit-credit-insurance, business office, medical records).

This is by no means a comprehensive survey of the number and types of diagnostic and therapeutic services a patient can receive while he is hospitalized or of the degree of involvement or relationships of the departments providing these services. It is merely an example of the many factors that must be coordinated during a patient's hospitalization.

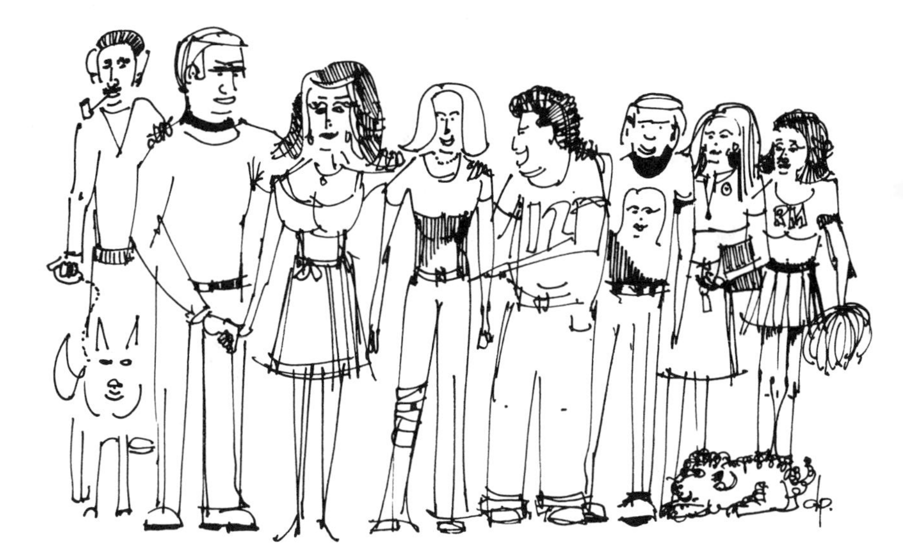

The Family

The direct and indirect effects of disease and trauma on the immediate family are overwhelming. Even the great joy involved in a successful treatment is emotionally draining. The atmosphere of the hospital is very important to the family's state. For each visit, admission, test, and discharge, three to ten family members and friends may be involved. The family still performs major nursing functions. Many European systems rely on the younger and older patient mix to help each other and thus meet emotional needs and expanding costs of care. Home care and programs that include high input by the family and volunteers have become a real alternative to high inpatient costs.

The most important point here is the environment offered to the public. Our manufactured items, designs, engineering systems, and programs must be thought through for the human scale and emotions. Planning without the sense of the individual user will result in failure.

New York University Medical Center Cooperative Care Center, Crafts Room

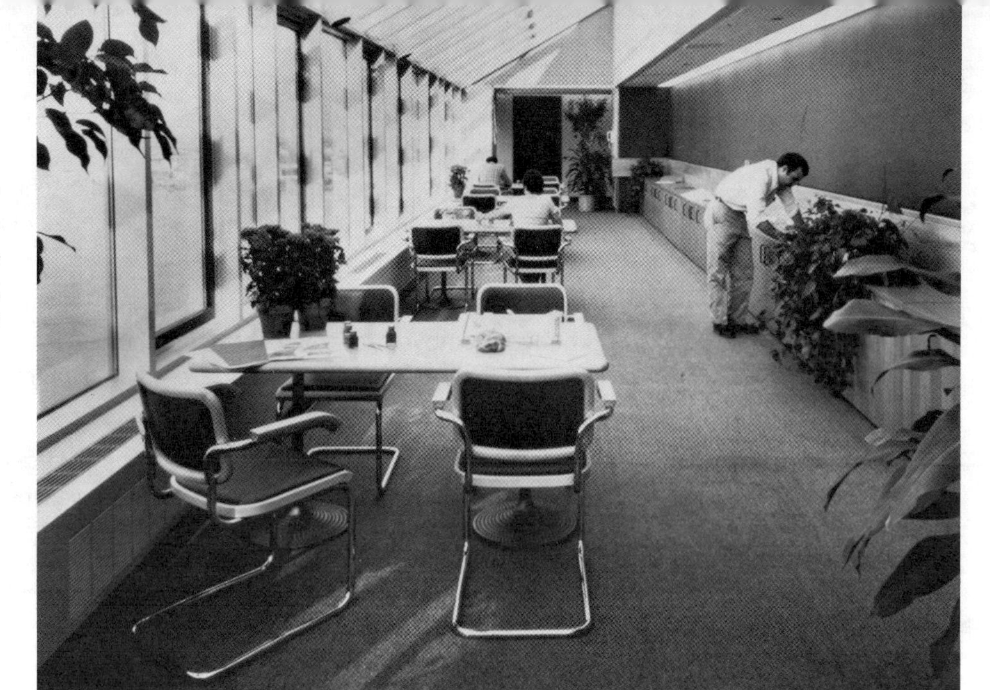

Patient room, extended care facility

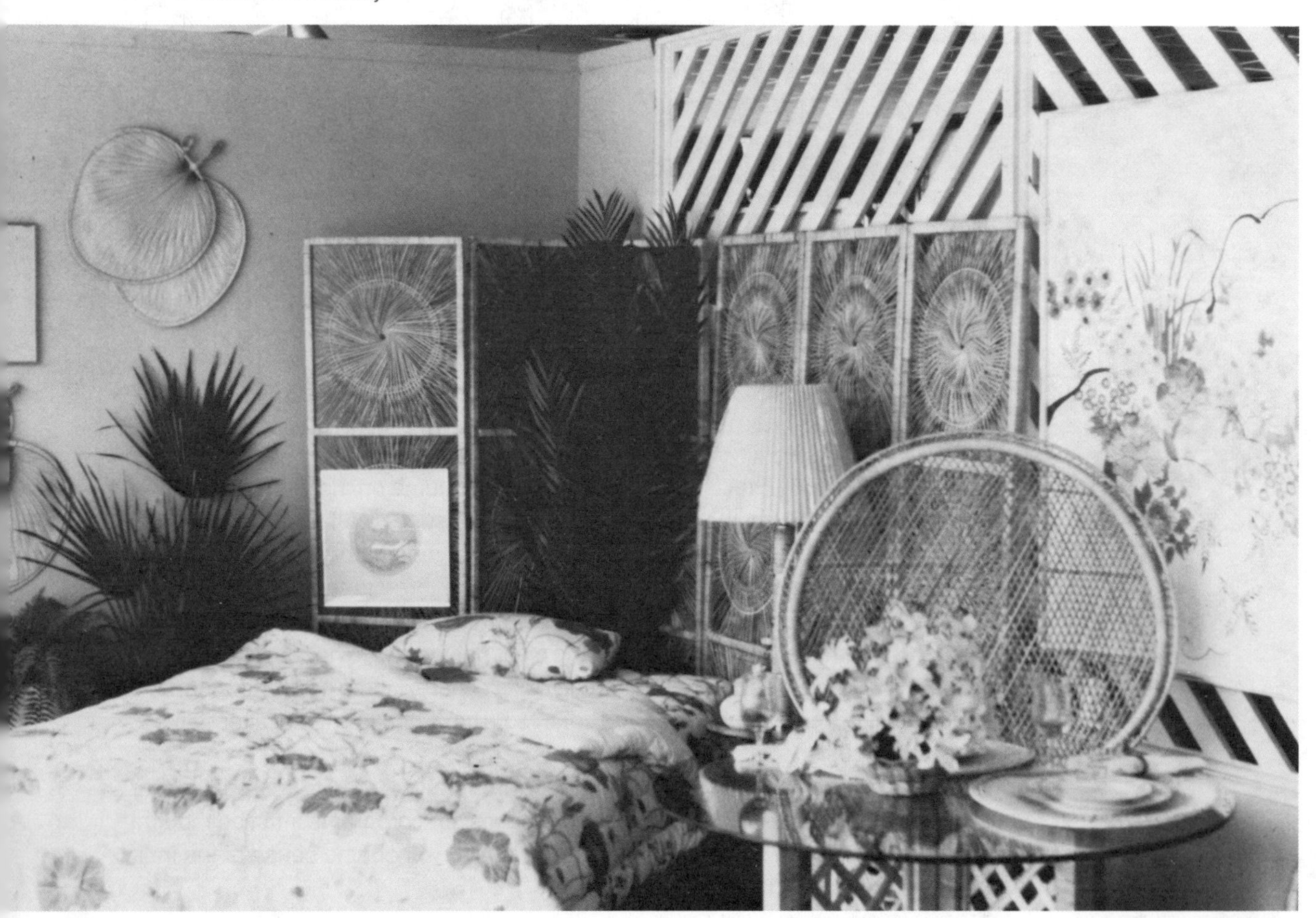

SCALE AND TASTE

Patient needs are based upon scale. The level of comfort involves a very small radius of space. Reach, light, view, and noise become the critical concerns of patients. All layout of rooms, design of lighting, levels of noise, comfort of mechanical systems, and use of color and contrast should be based upon these concerns. The tastes of the patient, family, and staff must also be a priority of design and planning. Emotional safety depends upon concern for this level of detail.

Interior design and visual graphics are also factors in patient comfort. Seldom does one see the sort of accessories found in a home designed for a medical facility. Lamps, flowers, baskets, linen, and art can have an incredible impact on the patient's emotions. This element of taste should be a part of the hospital design, especially in the patient areas.

Because it is impossible to judge and explain this level of development to a hospital board or even a planning committee, the responsibility for design falls on the administrator, the architect, and the design engineers.

Designing for the patient costs no more initially and it will boost public relations for many years.

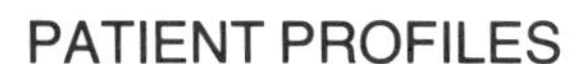

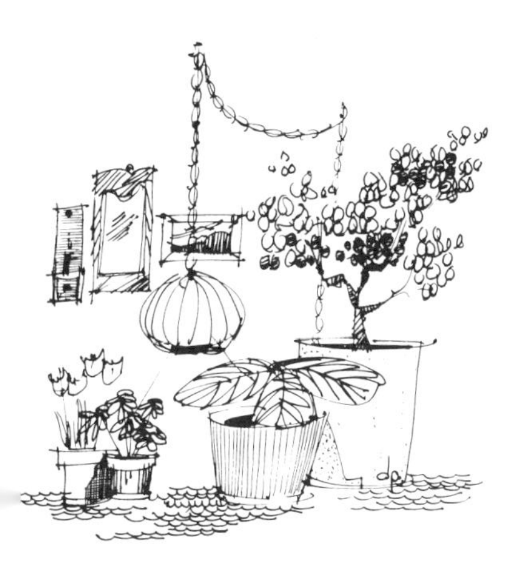

PATIENT PROFILES

Patient profiles represent patients' needs, tastes, and opinions on their hospital stay directly to the architects and design people. Profiles will not only directly affect the administrator, as a buyer of hospital products, but will establish the patient and hospital staff as a partnership that works together to achieve a good professional environment that ministers to the physical and emotional needs of the patient.

The last decade has seen a wave of consumer advocacy programs funded by the government. It is very important that this awareness of consumer needs be carried over to the hospital environment. Administrators, professionals, and students in the design field must be aware of the need to directly communicate with the patients and their families. Patient advocacy programs are already quite effective in some hospitals across the country. They are a valuable source of information to management. A great many patients over the years have told friends and relatives that hospitals as institutions reduce privacy, individuality, and more importantly, dignity. Patient advocacy programs, directly informed as staff members within a hospital, are helping to change these feelings. Hospital consultants on a national level can alleviate these inadequacies nationwide. With a patient profile system, reported patient needs can be analyzed in order to improve design standards. Whether a hospital and its board of directors has hired a consulting architect for a completely new facility or a phased renovation, the patient profile information is a valuable tool in design.

At the time patient profiling was being implemented, my father was hospitalized for the first time in his life, at age 65. His stay was in an established, 200–bed secondary facility on the East Coast. The facilities, professional care, and general atmosphere were of high quality. However, a number of constructive changes in the patient profile came about as a result of discussions with my father. Aside from the standard cry of the dehumanizing effect of the hospital gown, he talked about his comfort needs related to the bed, phone, and lights. I was shocked at the discrepancy between his needs and standard manufactured items. Another important fact was lack of privacy for visiting family members. In my last patient profile, patient dignity was repeatedly stated by the physicians as being the highest priority.

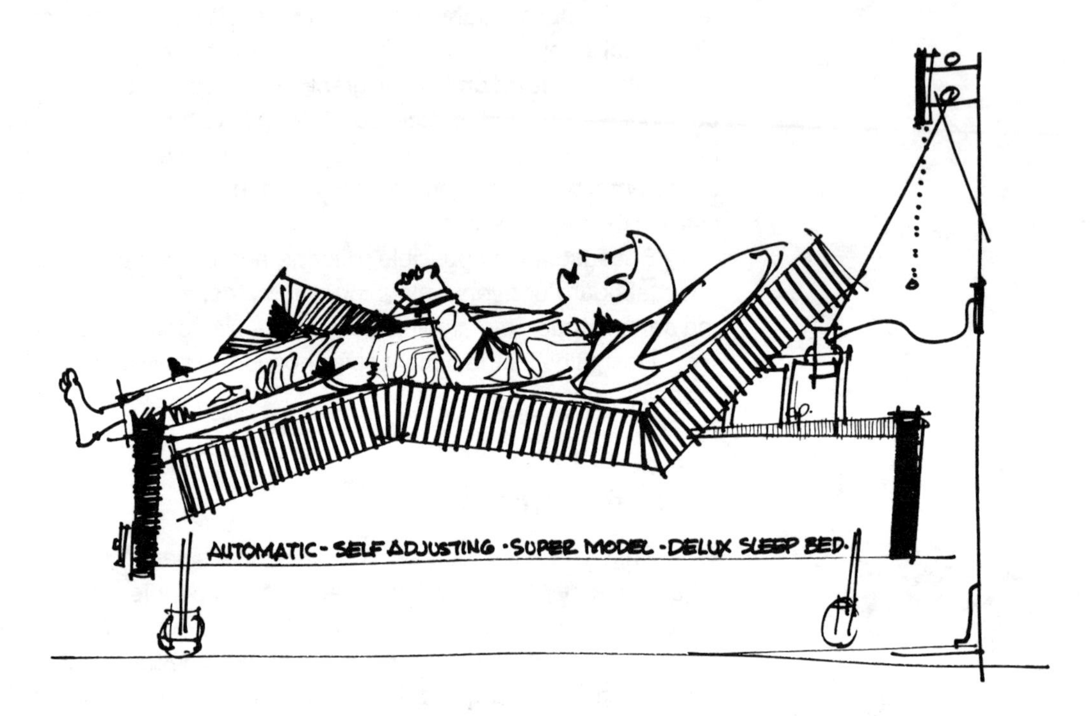

The following is a sample patient profile questionnaire and can be reworded or added to in order to meet the needs of the particular locale.

Sample Patient Profile Questionnaire

Age:______

Sex: M______F______

Admitted by Doctor______Emergency Room______Other______

How many people came with you?______

Did you arrive in a Car______Bus______Taxi______Other______

Did you have any problem knowing where to enter? Yes______No______

Do you think it is difficult to find things in the hospital?

Yes______No______

How many visitors do you have each day?______

Do you prefer a private room______Semi-private room______?

Can you control the lights in your room? Yes______No______

Do you want to?______

How many chairs would you like in your room?______

Do you use any other areas for visiting?

Lobby______Corridor______Waiting room______

What color do you prefer?______

Do you prefer large windows?______

Small windows______

Is the view from your room outside important? Yes______No______

Do you use the gift shop? Yes______No______

Do you use the coffee shop? Yes______No______

Do you need space for flowers? Yes______No______Other______

Did you bring a suitcase with you? Yes______No______

Should the sink be in the toilet room______Bedroom______?

Do you prefer a bathtub______Shower______Neither______?

How many meals a day do you prefer?______

Do you want a mirror in your room?______

Can you reach everything you need? Yes______No______

What items do you always need at your bedside?________________________

Where should the TV be located?________________

Should the hospital present health subjects on TV? Yes______No______

What type of furniture do you prefer? Contemporary______

Casual______Classic______

Can you make your bed position comfortable? Yes______No______

Do you ever use the chapel? Yes______No______

What service do you need that is not supplied?__________________________

How do you rate the noise level? Good______Fair______Poor______

What would you prefer on the floor? Tile______Carpet______

How would you change your room?____________________________________

What would you add?____

Do you need a handrail in the corridor in order to walk? Yes______No______

Would handrails make you feel safer in walking? Yes______No______

What services do you need at night?______

What would you add to the hospital?______

Do you prefer drapes______Blinds______Other______

The finished profile should be of interest to administrators, designers, consumers, and the federal policymakers in budgeting future funds. It is time our profession reflects on needs of patients themselves, not on what we perceive to be their needs, for "their" needs are truly our own.

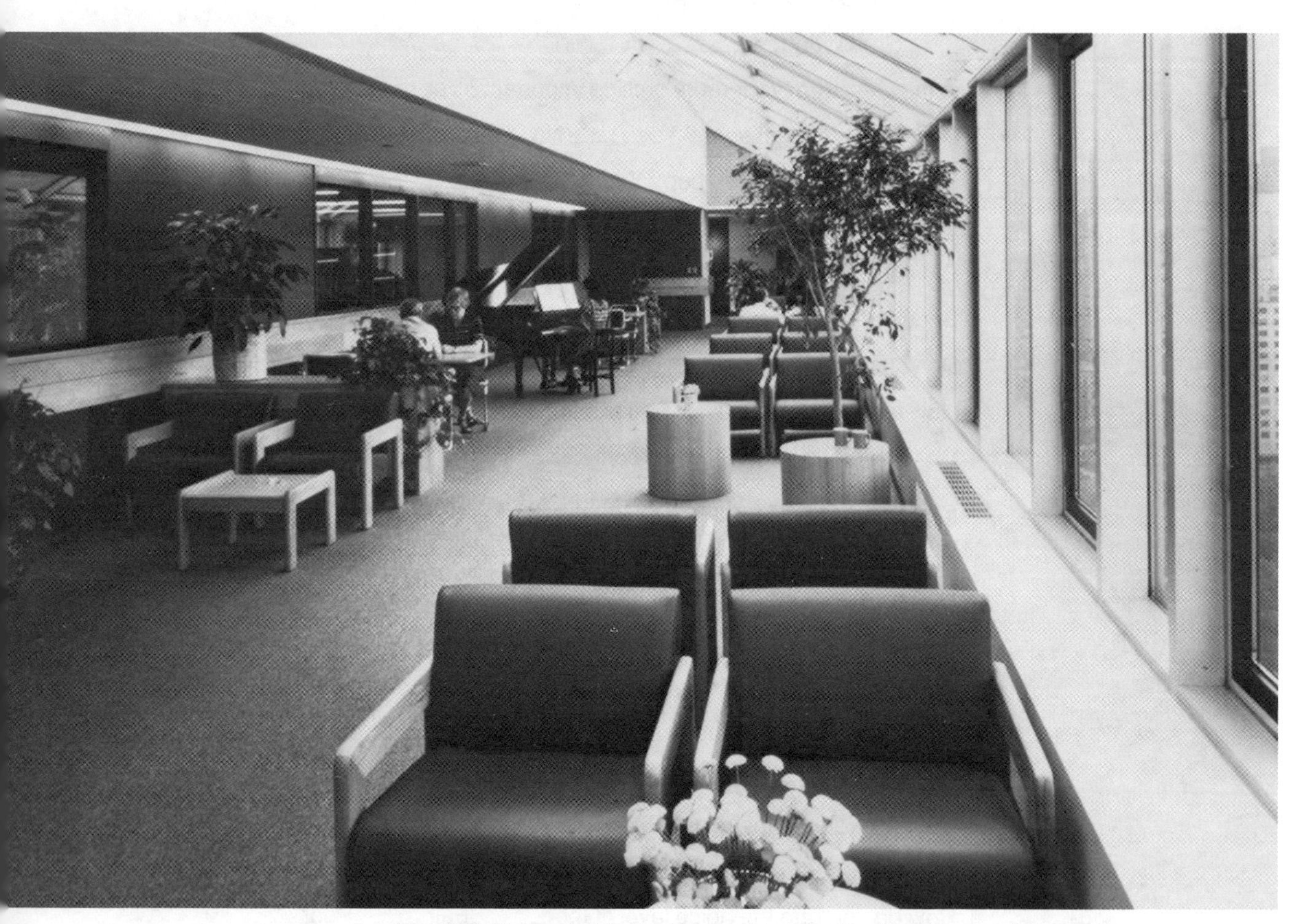

New York University Medical Center Cooperative Care Center, Recreation Room

VIII

department planning: administrative services

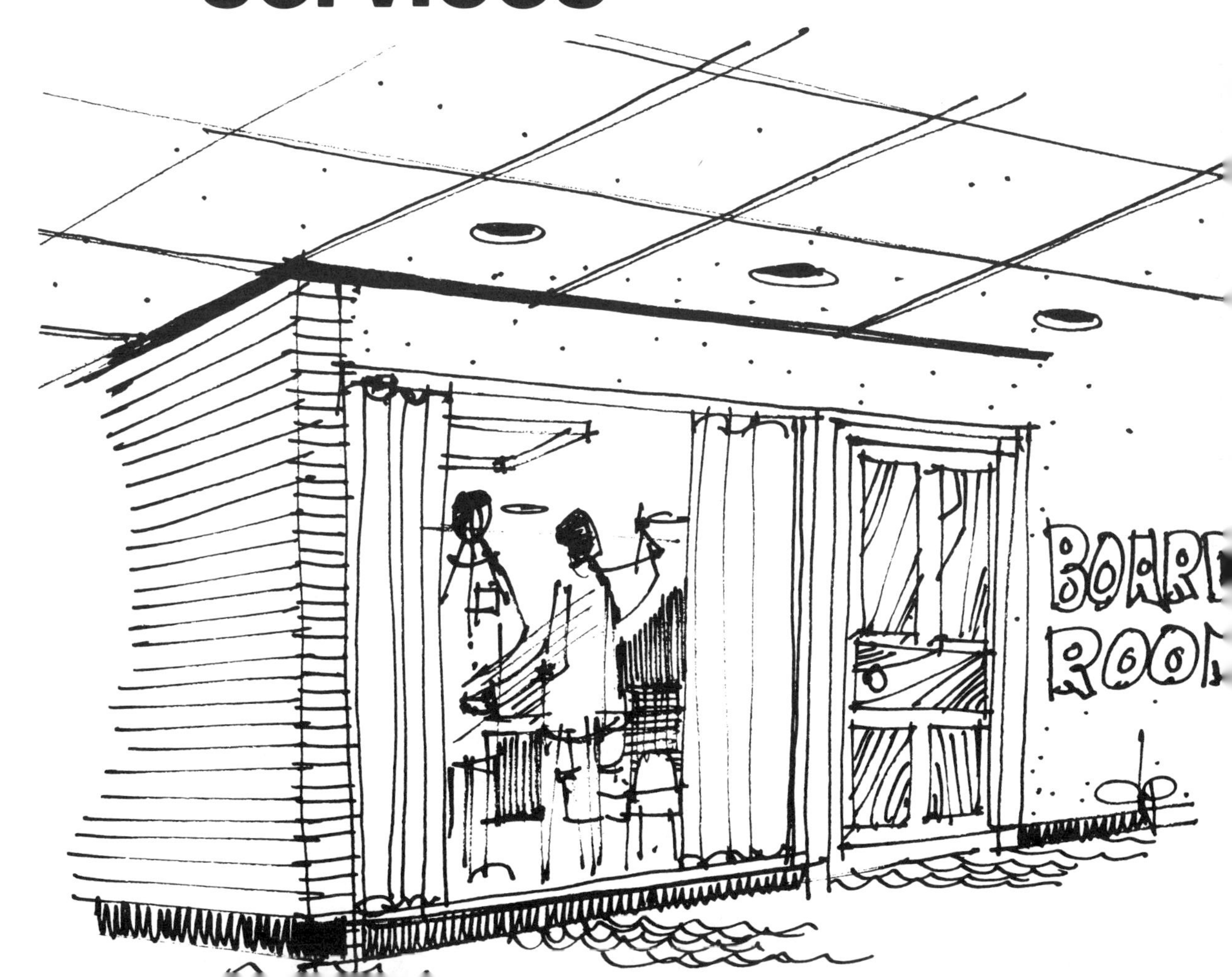

The modern hospital is no longer merely a refuge for the sick or poor, but a highly complex social institution functioning as a center for comprehensive health services. These services include prevention, diagnosis, treatment, and rehabilitation for acutely ill patients, long-term care patients, ambulatory patients, and, lately, patients in their homes.

In rendering these services, the hospital must maintain a high concentration of professional personnel and equipment. It must emphasize a high degree of utilization of personnel and equipment, and the capital investment. In addition, the hospital must correlate its activities with other health care agencies in order to reduce duplication. In the course of responding to these and other pressures, today's hospital has evolved into a multifaceted social organization. It is no longer isolated. It is now a vital component of the community and must interact with other social organizations.

The following table of administrative services gives an estimate of their relative size per bed and lists their order of treatment in the text.

Hospitals should be viewed as a social system that serves the interest of the patient. Management or control of this social system is through a human organization with established levels and lines of authority, responsibility, and communication. Each person has a definite role in the decision-making process. An organization may be managed best by permitting maximum freedom of decision making among its members. Implementation of institutional policies and objectives established by the Board of Trustees can best be accomplished, interdepartmental communications can best be facilitated, and decision-making can best be expedited if the major components of this social organization are physically adjacent to one another in an administrative services center.

Department	Gross Square Feet per Bed
Administrative suite and Board room	9.0
Finance	8.0
Data processing	5.5
Personnel	4.0
Admissions and discharge	4.0
Central switchboard and PBX	1.0
Meditation areas and chaplaincy	2.0
Medical library	2.5

ADMINISTRATIVE SUITE

The pivotal element of the administrative services center is the administrative suite, including the offices of the administrator; the assistant administrators for financial management, administrative services, and planning; the administrative assistants; and the director of community relations.

In direct charge of the hospital and responsible to the governing board is the hospital administrator. The administrator is responsible for interpreting and administering the policies of the board and acting as technical advisor and liaison officer in policy formulation. Furthermore, he is responsible for the management and supervision of all hospital operations. The hospital administrator is responsible for:

—transmitting and interpreting policies, rules, and regulations affecting all hospital activities and personnel

—establishing procedures for systematic performance of hospital duties

—coordinating activities of all departments

—acting as liaison between the governing board and the medical staff

—providing for equipment and facilities consistent with community needs and goals of the hospital

—ensuring that high professional standards of patient care are maintained

—formulating and maintaining a program for good community relations

—maintaining sound financial structure for hospital operations, including the preparation of the hospital budget for approval by the governing board

—preparing periodic reports to the governing board indicating progress and activities of the institution

Administration Suite, Interdepartmental Relationships

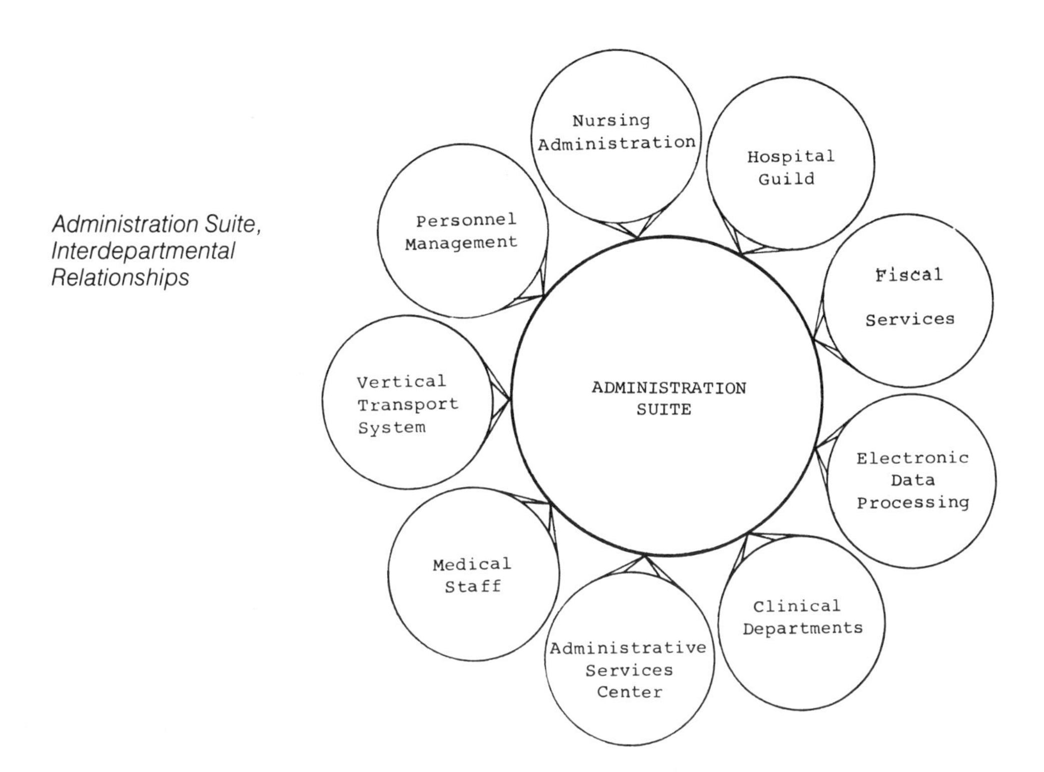

Location. The administrative suite should be located at a focal point of the hospital, within easy access of the main entrances and lobby, but not directly available to the general public. The suite must be accessible to key persons of the public, medical staff, hospital personnel, and administrative staff. It should be as close as possible to the other departments in the administrative service center.

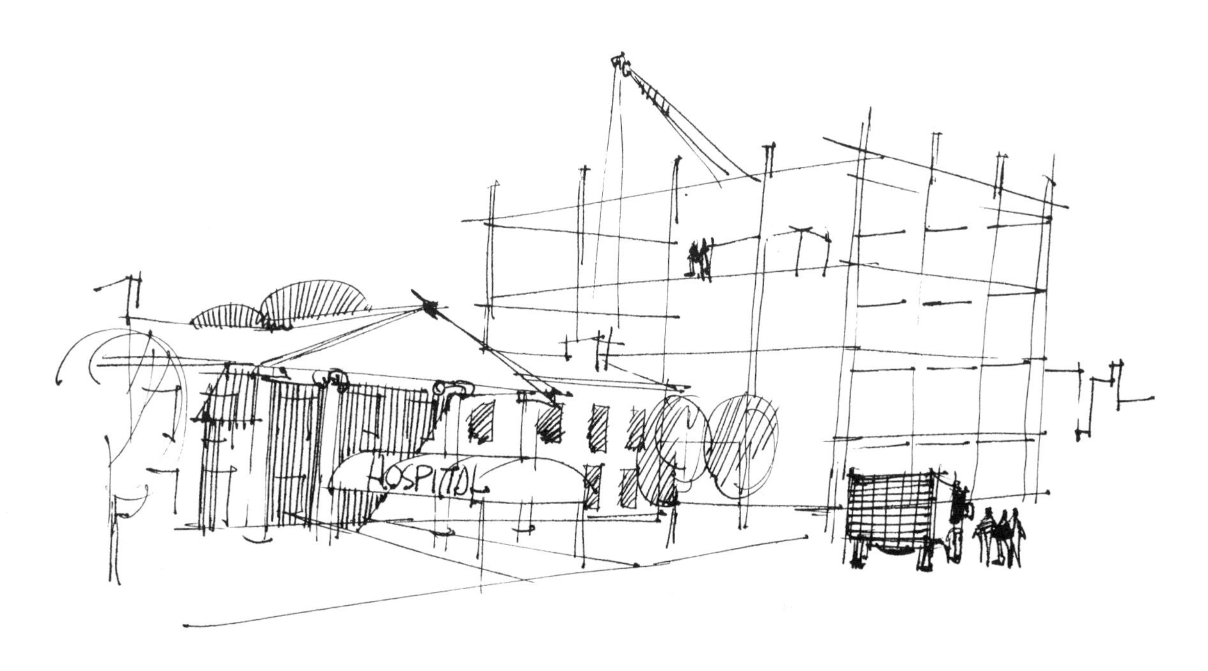

Design. It is recommended that floors be carpeted throughout. Vinyl wallcovering or wood paneling, used with discretion, is attractive in an administrative area. Furnishings and decor should be chosen to complement the activities of the suite. Office landscaping is recommended for secretarial and other open spaces. Furnishings chosen for individual offices should coordinate with the style used in open areas.

Intradepartmental Relationships. The administrator's office should be planned with an entrance from the administrative suite via the executive secretary's area and with an unmarked entrance onto a public corridor so the administrator can enter or leave without public notice. The executive secretary's area should be immediately adjacent to the administrator's office. No one should be able to enter the administrator's office without first stopping at this area.

Administration Suite, Intradepartmental Relationships

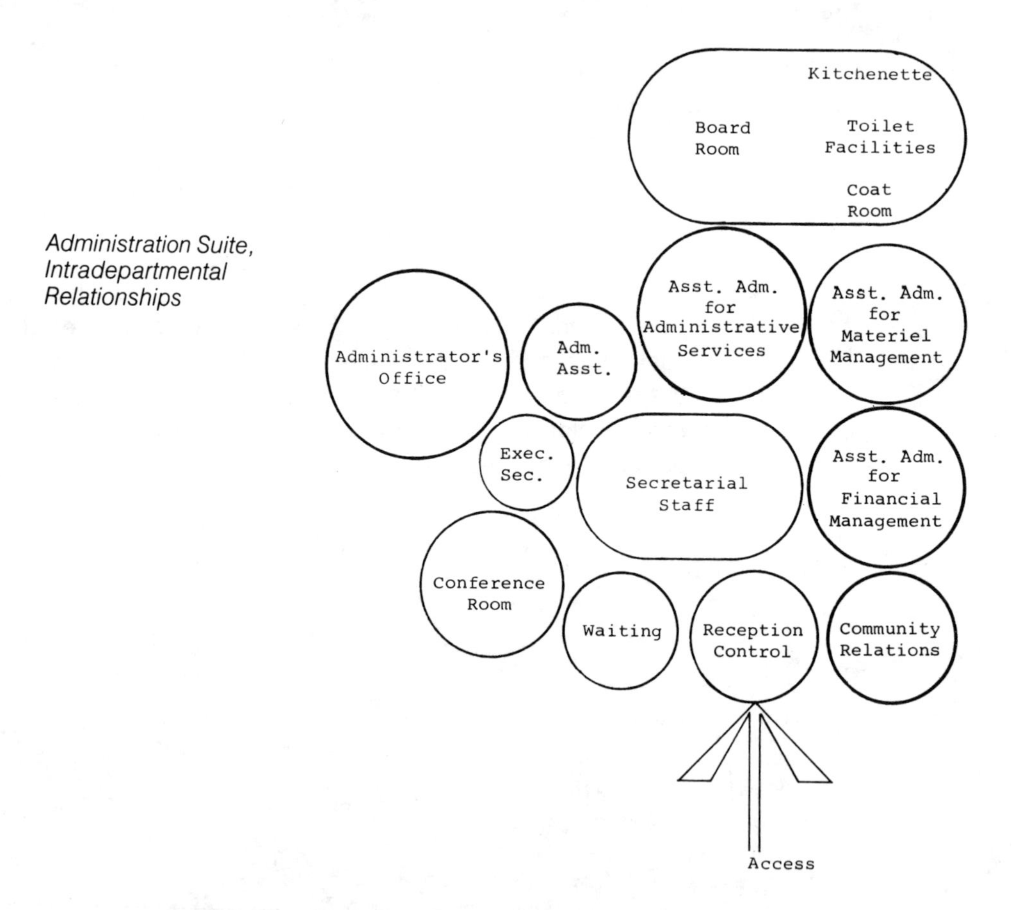

The administrative assistant's office should be included in the suite close by the administrator's office, as the assistant usually performs in a staff capacity to the administrator. The office of the assistant director for administrative services should be adjacent to the administrator's office; the office of the assistant director for planning should be within the administrative suite. The former aids the administrator in

Floor plan, administrative services area. Annie M. Warner Hospital, Gettysburg, Pennsylvania

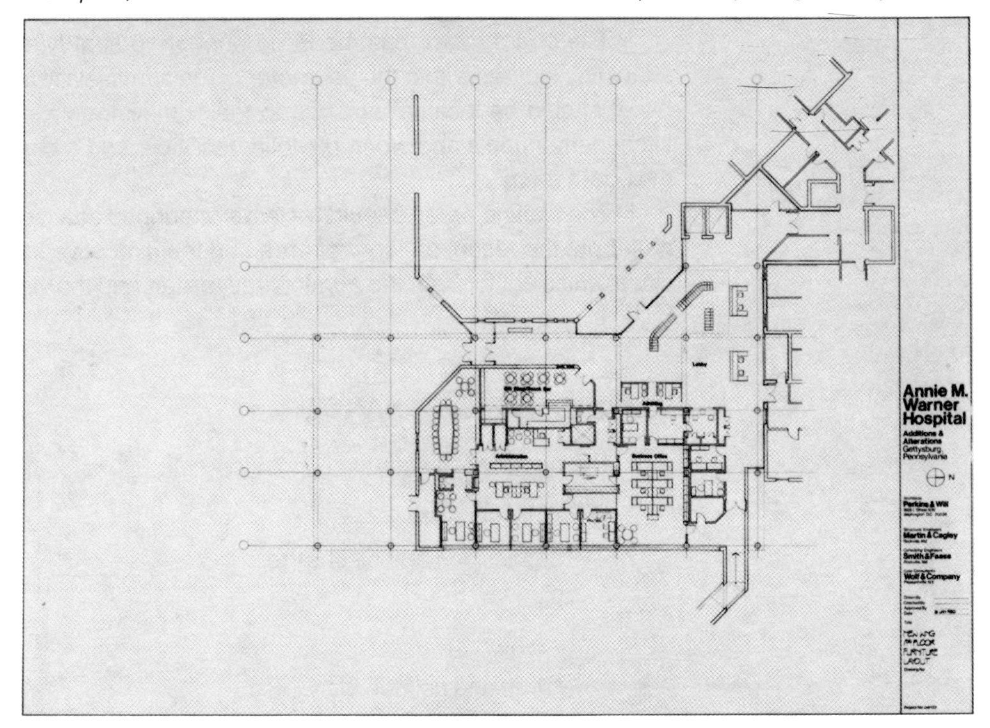

the daily operation of the facility, and the latter coordinates the complex activities of certificate-of-need requirements, long-range planning, and short-range renovations.

The office of the assistant director for financial management must also be included in the main administrative suite. In a large hospital, it is not possible for the administrator to devote the necessary time to detailed fiscal planning in addition to coordinating all other facets of hospital activities. Putting the financial manager (comptroller or director of finance) in the administrative suite is vital for providing the administrator with current financial data and fiscal advice.

The reception-control area is the main entrance into the administrative suite. It should accommodate four persons, including secretaries and clerk-typists for the administrative team. The reception–control area should therefore be adjacent to the three assistant director's offices. It should also be adjacent to the executive secretary's area, allowing the executive secretary to supervise this supporting secretarial staff.

The office of the director of community relations should be accessible, via the reception–control area. Placing community relations in the administrative suite allows easy access to hospital management, and vice versa.

A conference room, large enough to accommodate the department's senior staff, must be included in the administrative suite. There should be immediate access to the offices of the administrator and the executive secretary. A sofa or easy chairs should be placed near these doorways. If possible, the conference room should have an unmarked entrance from a public corridor.

The board room must be large enough to seat twenty to thirty persons and should be located within the perimeter of the administrative suite. If this is not possible, it should be located as close to the administrative suite as possible. A small kitchenette, men's and women's toilet facilities, and a coat room should be part of the board room.

The waiting areas should be large enough to seat several visitors; be located near both the reception–control area and the executive secretary's area; include a closet sufficient for both the administrative staff and the visitors.

DEPARTMENT OF FINANCE

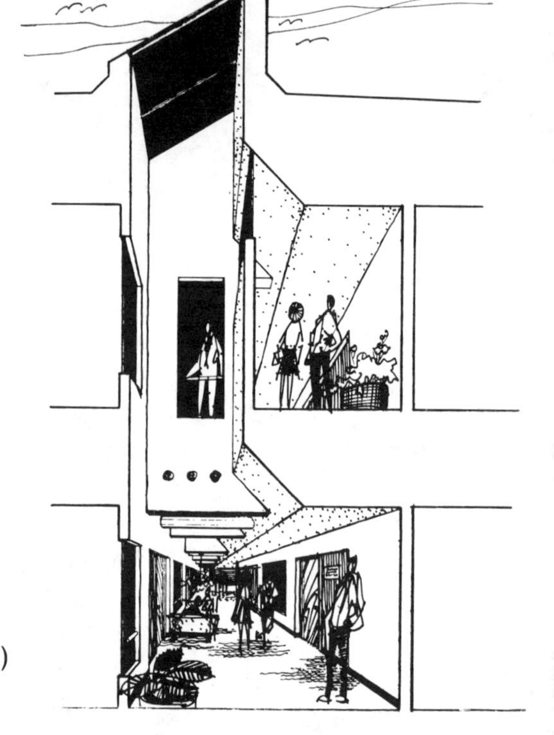

The department of finance includes:

1) Patient services
 —admissions and discharge
 —billing
 —cashiering
 —credit and collections
2) Accounting services
 —auditing and statistics
 —general ledger
 —accounting
 —special accounts
 —data processing control
 —budgeting
 —accounts payable (including payroll)
3) Finance services
 —planning
 —forecasting
 —advising
 —evaluating

Location. The department of finance suite should be centrally located and be close to patient and staff elevators. Ideally, it should be close to, but not located in, the hospital lobby. Because this department relates directly with all administrative departments, it should be located within the administrative services center and convenient to the administrative suite.

It is imperative that the department of finance and the data processing department develop and utilize optimum communication and control systems because of the nature and high volume of the work that flows between them. Good data transportation and communications systems (whether manual, electronic-telemetry, or pneumatic tube) should be developed between all clinical and administrative departments and patient care areas and the department of finance.

Design. The department of finance should be designed for maximum internal flexibility. Use of large, open landscaped areas should be encouraged, with minimal use of contained modules. This permits adaptations of the space as required by changes in accounting practices, third-party regulations, increased use of computers, or changes in personnel requirements.

Intradepartmental Relationships: Patient Services. All elements of patient services relate to one another. However, selected elements such as data processing and admissions may be decentralized to benefit patient flow without disrupting work efficiency.

The cashiering function is decreasing in importance within the department of finance. All handling of cash should be under the same supervision and control. Nonetheless, cashiers must be conveniently located for those who pay direct charges. The principle cashiering unit should be adjacent to the credit, collection, and billing areas. Subsidiary cashier units should be located in the ambulatory care areas (to serve emergency and ambulatory care patients), in admissions, and in the cafeteria service line.

Cashiering booths should be placed behind glass or plexiglass windows and each booth should be equipped with a cash drop-in safe. The main cashiering unit should include a safe for patient valuables and at least one booth designed to serve wheelchair patients. The safe itself should be a large walk-in safe containing a small safe for cash and papers and lockable cabinet for storing patient valuables. This area may also include a fireproof vault for storing duplicate disk drives for electronic data-processing. The principle cashiering unit should be provided with a supplies-records area for copies of inpatient accounts, prorated insurance data, and a copy of the most recent trial-balance of outstanding accounts. A waiting-room should be provided in the lobby for patients and their families waiting to pay bills in order to prevent an overflow into corridors or other hospital units.

Credit and collections should be adjacent to the principal cashiering unit and the billing area. It must also be easily accessible to patients via the main entrance and the vertical transport system. A reception control area should be located in front of the clerical staff at the entrance to this unit. It is important that well developed communications and control systems be established linking credit and collections with the accounting unit.

The credit manager's office should be accessible via reception-control, though it should be the office farthest away and immediately adjacent to the clinical staff area. The assistant credit manager's offices should be located near the clerical staff area and immediately adjacent to the credit manager's office. Interviewers' cubicles should be located near reception-control and immediately adjacent to the assistant credit manager's office. The cubicles should be soundproof, floor-to-ceiling modules.

The clerical staff area should be an attractively decorated open area adjacent to reception-control, the credit manager's and the assistant credit manager's offices, and the interviewers' cubicles. The billing area should be an open landscaped area, with desks grouped by billing element, such as Medicare, Blue Cross, and so on. The billing area should be contiguous with, or adjacent to, the clerical staff area of credit and collections and the audit and statistics area of accounting services. Files used by each of the billing elements should be contained within or immediately adjacent to the various work areas.

Intradepartmental Relationships: Accounting Services. Reception–control should be located at the main entranceway into this suite. The assistant comptroller's office should be located near the reception–control area and all accounting functions. The accounting manager's office should be centrally located in an open landscaped area with functional elements grouped together. Functional elements include:

1) Audit statistic area
   —accounting clerk
   —clerk typists
2) Data processing control area
   —data coordination space
   —audit clerks
3) Payables area
   —accounts payable personnel
   —payroll personnel
4) Budgeting area

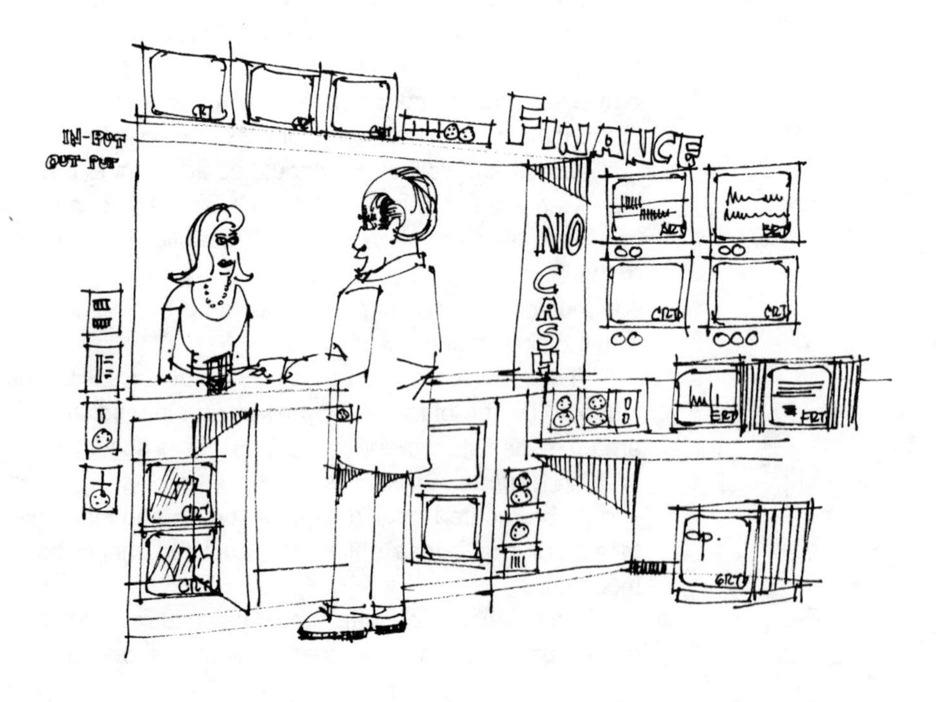

A conference room should be centrally located convenient to all functional areas of the department of finance and sufficiently large to be used for departmental meetings, for special work sessions, and by auditors from Medicare, state and county organizations, and other groups.

The archives storage area should be designed for storage of patient records (prior to microfilming), purchase invoices, and payroll records. This area may be located in a remote area of the department or may be removed entirely if space is not immediately available. A supply storage area should be included for storage of necessary office supplies and special forms required for various billing and office activities. The coat room should be centrally located and sufficient for all accounting services personnel.

DATA PROCESSING

The functions of the data processing department include:

—programming

—systems analysis

—keypunching

—accepting data (input)

—processing data

—printing reports (output)

—storing data

—collating printed reports

—preparing reports for distribution to user departments

Location. The data processing department should be centrally located within the administrative services center. This department should be close to the vertical transport system for expedient transportation and distribution of input and output materials between EDP and all user areas. It does not need to be in a prime area, but a design that includes a glass wall allowing visibility into the department from a well-traveled visitor hallway would promote public and employee interest. Properly planned and administered departments are designed to help management hold down hospital costs and provide new or better services at minimum costs. The use of computers in the hospital should be presented to the community as a modern, progressive management tool for comprehensive patient care.

Intradepartmental Relationships. The EDP director's office should be convenient to all processing areas and accessible via a public corridor, as well as via the reception–control area. The reception–control area is designed to include: a secretary-receptionist, a waiting area large enough to accommodate two to four persons, and a control and distribution center for incoming data and outgoing reports. No one should be able to enter or leave processing areas without passing through this control point.

A programmer-analyst may spend time outside his office interviewing, collecting data, and studying systems. Other departments may send personnel to the analyst's office for interviews and discussions on proposed or ongoing systems and programs. The programmer-analyst area should, therefore, be removed from main processing areas and have easy access via a public corridor. Accommodations should be made to include a computer reference library in this area.

The keypunch area needs to be close to reception–control, sorting, supplies storage, and the central processing areas. All work received by keypunch should come from reception–control. Because some of the punch cards generated in keypunch may need to be sorted before entering into the central processing unit, the card sorting area should be immediately adjacent to both the keypunch and the central processing areas. Storage area for punch card supplies should be convenient. In the sorting area cards are put into a defined sequence on a key or control field. It is not uncommon to sort records on magnetic tape using the computer; thus, the need for a card sort and sorting area will depend greatly on the nature of computer programs and on the tape and disk limitations.

The central processing unit is the main storage and control device for the electronic processing system. It holds program instructions for a job and data for processing during the job. This control unit is the decision maker and the calculator. The tape-disk drive area and the printer should be together with this unit in a large open area for operator efficiency.

The printer area contains the printer unit which provides output from the processor in the form of printed reports. Space must be allocated for two tape drives and two disk units. These units are the input processing and output storage components of the computer system. The collating area consists of work tables with collating and bursting equipment for integrating or decollating printed reports for distribution to users.

Cards, and paper for the printed reports, should be stored at the same temperature and humidity as that in which they will be used for at least forty-eight hours before use to assure processing efficiency. The storage area should contain fireproof facilities for storing magnetic tapes and disks.

PERSONNEL

The director of personnel must be aware of the philosophy and goals of the organization and have at hand overall cost figures, personnel needs for present and long-range positions, and information systems that will supply him with turnover statistics, trends in the labor market, skill inventories on employees, job classifications, and so on. Once the information on the individual organization and the individuals within the organization are available to the director of personnel, it becomes possible to manage the organizational and individual needs.

Considerable thought should be given to using a computer if a personnel department is to develop the information systems necessary to meet its philosophies and objectives. These systems must be carefully designed to yield maximum benefit and to supply data for analysis, interpretation, and decision-making. Careful consideration should be given to the available hardware and software packages so that appropriate combinations are selected to meet the individual hospital's needs.

Functions. The personnel department is responsible for:

—coordinating the needs of the hospital with the needs of its employees

—recruiting and screening job applicants

—orienting new employees

—developing training methods

—administering wages and salaries, including development of employee job sheets and work specification

—developing and implementing fringe benefits programs

—maintaining personnel files

—negotiating in union disputes

—establishing health and safety programs

—finding out causes of personnel problems and turnover

—managing development programs

—administering a supervisory training program

—overseeing employee health programs

The elements of the personnel department are:

—the director's office

—the assistant director's office

—the reception–control area

—the clerical staff area

—testing area and workshelves for applicants

—waiting area

Location. There is heavy traffic from job applicants and usually relatively light traffic from hospital personnel to this department. A street-level entrance to the personnel department should be planned. The department should be easily accessible to potential applicants, but the stream of these applicants should not interfere, or coincide, with the regular flow of hospital traffic. Because of the close working relationship between the director of personnel and the hospital administrator, the personnel department should be adjacent to the administrative suite.

Since the personnel department is usually the first impression of the hospital that the prospective employee receives, this department should be carefully planned. The lounge and its furniture, the offices and their decor, the equipment, and so on should reflect the overall image and philosophy the hospital wishes to impart.

ADMISSIONS AND DISCHARGE

Admissions and discharge calls for close cooperation between many departments of the hospital. The current trend is toward "pre-admission" procedures to improve the patient's transition from the community to the hospital. Patients are usually admitted to a hospital through the emergency service, from the community as ambulatory cases that are considered "elective," or from the outpatient department as "urgent" cases. While pre-admission is not possible with emergency cases, planning should always be towards integrating services to handle all admissions as quickly and efficiently as possible.

Admissions sets the stage for an uninterrupted program of care by providing the medical staff with essential information regarding the patient's background and preliminary diagnosis. Physical facilities and equipment are only a part of such a process. The hospital's policies relating to control of admissions, hours of discharge and reporting, and so on combine to make the operations function efficiently or inefficiently, and should be carefully designed.

Discharges, due to the increased role of third-party payers, have become a simpler procedure. Rarely does the patient have to stop at the business office to pay the bill as in the past. Whenever possible, procedures should be adopted to eliminate this time-consuming step and allow the patient to move from his room to his transportation home as smoothly as possible. It is recommended that this traffic bypass the front door of the lobby.

Location. Admissions in a large hospital is usually a strategically located, self-contained department or subdepartment. Ideally, it should be near an outside en-

Admissions-Discharge, Interdepartmental Relationships

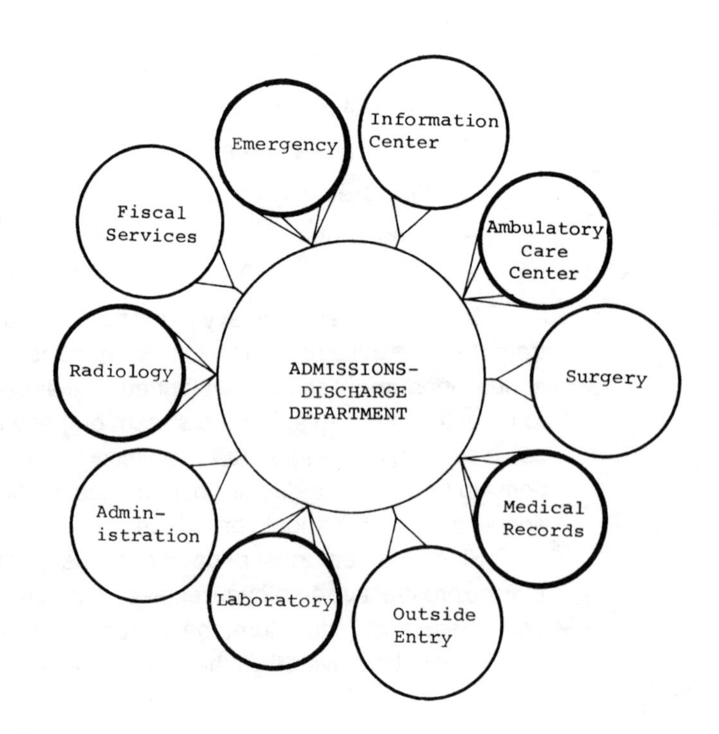

trance and adjacent to emergency service, outpatient service, medical records, laboratory, and radiology. It must have good access to, or communication with, the business office, operating room, administration, and information center.

Design. The proposed allocation of space involves four basic concepts that should be clarified:

—There are many disadvantages to admitting and discharging patients through the main lobby or in the midst of heavy traffic patterns. Ideally, these two functions should use a separate entrance with planned traffic patterns.

—The admission of a patient should be as free of emotional trauma as possible. A minimum of delay should occur between his arrival at the hospital and his being established in his room.

—Discharge, which should be a pleasant occasion, often becomes traumatic, due to delays, lack of information, confusion, poor planning, and so on. This results in a poor last impression of the hospital.

Admissions-Discharge, Intradepartmental Relationships

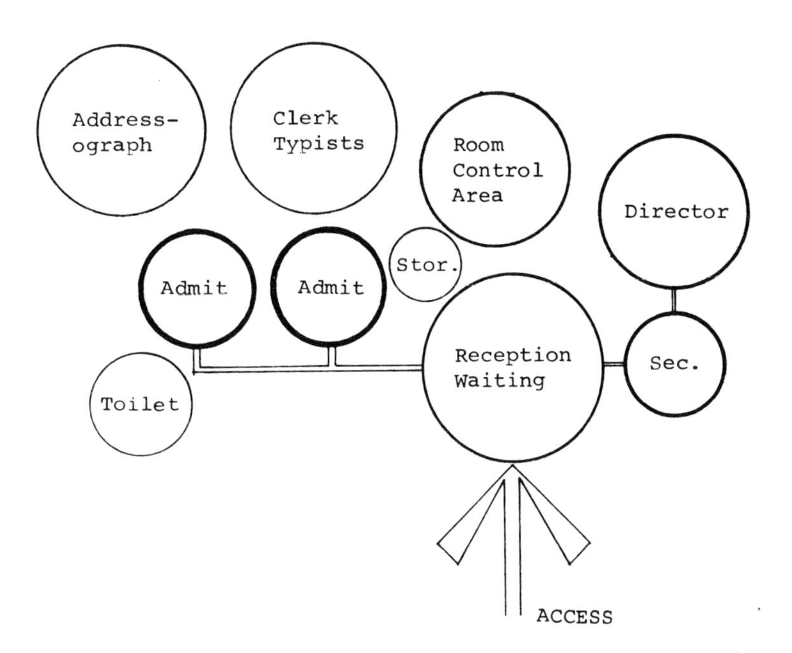

—Admission and discharge should take place in a pleasant, comfortable area that assures the patient of individual attention and privacy. Special consideration should be given to decor, material, and so on to create the image wanted by the hospital.

CENTRAL SWITCHBOARD AND PBX

The telephone company has specific space requirements not only for its equipment, but for ancillary services as well. In addition to telephone equipment, and closely related to the operation of the telephone service, are other communications systems such as the radio-paging system, and so on. There is often a tendency to overload and complicate the equipment and tasks of the switchboard because it is a focal point of hospital activities and it is continuously staffed. In planning this area, one should try to minimize the number of devices and tasks assigned to the telephone operators so as not to jeopardize their efficiency.

Location. The telephone facilities should be located within the hospital structure, but specific location is not functionally critical. They should not, however, be located in a main traffic area or where there will be excessive noise to disturb the operators. The telephone equipment room should be readily accessible to repairmen; they should not have to traverse the operator's work area or other areas of hospital activities. The areas should be well ventilated, and the equipment room should have a high level of illumination. Careful attention should be given the telephone operator's room to assure proper lighting levels, without glare, and to control the noise level, which would contribute to operator fatigue.

Intradepartmental Relationships. An office work area will be provided for the communication supervisor. One operator's post in the switchboard room should be designated the patient information center and receive all calls regarding patients' conditions. In addition, visitors coming to the main lobby will use house phones to request the room number of the patient they are going to visit. This procedure eliminates calls made from the switchboard to patient information, insures that confidential patient information will not be discussed in a public area, and frees personnel at a lobby information desk to concentrate on giving directions and generally assisting people who come to the hospital.

There should be a lounge (with toilet) available so telephone operators do not have to leave the unit. The lounge would also permit frequent rotation of duties to avoid operator fatigue and tension. The area should be provided with a refrigerator and a hotplate for fixing coffee and other light nourishment on breaks. There should be a combination sitting and sleeping arrangement to provide for emergency conditions when operators may not be able to leave their post.

MEDITATION AREAS AND CHAPLAINCY

A chapel, or nondenominational meditation room, should be accessible to the public, to the staff, and to inpatients. A small supporting space for religious equipment should be near, and, depending on the site of the facility, a chaplain's office should be supplied.

MEDICAL LIBRARY

A medical library should be located near the physician's entry, with space for library tables and book storage.

IX

department planning: support services

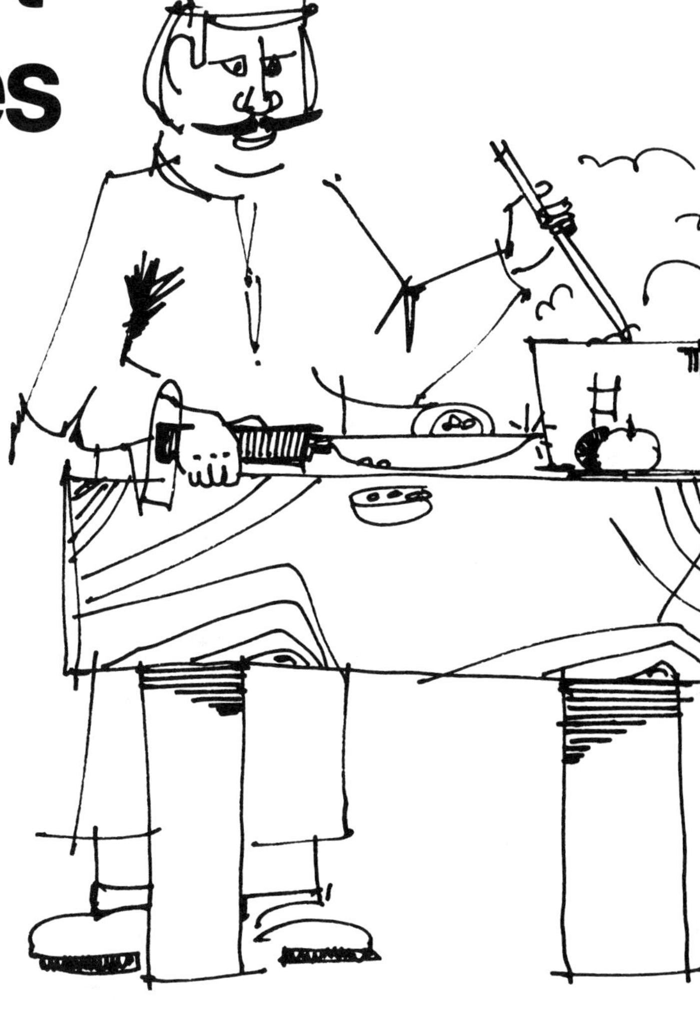

Those without experience in the operation of health care facilities may only think of hospitals as doctors (medical services), nurses (nursing services), and bill collectors (administrative services). Those who are familiar with the day-to-day operations of a health care facility realize, however, that without the less glamorous and less conspicuous operations known as support services (housekeeping, central stores, laundry–linen, etc.) the health care facility as a whole simply could not operate. The space dedicated to support services and the programming of that space is, therefore, a major consideration in the programming, design, and construction of any health care facility.

HOSPITAL AUXILIARY

In one form or another, the auxiliary or hospital guild is nearly as old as the hospital, and contemporary hospitals of all sizes and scopes are enthusiastically encouraging the development of auxiliaries with increased activities and services. It is highly desirable that the membership of the hospital auxiliary represent a cross-section of the community. Men, women, and teenagers should be encouraged to participate in programs.

The hospital auxiliary performs duties and provides amenities that contribute to the comfort and pleasant environment of the patient. It also operates and staffs the following:

—gift shop

—coffee shop

Department	Gross Square Feet per Bed
Hospital auxiliary	4.0
Dietary	30.0
Housekeeping	5.0
Materials management	5.0
Purchasing	2.0
Central stores	35.0
Central supply, including Central sterilization decontamination	12.0
Laundry—linen	12.0
Medical records	9.0
Public areas	15.0
Circulation	135.0–150.0
Engineering and maintenance	60.0
Pharmacy	7.0
Employee facilities (may be placed with departments)	9.0
Public relations	1.5
Security	2.0
Education-in-service	6.0
Archives	10.0

—book truck

—information desk

—mailing services

—special projects

—flower delivery

—waiting room attendants

—recreational therapy program

—patient service programs (in pediatrics and physical therapy)

—candy striper programs

The auxilary is organized by the authority of the governing board of the hospital and its bylaws must be approved by the board and the hospital administrator before becoming effective. The director of the auxiliary usually reports to the governing board through the hospital administrator. The auxiliary should work closely with administration to fully understand the objectives of the hospital and how they may best serve the institution.

Location. The auxiliary may work with every department as requested by the hospital administration and respective department heads. Centralization is, therefore, recommended. The auxiliary's areas should also be readily accessible to the general public, located if possible in or near the main patient and visitor entrances.

Hospital Guild, Interdepartmental Relationships

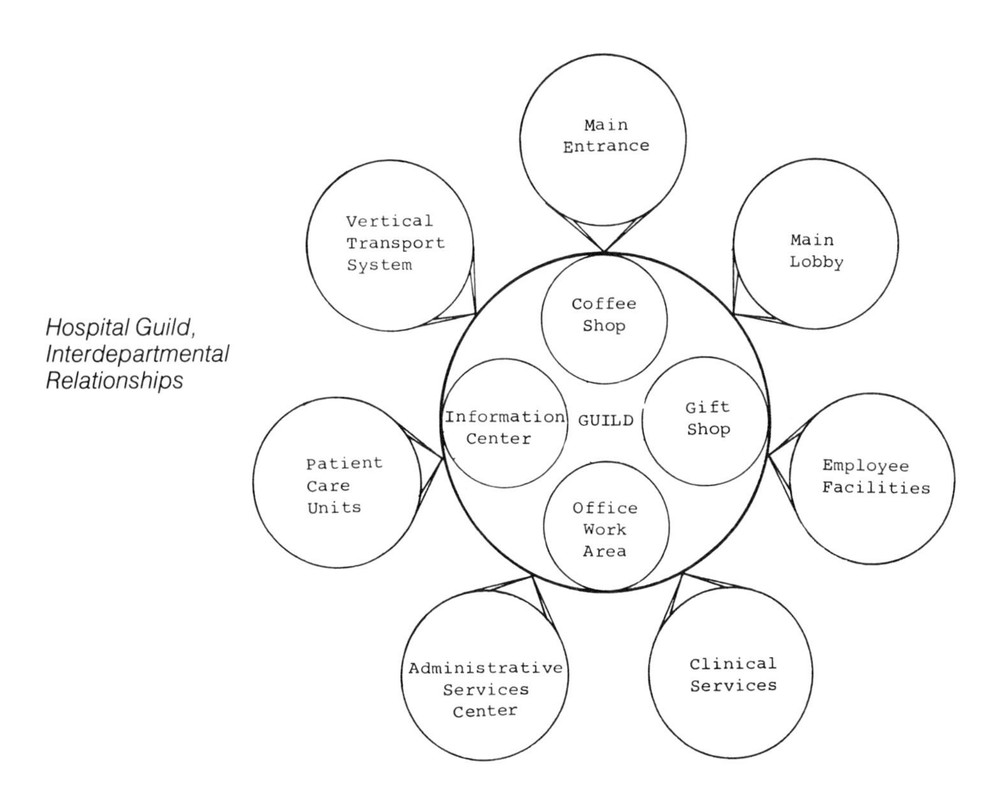

Easy access to administrative services (especially the community relations director) is desirable because of the auxiliary's numerous contacts with social and civic groups.

Design. The overall impression of the hospital is set for the visitor immediately upon entering the facility. The hospital auxiliary area includes the office area, coffee shop, gift shop, and necessary storage areas. The decor of the coffee shop and gift shop should be consistent with the image the hospital desires to impart to the public. Service in the coffee shop and gift shop often sets the pace for the family member who will later visit the patient. The irritated customer in the coffee or gift shop will complain at the patient's bedside and will look for errors in hospital service provided to the patient.

The coffee shop should serve more than sandwiches to visitors: it should serve hot meals. It should be designed for rapid turnover of guests so it will not become a lounge area for hospital personnel. The design should be the counter type found advantageous in restaurants operated by large chains. The type of seating used at the counters of these nationally franchised restaurants is also recommended. The low, wide, nonswivel seats will accommodate not only healthy visitors, but also the ill and handicapped. These nonswivel seats also protect against falls and injuries.

Intradepartmental Relationships. A reception–control area with desk, sofa, and chairs should be located at the entrance to the hospital auxiliary area. Various activities evolving from this area can be directed from this point. Potential volunteers can complete applications or await their interviews here. A registration area for logging hours of volunteers is included in this location. The director's office should be large enough to accommodate the director and one or two interviewers at any one time.

The conference-work area, which may be a continuation of the reception–control area, should be large enough to accommodate a large table with ten to twelve chairs. The walls of this area should have shelves for books and magazines for the patient book truck or library.

The gift shop should be contiguous with the coffee shop to maximize sales in both areas. It should be located on the main visitor traffic route into the hospital, adjacent to the lobby and public areas. It also should be convenient for the hospital staff.

The gift shop storage area should be planned for additional sales items and storage of gift carts for selling items on the patient units. This area should be immediately adjacent to the gift shop.

DIETARY

Food service is one of the most important services in any health care facility. Good dietary service must be based upon optimum nutritional requirements and contribute to the care and recovery of patients and the well-being of hospital staff. The delivery of food to patients and personnel should likewise be aesthetically pleasing in order to enhance acceptance and to favorably influence morale.

The various elements of dietary service include:

—dry storage and refrigeration areas

—food preparation areas (including salad area, baking shop, special diets area, and production area)

—tray assembly and cart storage areas

—dishwashing area

—cafeteria (scramble bank and seating)

—private dining rooms

—administration areas (administrators and dietician's offices, clerical areas, and employee facilities)

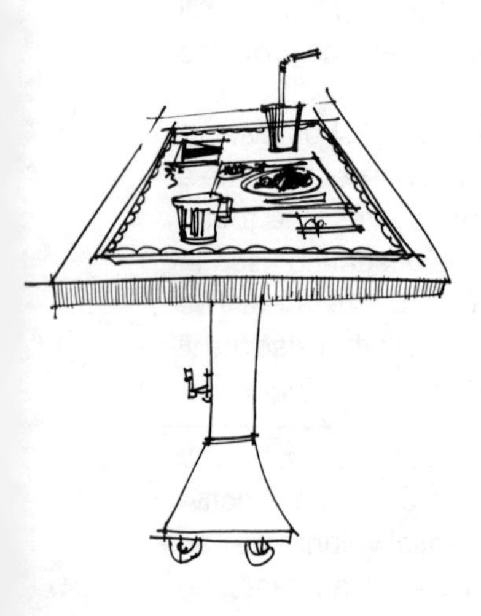

Functions. The following are traditional functions of a food service:

—planning, organizing, and scheduling meals

—controlling quality and service

—buying to specification

—receiving stores and checking their quality and quantity

—storing food

—producing food

—portioning, assembling, and distributing food

—evaluating services, menus, and waste

—record-keeping

—educating patients, employees, and professional staff

Several systems are available for food production and distribution. Dietary services in a hospital may be provided via conventional or convenience systems, or a combination of both. Food services may be centralized, decentralized, or a combination of both. Advantages and disadvantages will attend any system. In general, the facility must be designed for a particular method in order for it to be most efficient and successful.

Conventional food service is a restaurant-like food processing system in which large quantities of food are prepared according to menu-planning recipies utilizing mainly bulk raw foods and canned or frozen food stuffs. Conventional kitchens often have a butcher shop, bake shop, and a specialty diet area. A single chef is responsible for all food preparations.

Convenience food service utilizes a wide variety of partially or fully processed (precooked, preportioned, frozen) entrees and platters in meal preparation. Total reliance on fully processed meals eliminates the need for ranges, ovens, steam kettles, and boilers in the hospital kitchen. Instead, microwave or reconstitution-convection ovens are used to heat foods for immediate use.

Conventional or convenience food services can be either centralized or decentralized. In a centralized service, food processing and tray preparation (and in the case of a conventional centralized service) heating, and placement into hot-cold carts for immediate distribution, all occur at a single location. Decentralized food service is more complex.

Table 9.1. General Comparisons Between Conventional and Convenience Systems

Conventional	*Convenience*
Requires a major capital investment	Requires more refrigerators and freezers
Requires more space and personnel to serve equivalent numbers (see Table 9.2 for HHS guidelines)	Greater potential for quality and for portion control, thus spoilage tends to be less
	Per meal costs tend to be higher
At present, can provide greater menu variation	

Table 9.2. Guidelines Set Up by the Department of Health and Human Services for Dietary Department Size

	Number of Meals per Gross Square Foot	
Meals per Day	*Conventional*	*Convenience*
0–250	.06–.11	.06–.17
251–550	.08–.18	.15–.26
551–950	.11–.24	.20–.35
951–1,800	.13–.28	.23–.42

In a conventional decentralized food service, bulk, hot and cold, processed food could be delivered to local subkitchens for tray preparation and delivery. Or, only food storage could be centralized with all preparation and distribution occurring at local kitchens. Or, finally, all dietary procedures, from purchasing to distribution, could occur at local kitchens. A convenience decentralized food service could use central storage and local heating or total decentralization. See Table 9.1 for a comparison between conventional and convenience systems.

Comparisons of the various systems are inconclusive and a final choice depends very much on the attitudes of the people involved. In other words, the best system is the one whose problems and disadvantages are most easily handled by a particular institution at a particular place and time.

Dietary Department, Interdepartmental Relationships

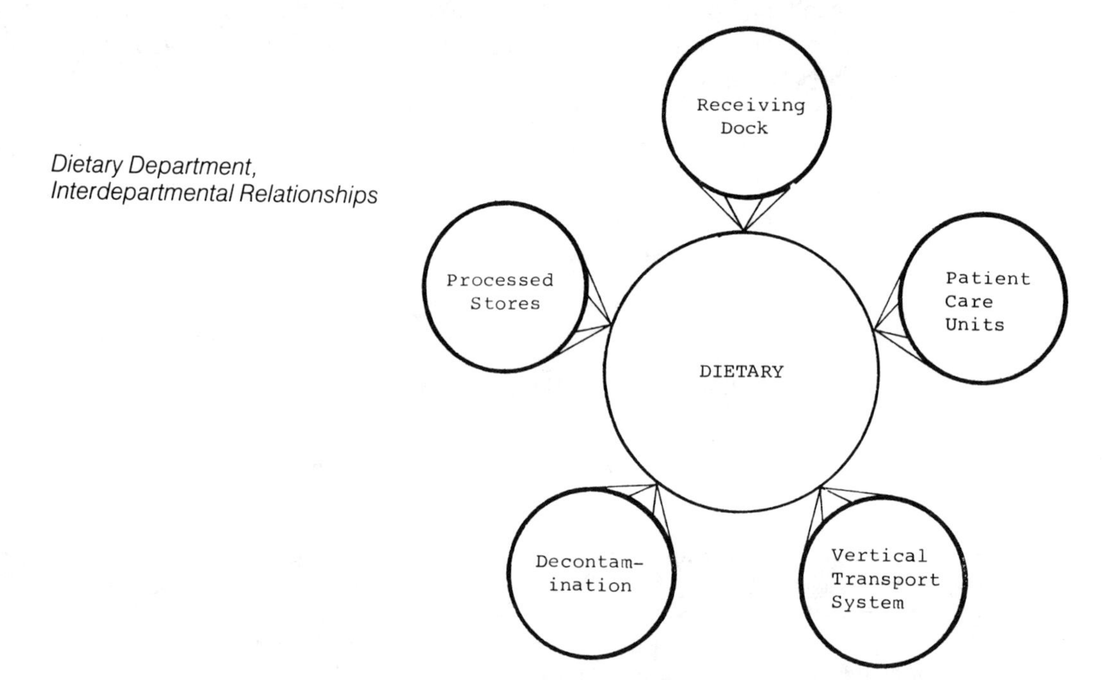

Location. The dietary department should be located within or adjacent to material-handling systems. The storage areas should be close to the receiving dock. The dietary department must also have easy access to the vertical transport system serving the patient care units to facilitate delivery of dietary supplies and patient meals and the return of used utensils. The dining room and cafeteria areas of the dietary department should be convenient to elevators for hospital staff.

Design. Before design is considered, the following planning assumptions must be made:

—The number of patient meals should be based on an 85 percent occupancy, with a ratio of full-time-equivalent personnel of 2.5 per bed. Approximately

10 percent of hospital personnel will be served breakfast, 50 percent lunch, and 40 percent dinner. Visitor meals are estimated at 20 percent of patient load for lunches.

—Cafeteria service will be available for ambulatory patients, personnel, and visitors; the vending area and coffee shop may also serve this need.

—A selective cycle menu will be used for all patients, personnel, and visitors, with a choice of entree, vegetable, salad, and dessert for lunch and dinner.

—Infant formulas can be prepared in the nursery.

—A centralized dishwashing system that meets local health standards must be used.

—Seven days' worth of refrigerated foods will be stored, and thirty days' worth of dry foods will be stored.

Work areas should be carefully planned for each unit of dietary service. Food service areas and equipment should be designed and arranged so that personnel can perform tasks efficiently and economically. Work flow should proceed in a single direction (in either a straight or circular path) to avoid crisscrossing and backtracking. Such a design will insure that food service is performed in the shortest time possible from receiving and storage, through preparation and distribution, to cleanup and waste disposal.

Dietary Department, Intradepartmental Relationships

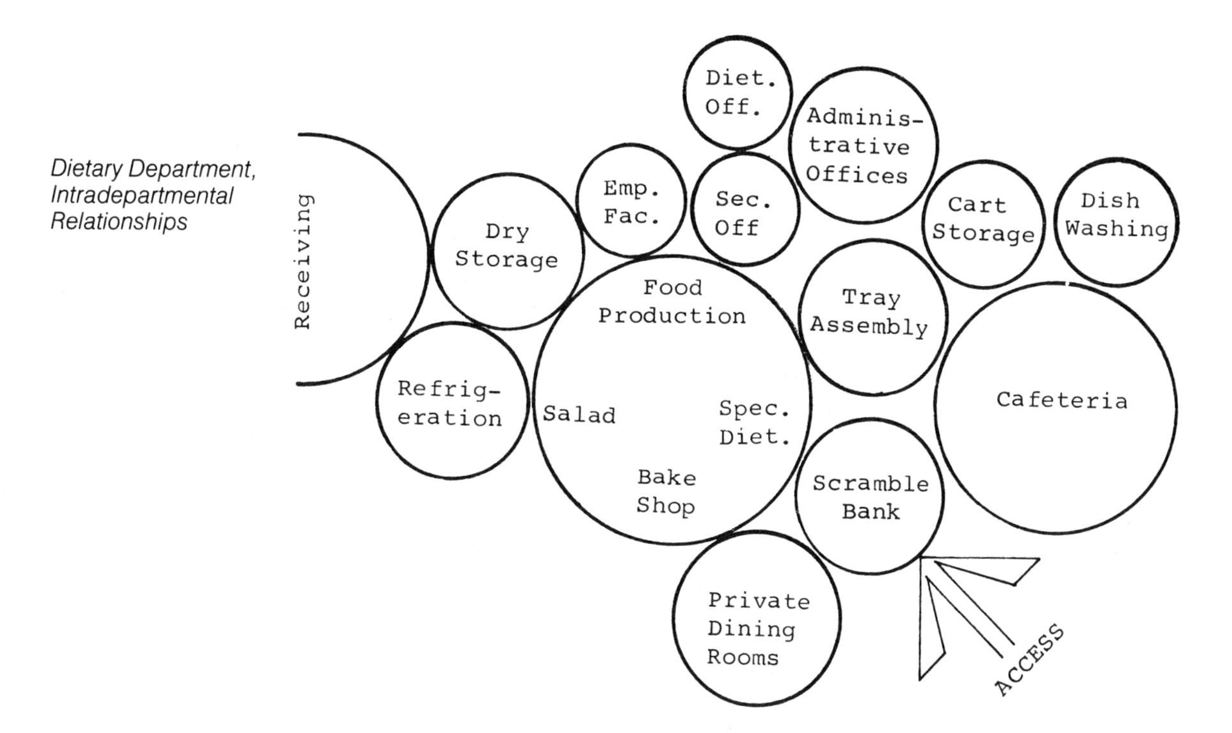

A centralized tray service should be located near the preparation and cooking area and mobile food storage units should be arranged at right angles to the serving line. The maximum elapsed time between food service and the patient should be aboaut six minutes; therefore, the tray distribution system should be convenient to vertical transportation and the cart storage area should be adjacent to the distribution area. Facilities for washing dishes should be separated from other food service functions, but should be convenient to the cafeteria and to both the horizontal and the vertical transports used for patient trays.

The cafeteria should be designed for self-service operation and the food preparation area should be close to the serving area. Storage space for empty trays must be provided in the dining area, as well as space for the coats and paraphernalia of personnel, visitors, and ambulatory patients.

Office space for administrative personnel should permit observation of the food service operation and should be accessible without travelling through food production areas. Throughout the food service area interior walls should be smooth, nonabsorbent, light colored, and washable. Ceilings should be of accoustical tile and floors of hard, smooth, nonabsorbent and easily cleaned material. Special attention should be given to lighting, ventilation, temperature, and humidity.

HOUSEKEEPING

Good housekeeping is paramount in providing the optimum environment for patient care. Maintaining a clean and sanitary hospital is important not only because of its psychological and physiological impact on patients, visitors, and staff, but also because it is economical. A properly maintained building has a potentially longer and less expensive service life than a poorly maintained one. Also, though the housekeeping department constitutes a minimum percentage of the hospital operating budget, the effectiveness of this department contributes largely to the overall efficiency of all other hospital departments. Employee morale and productivity, for instance, are enhanced by a clean, attractive, and orderly work environment. Because it is often difficult for lay people to judge the practice of medicine, the reputation of the hospital may well be based on its appearance. Good housekeeping is, then, an asset in community relations.

Newer trends in housekeeping management and services include the use of housekeeping management consultants, contract housekeeping management services, contract total housekeeping services, and contract window washing. Each hospital must weigh these trends against an in-house service.

Changes in building material and design also affect housekeeping functions, operation, and design. The following are examples:

—central vacuum systems

—vinyl tile flooring

—poured vinyl floors

—seamless plastic paneling in bathrooms, showers, janitorial closets, and so on

—fiberglass, modular bathroom facilities

—vinyl wall coverings

—carpeting of floors and walls

—double glazed window units with internal blinds

Functions. The housekeeping department is responsible for daily and periodic cleaning of patient care, clinical, and office areas of the hospital. This must be done to control infection, to help preserve the physical facilities, and to make the hospital more aesthetically pleasing. Housekeeping also maintains a safe, orderly, and functional arrangement of the furnishings of the hospital. Preventing the spread of infection is as much a responsibility of the housekeeping department as it is of direct patient care departments. Thus, housekeeping is part of a larger unit that can be referred to as environmental sanitation. For this reason housekeeping has a representative on the hospital infections control committee. Since the spread of infectious diseases and the prevention of infection are so important, many hospitals are restructuring the housekeeping department as a department of environmental sanitation for greater emphasis on this major responsibility.

Housekeeping, Interdepartmental Relationships

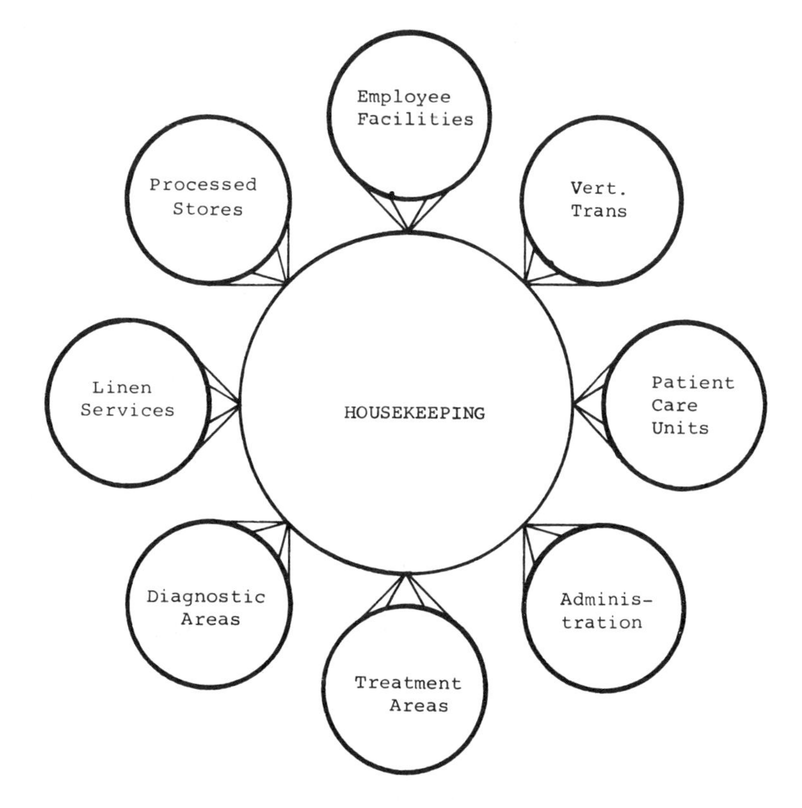

Location. Housekeeping serves all institutional departments and units, and therefore should be as centrally located as possible, but it can be in a non-prime area. It should be near the vertical transport system, processing stores, decontamination, and linen services. Centralized employee facilities should be convenient to this department.

Design. The housekeeping department is designed to function as a decentralized department, with supervisors physically located in the areas where their personnel are assigned. Housekeeping closets with floor sinks and shelves for supplies should be provided throughout the hospital. Housekeeping carts should be stored in the closets when not in use. Supplies for use by janitors and maids should be delivered directly to housekeeping closets on a routine basis. Equipment and carts should be chosen with the knowledge that they will periodically pass through the decontamination department for cleaning and sterilizing to control infection.

Intradepartmental relationships. The director's office should have an entrance through reception–control and a doorway into a conference area. Reception–control is located at the entrance to the housekeeping department. The conference room should be adjacent to the reception–control area and the director's office for use by the director and supervisors. A storage area for patient and office furniture and housekeeping supplies should be adjacent to reception–control. The paint shop is responsible for finishing and baking beds, cabinets, and so forth. It should be adjacent to the storage area and near an exterior wall so it can be easily vented. Housekeeping closets should be located throughout the hospital and should contain shelves for supplies, space for a maid's coat, and space for other portable equipment.

MATERIALS MANAGEMENT

The most often overlooked systems affecting production of quality patient care and efficient service department operation have been those of materials handling and distribution. Due in part to their lack of "drama," when compared to "direct" patient care or treatment and diagnostic procedures, these necessary adjuncts to patient care have, unfortunately, been relegated to the bottom of most priority lists.

The fact remains that increasing demands for new techniques and services, increasing size of hospitals, changing mix of hospitalized patients (to a higher proportion of acutely ill), and shorter hospital stays have resulted in more requirements for materials and their disposal, more traffic in the transport facilities and hallways, more noise, more confusion, and more danger of cross-infections. In short, the existing material-handling and distribution systems have reached a point of chaos, a nightmare for cost-conscious, efficiency-minded administrators.

Design. This is the ideal time to take corrective steps. New designs and plans should consider and accept the following principles: There is a total cost to any item supplied to a patient or service, what it costs to purchase, to receive, to process, to store, to handle, and to get rid of waste. Common handling denominators in hospital operation (linens, food, records, supplies, and wastes) have in common such things as weight, cube, quantity, and flow rate. There is a need for a central authority to control, correlate, evaluate, modify, and plan logistics for all components; thus, a director of materials management is recommended. This person is responsible for all hospital material, including purchase, receiving, storage, processing, and distribution to the ultimate user, as well as for a waste retrieval program. This director should be a member of the administrative staff and involved in overall planning, decision-making, and policy formation.

The components of the envisioned system are basically purchasing, receiving, bulk storage, processed storage, central sterilization, decontamination, and dispatch. Other processing areas of this system include dietary, laundry, printing, mail room, and pharmacy. These may or may not be under the manager's administrative control, but the manager should control the distribution of the processed items from these departments. They should be as close together as possible and designed to flow into the main distribution channel.

Components of the distribution system play an important role in the overall effectiveness of the system. Early administrative decisions on type of distribution equipment, or combinations, are always vital to planning a department's function and operation, but they are paramount in a materials-handling system. Selection should be based on cost, but consideration should also be given to reduced employee travel time, reduced steps in material flow, and number of employees necessary for each component.

Elevators are used to move bulk items, patients, visitors, and hospital personnel. Certain elevators should be designated for distribution of materials and retrieval of wastes, others for visitors, and still others for patients and hospital personnel. The visitor's elevators should be large enough to accommodate patients. These divisions would eliminate the current undesirable mixes of functions and expedite movement of patients, personnel, and material.

A manual cart system of delivery and collection reduces handling of items. It offers a better cost control system for supplies, reduces storage space in the user area, and minimizes overall inventory. In selecting carts, one should consider standardization by dimension, weight, and design for maximum flexibility of use. In addition, the cart design chosen should be adaptable to automated cart transport systems.

A variety of automated transport systems is being installed in hospitals. Each has advantages and disadvantages to be considered, but they are generally a step in the direction of improved material-handling and distribution. They form the nucleus for incorporating known departmental systems into one complete system that reduces the number of employees and employee travel time and offers flexibility in operational programs. If present funds will not allow the inclusion of an automated transport system, space should be allowed for future installation of such a system.

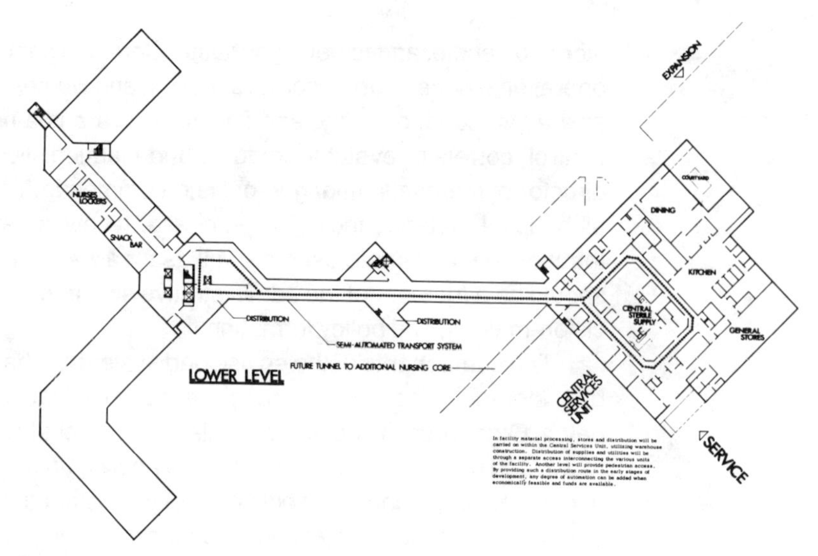

Automated material-handling system

The pneumatic tube system is ideal for handling small objects, such as "stat" (immediate) pharmaceuticals, laboratory specimens, requisitions and other paper reports that can be rolled and placed into a tube. New models are large enough to hold flat patient records, even X-rays. Models are also available for bagged laundry and trash. Improved pneumatic systems can also deliver fluids such as intravenous solutions and liquid pharmaceuticals. Advantages of the pneumatic tube system are the speed of request, transmitting, and delivery and the low employee travel time. This system is only recommended for convenience, as it may not prove to be cost effective.

Other worthwhile systems are overhead laundry systems, dietary conveyor belts, conveyor belts to trash compactors, and so on. Proper placement of equipment, such as dishwashing systems, sterilizers, and cartwashers, also serves to eliminate transport time and handling. Some equipment can be located centrally between two areas of use to reduce employee transit time.

The computer is often overlooked as an element of the materials distribution or handling system. Computer tie-in and printout facilities can make an important contribution to the overall system in such areas as inventory control, reorder and invoice production, cost records, and distribution logistics. The communication system should correlate with, enhance, and expedite the distribution system, as well as improve hospital communications.

PURCHASING

Efficient purchasing control can obviate one of the most common financial drains on hospitals—loss of material—and can contribute significantly to patient care and employee utilization by assuring economical but quality supplies, equipment, and services. In order to maintain the necessary inventory levels and keep abreast of changes in materials available, it is imperative that one department be totally responsible for these functions. In the past, service departments, such as dietary, or central sterile supply, maintained their own inventory and control. Their orders were given out independently, and purchasing, as a hospital function, was concerned more with general patient items and acknowledgment of these service orders. Now, with the centralization of supply functions and the increased scope of materials available, it is essential that purchasing be given total control over what is needed (based on requests), how much to purchase (based on use-experience), how often to restock (based on storage availability).

The purchasing department is responsible for:

—developing specifications

—initiating orders based on requisitions from other departments

—advising the administration on equipment available, when to replace existing equipment, and solutions of supply-related problems

—maintaining proper records

—maintaining inventory control through automated storage management

—researching sources of improved equipment, materials, or systems

A central purchasing department would, then, provide centralized procurement for all supplies, equipment, and material used within the hospital and, with the help of the various hospital departments, determine present and forecast future hospital needs. Many purchasing departments are using computers as a tool for inventory control and the maintenance of a smooth restocking system. Through the effective use of computers, total inventory control can be implemented, including:

—cueing reorder cycles and volumes

—determining and evaluating long-term inventory needs

—implementing cost control through expense-budget comparisons over designated periods of time

—maintaining, and supplementing as necessary, accurate records for every user-department

—evaluating items through rapid comparisons of manufacturer claims versus actual results

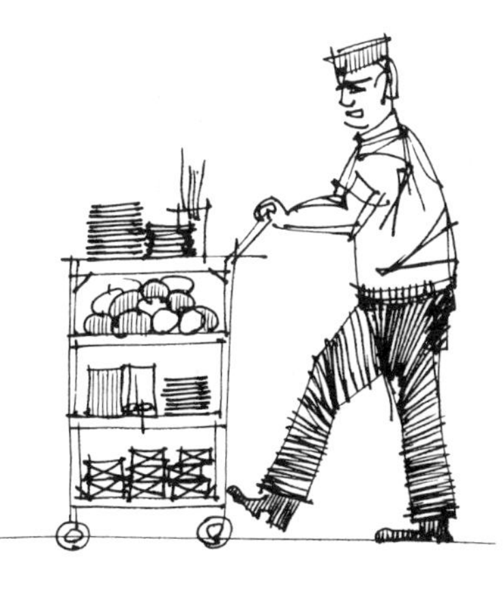

Location. The purchasing department should be located either adjacent to the receiving dock, bulk stores, and processed stores or in the administrative services center. Access should be readily available from outside parking, allowing salesmen to go directly to purchasing without interfering with established hospital traffic. One or two parking slots near the receiving dock or main entrance for this use would be ideal.

Purchasing, Interdepartmental Relationships

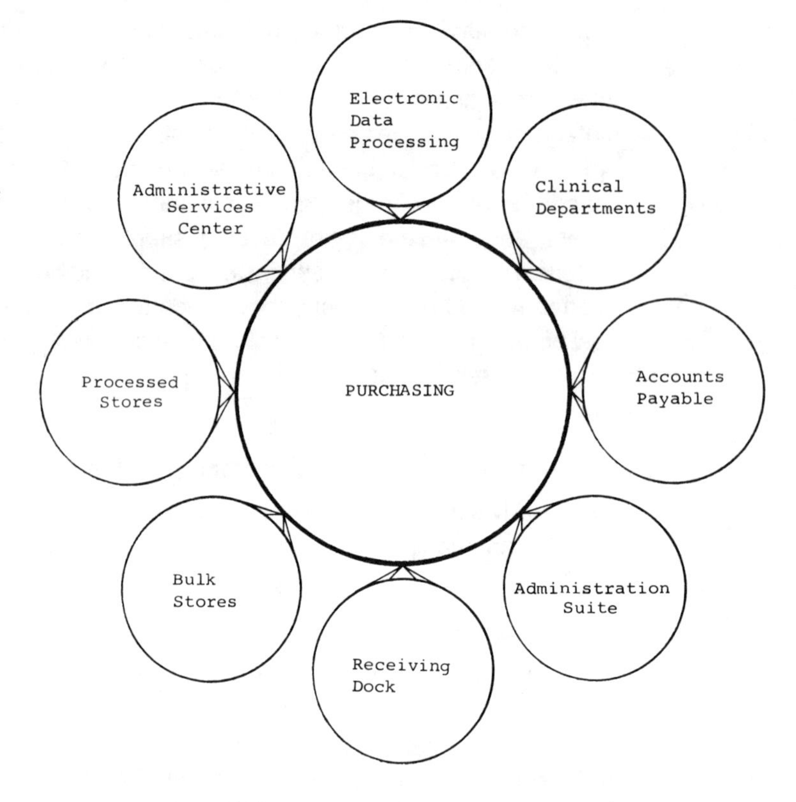

Intradepartmental Relationships. Good communication and distribution systems must be developed between hospital administration, the accounts payable function of the comptroller's department, electronic data processing, and the purchasing department. All hospital departments, whether clinical or administrative, must have access to purchasing through a requisition system for items not usually stocked. All purchases must be made through the purchasing department.

CENTRAL STORES

In order to control the receiving and distribution of all supplies, the departments responsible for these duties have been gathered under the general title "stores." Basically these departments can be considered the warehouse areas of the overall supply system. There has been an increase in the use of two new concepts in material-handling: prepackaging and automation. Prepackaged and disposable goods (such as larger bulk modules of in-use items) are packed by similarity of service or use, requiring more floor space and general circulation area. Automated transport systems require more space for the movement of automated carts. The role of the computer in maintaining a controlled inventory should not be overlooked.

Functions. Central stores is responsible for receiving, breaking out, storing, and distributing supplies used in the hospital. At the receiving dock supplies are received and checked or weighed in. Bulk supplies are stored as delivered or are broken out into use modules to be stored or sent directly to user departments. Centralizing all storage and processing of hospital supplies increases the functional use of space, but decreases the total square footage required.

The amount of paper work necessary in larger hospitals makes it feasible to print forms in-house, rather than contract work to outside printers. The print shop should be located near the receiving dock and processed stores area so that the same transport system can be utilized for distribution. The mail room, a storage area for in-house printing, and a documents archive may be included in this area as basic institutional supply functions.

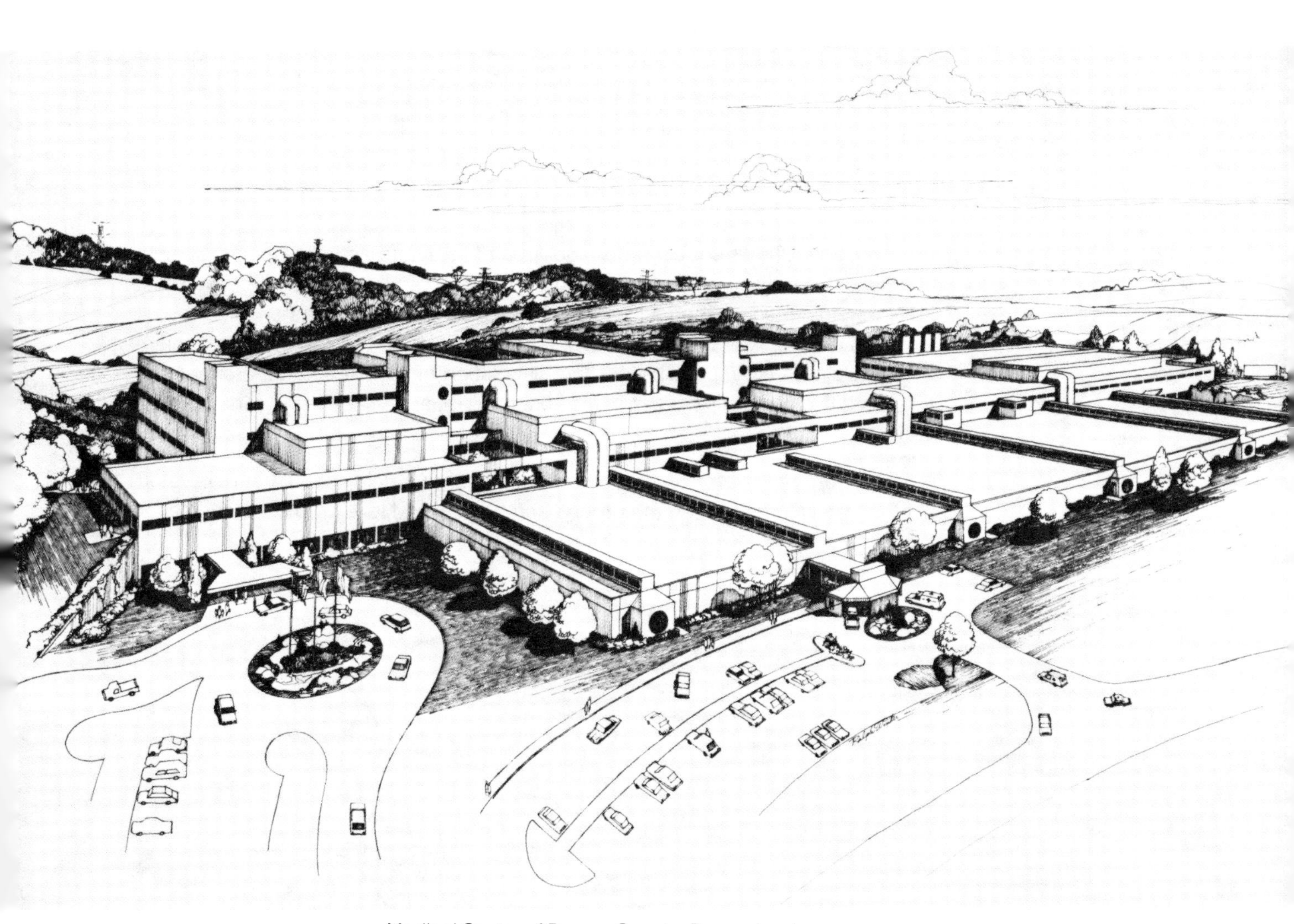

Medical Center of Beaver County, Pennsylvania

Stores, *Interdepartmental Relationships*

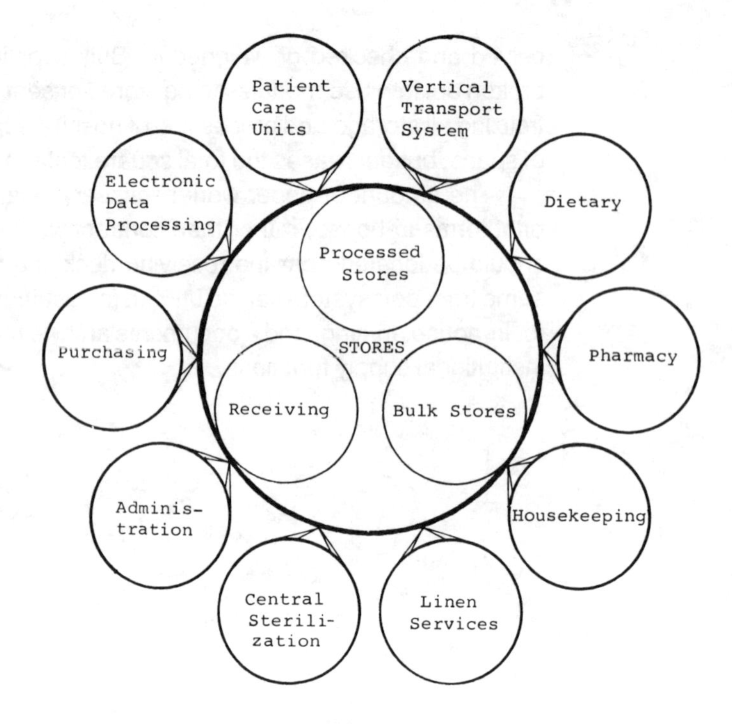

Location. Stores should be on the ground level and as far away as possible from all other traffic areas. A truck service court big enough to handle the largest truck that might serve the facility must be provided, and the area should be built along an exterior wall to provide for a receiving dock and to allow for expansion. Because stores is responsible for the distribution of supplies and material to all administrative and clinical areas of the hospital, it must be close to the vertical transport system.

Intradepartmental Relationships. The receiving dock should be elevated approximately three feet off the ground and have a load leveler to compensate for

Stores, *Intradepartmental Relationships*

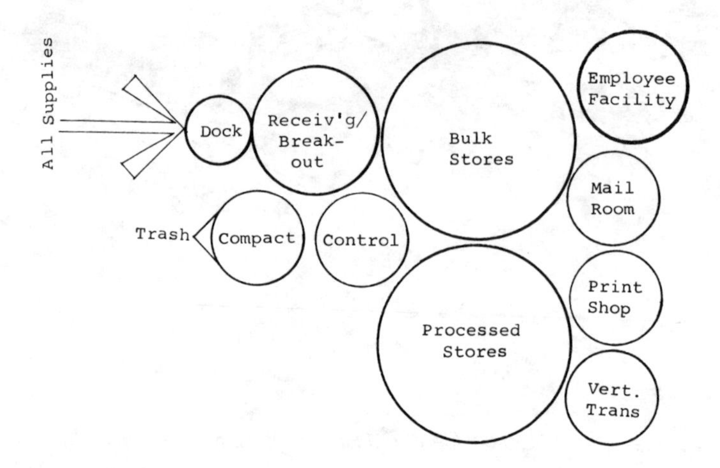

variations in truck heights. It should be wide enough to accommodate semi-trailer trucks and it must be covered. The receiving office, enclosed in glass, should be adjacent to the receiving dock in order to manage the delivery area. The receiving breakdown area should be adjacent to the receiving dock, receiving office, and bulk stores for breaking down material delivered and for verifying purchase orders and delivery invoices prior to further processing. A floor scale should be included here.

Bulk stores includes the pallet warehousing of bulk supplies and the storage of oxygen and anesthesia and chemicals. State and local building codes and national fire safety codes must be followed. Processed stores contains items stored in use modules, ready for issue. It should be warehouse type space with flexible shelving throughout. Items should be stored by use or service, or both. The sterile storage space for medical-surgical packs, trays, and supplies should be separated, if possible, from the general flow of activities in the area.

The control area (dispatch center) is a clerical area for the control of requisitions and the distribution of supplies. Special accommodations must be made to inventory medical equipment in use. The supervisor's office should be a glass-enclosed space, sufficiently large to accommodate the supervisor and, on occasion, several of his staff for conferences.

The mail room should be large enough to provide slots for sorting departmental mail. The slots themselves should have access from both the mail room and outside corridor, with locks on the corridor side. A scale and work table are necessary for outgoing mail, and a pneumatic tube station should be provided. The print shop should be large enough to accommodate the equipment and supplies necessary to fulfill the objectives of the stores department. Equipment may include electrostatic duplicators, copiers (Ditto machines), mimeograph machines, and offset lithography. Employee facilities should include male and female toilets in the stores area and, if employee locker and lounge facilities are not centralized, space must be allocated within stores for such purposes.

CENTRAL SUPPLY

The elements of central supply include:

—sterilization
—storage and equipment
—offices
—materials handling
—clean processing
—storage of sterile supplies
—linen processing
—cartwash
—employees' lockers
—toilets

—vertical transportation
—trash room or system
—janitor's closet
—wire closet
—instrument processing
—instrument storage

The major responsibilities of central supply include:

—storing and distributing all disposable sterile supplies
—storing and distributing all patient charge items
—cleaning and storing portable medical equipment
—reprocessing, storing and distributing patient bedside items
—reprocessing all instruments and equipment for surgery and delivery

Location. Central supply may be located in one of a number of locations. It could be adjacent to the surgical suite (or combined surgery-delivery suite) and primarily function as the distribution and processing center for sterile supplies while also processing the instruments and packs for surgery. It could, however, be integrated with a centralized materials-management system and operated in conjunction with purchasing to distribute all supplies used in the hospital. In this arrangement, central supply might not be adjacent to surgery, but would have a direct clean-and-soiled transport system to deliver reprocessed and sterilized supplies to the surgical suite. Or central supply could even be a separate department from general stores, purchasing, and receiving with transportation links to the surgery-delivery suite and the patient care units.

Design. Supplies to the patient and surgery units can utilize various approaches. Exchange carts can be used to deliver supplies to the departments and patient units. This system is based upon a predetermined amount of sterile supplies packed on a portable cart: the cart is delivered to the patient or department station for use at that location; a new cart is exchanged at programmed-use intervals. Nurse server concept can also be used to supply patient units. All patient charge items are then stocked from a central supply cart at the patient's room; custom carts are supplied to the departments. Floor stocks can also be maintained in departments and in patient units. In this approach central supply stocks patient floors and departments with programmed inventory items that are distributed as required on the units.

All the systems mentioned require a central supply flow pattern within the department, and the space needs and layout are determined by study. A major space determinant can be the introduction of automated systems within central supply. Such systems may be overhead rails, floor guides, conveyors, or various complete stat systems.

Soiled Processing →	Sterilization →	Clean Processing →	Distribution
Supplies	Clean packs	Linen	
Soiled carts	Instruments	Sterile supplies	
Soiled dishes	Solutions	Processed packs	
		Clean carts	

CENTRAL STERILIZATION

Central sterilization is the area into which patient utensils and medical-surgical supplies are received from the decontamination department and are further processed for reuse throughout the hospital. For many years, central sterile supplies related only to surgical suites. Other departments reprocessed and cleaned their own equipment and material. Present thinking combines all sterile processing into central sterilization.

Centralization of sterile processing provides:

—greater economy by putting expensive processing equipment in one area

—greater uniformity by standardizing supplies, equipment, and techniques of operation

—more efficient utilization of personnel by training workers in precise processing procedures

—sterile processing of medical-surgical supplies under controlled conditions, thereby contributing to total environmental control in the hospital

Functions. The basic function of central sterilization include:

—receiving and sorting decontaminated material from the decontamination department

—specialized cleaning of equipment and supplies

—inspecting and testing instruments, equipment, and linens

—assembling treatment trays, sets, and linen packs

—packaging all material for sterilizing

—labeling and dating material

—sterilizing

—participating in supply and equipment research in an effort to provide the most suitable material for patient care

Location. Because central sterilization provides a purely processing function following decontamination and preceding storage and distribution, it must be adjacent to decontamination and processed stores. Central sterilization should also be near linen services so that linens for medical-surgical packs, sets, and trays will be readily available.

Central Sterilization, Interdepartmental Relationships

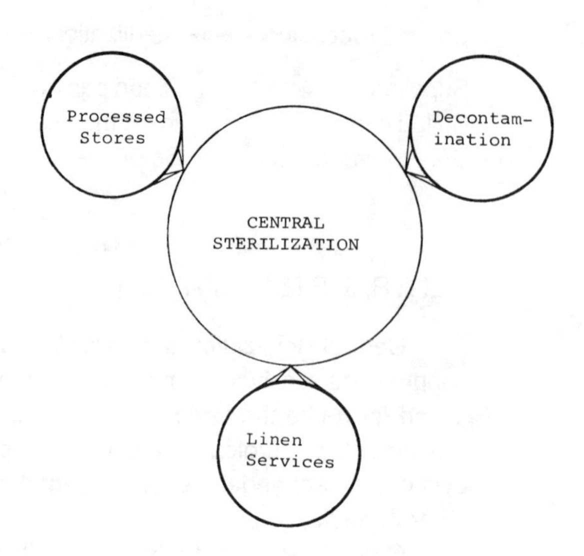

Intradepartmental Relationships. The supervisor's area should be removed from the flow of activity within the area, but able to see processing areas. The control area receives processed materials from decontamination, linen service, and processed stores. It controls processed materials sent to processed stores for distribution to user departments. The sorting area prepares decontaminated instruments, equipment, and supply set-ups for the assembly area. Personnel in this area will inspect instruments and equipment to assure that they are in good working condition. The assembly area includes work stations for assembling specific medical-surgical treatment packs, sets and trays. Workbenches with multiple drawers for instruments and supplies are necessary. Employees should be seated while working. It is recommended that specified packs and sets be assembled only at specified work stations. The linen pack area requires large work tables and a special inspection table for examining linen wrappers for minute instrument holes.

The terminal sterilizing area contains high vacuum steam and gas sterilizers. Ample floor space is required for carts into which items are loaded for sterilization. Aeration is needed following gas sterilization. After being sterilized items are packaged, labeled, and dated before being distributed through processed stores.

The supplies storage area consists of backup instruments and parts for general sterile processing. Cabinets and shelving are appropriate.

Linen Pack Area
Supplies Storage
Terminal Sterilizing
Assembling
Director's Office
Sorting
Reception Control

Central Sterilization, Intradepartmental Relationships

DECONTAMINATION

The decontamination area is the central point in the hospital's reprocessing supply system. All soiled items used throughout the facility, from patient utensils to wheelchairs, pass through this area, where a determination is made as to whether the item should be reused or discarded. The importance of the decontamination area as an infection control center has increased drastically in the past few years as a result of the rising costs of supply reprocessing, the development of new techniques for reprocessing, and the lack, in many cases, of personnel qualified to work in this department. In order for any reprocessing system to work effectively, it is paramount that the decontamination department be designed well; inefficiency here affects the whole system.

Functions. The basic function of the decontamination area is to receive soiled goods from all hospital departments, sort these goods according to service, and begin the cleaning and sterilizing cycle appropriate for them.

Soiled laundry linen is received, sorted, and entered into laundry processing. Patient utensils and medical-surgical instruments are sorted, racked, and passed through washer-sterilizers to the central sterilization area. Soiled items from the dietary department are received; dishes are racked and sent through a dishwashing device, reaching the kitchen washed, sterilized and ready for reuse. Flatware is sent through washer-sterilizers and received in the kitchen. Any trash is removed, placed in a pulverizer, and conveyed to the loading dock for removal.

Decontamination, Interdepartmental Relationships

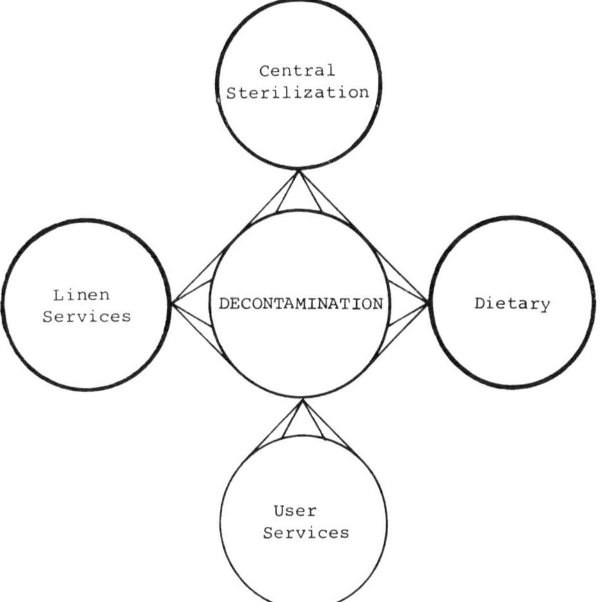

Location. The location chosen for decontamination is strategically important to the goal of rapid, efficient reprocessing of soiled supplies. Mandatory adjacencies are the dietary department, linen department, and central sterilization. Decontamination should either contain the soiled return shaft of the vertical transport system or be immediately adjacent to the elevator designated for return of soiled items.

Design. Because of the work done in the decontamination area, there should be no entranceways between it and any of the hospital service departments. Processing machines should be of the pass-through type. Soiled items are put into the machine on the decontamination side, and the cleaned items are removed in their respective areas. Only soiled items are in decontamination. Only decontaminated, cleaned items are received in dietary, central sterilization, or linen services. For this reason, decontamination personnel should be provided with their own shower, toilet, and locker facilities.

The physical plan of the decontamination area should take into account the rate of return of soiled items and the equipment necessary to process them. The basic components required are washer-sterilizers, sorting-working stations, cartwasher, and trash disposal unit. The general soiled items are put on racks at the work stations and then processed through the washer-sterilizers. Dirty dishes are racked and passed through the dish-processing unit. All laundry is loaded into washer-extractors. Garbage and trash should be placed in a pulverizer at the work station and conveyed to the loading dock for compacting and removal though other methods of trash disposal may be considered.

The planning of equipment and work areas is directly related to the rate at which soiled items are returned for processing. This rate of soiled return is not related solely to the bed count of the hospital. It is based on bed count, ambulatory patient load, utilization of disposables, dietary load, and reprocessing required by all user departments. No rule of thumb is possible when looking for a rate of return. The overall efficiency of decontamination is dependent on the reprocessing machinery. The key is the reprocessing rate of the washer-sterilizers.

The reprocessing rate controls the rate at which soiled items can be received in decontamination for reprocessing, the number of work stations needed, the number of conveyors needed between work stations and washer-sterilizers, the amount of overhead rack storage areas needed, the holding space for carts containing unracked soiled items, the cartwashing sequence, and space for holding empty soiled carts prior to washing. These factors must be considered in the design of a decontamination area:

—volume to be processed per department per day

—number of hours in use (shifts)

—number and capacity of processing machines

—efficiency of machinery

—method and rate of racking

—capacities of various holding areas

—scheduling of return of soiled items

The finishes used in the decontamination area should be selected for ease of cleaning, water resistance, and durability. Lighting should be 30 foot candles in general and 100 foot candles at work stations. Overall electrical requirements will also depend on the machinery selected.

In order to reduce the chances of cross infection via airborne organisms, it is recommended that the entire area be under negative pressure and that its air be completely exhausted.

Decontamination, Intradepartmental Relationships

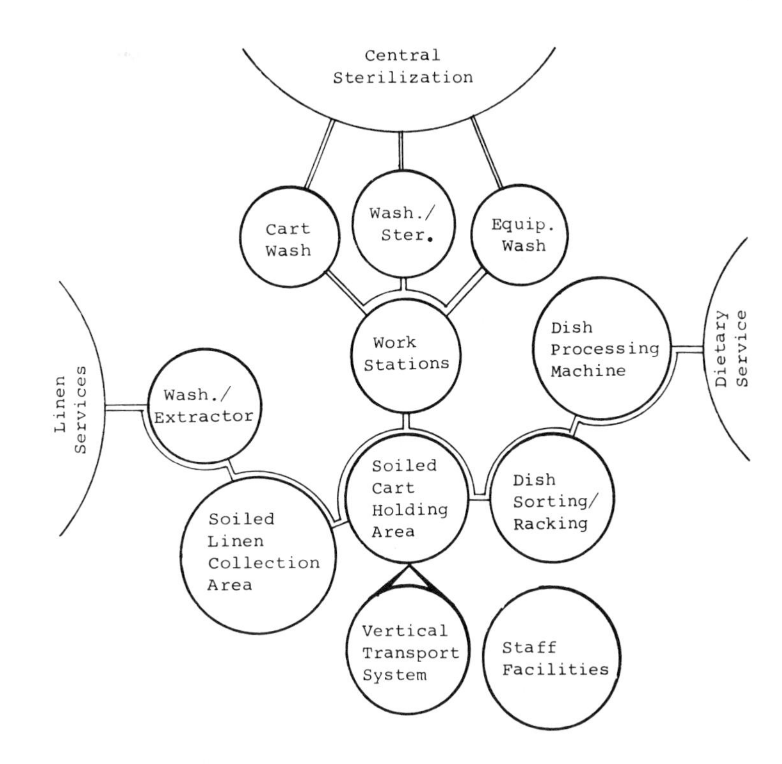

Intradepartmental Relationships. Essentially, decontamination is one large workroom divided as follows:

—Soiled cart holding spaces for holding soiled items on carts as received from user departments. These carts are received either from the vertical transport system (soiled return shaft) or from an elevator designated for soiled item return.

—Work stations are areas at which carts with patient utensils or medical-surgical instruments are unloaded and prepared for processing.

—Washer-sterilizers are loaded, manually or automatically, with racks of items ready for reprocessing.

—Soiled linen is removed from carts, weighed, and presorted by type for processing in the soiled linen collection-presort area.

—Washer-extractors are loaded with presorted soiled linen.

—The dish sorting and racking space is similar to normal work stations, but it handles only dishes and other dietary items.

In addition, the following elements are required:

—A cartwashing room, manual or automatic, devoted solely to cleaning and sterilizing all hospital carts. In either case, the space allowed should be sufficiently large for machinery necessary to convert to automatic cartwashing in the future.

—The equipment washing room is similar to the above, but is used for large hospital equipment that cannot fit into normal washer-sterilizers. If desired, it can be combined with the cartwashing room while both operations are manual.

—Staff lockers and toilets must be completely separate from other employee facilities in order to prevent possible contamination of other personnel and areas of the hospital.

In addition to the specific work areas indicated above, space must be provided for circulation throughout the main workroom.

LAUNDRY–LINEN

Criticism of linen services, by both patients and personnel, is one of the most frequent complaints heard by hospital administrators. The major share of such criticism can be and should be avoided by a properly planned laundry and linen services system that meets the individual hospital's objectives.

The laundry–linen services department of a hospital does far more than basic laundering and distribution. Quality linen and laundry services should contribute to quality patient care, improved control of infection, improved patient and employee morale, and improved community relations.

Today one can choose from a variety of linen and laundry processing systems or create a custom system by including components from several. All have advantages and disadvantages that must be evaluated carefully before a final determination is made. The basic alternative, processes briefly described, are as follows:

—*Shared laundry* operations are usually described as laundries built by contributions of capital and operating funds from a group of hospitals or health institutions in a community. They are operated on a nonprofit basis. The objective is to reduce costs by making optimum use of modern equipment and processing techniques, mass production, linen standardization, and reductions in number of personnel. It may include linen purchasing, linen rental service, mending, laundry processing, and linen distribution.

—*Commercial laundry* contracts with a private laundry may include linen rental service, laundry processing, mending, and linen distribution. Usually it includes only laundry processing, unless the laundry specializes in service to health care institutions. The major benefit is the elimination of capital investment in laundry equipment. Spiraling costs, excessive inventories, delivery problems, and increased wear because of extra handling are some of the problems associated with the use of contract linen services. Costs, however, are usually chargeable to patients and third-party payers.

—*Traditional in-house laundry* includes all linen and laundry services within the institution. The efficiency and cost-effectiveness of an in-house laundry depends upon the equipment and textiles used, the availability of personnel, and the quality of laundry management. Many administrators believe that a properly administered in-house laundry is far less expensive than any alternative. A smaller linen inventory is normally required for an in-house operation, and an internal system tends to be more responsive to changing and emergency linen needs than an external system. In-house laundries do, however, require a heavy outlay of capital for space and equipment, and the latter tends to become obsolete in a short time due to technological improvements. The current trend toward leasing equipment can lessen the problem of obsolescence and can allow costs chargeable to patients to be identified.

—*The continuous-flow laundry system,* particularly the Renfrew-Poensgen Flowline system and the Ametek Contro-Flow systems, is in use in some hospitals here in the United States as well as abroad. These systems are designed to reduce the number of personnel required for laundry processing, minimize linen handling between laundry operations, and eliminate the need for special construction for vibration-creating equipment. The American Institute of Laundering has rated this type of system as excellent. Continuous flow laundry systems appear to offer a valuable alternative to other laundry-linen equipment systems.

—The no-press garment finishers use specialized equipment designed to simplify the processing of polyester-cotton garments and uniforms. They utilize an automatically controlled humidity-temperature system to obtain a fine, finished, wrinkle-free product.

—Dry cleaning is considered by many laundry experts to be the best and most economical cleaning method for polyester-cotton blends with resin finishes, for polyester-cotton blends with metal fiber, and antistatic 100 percent nylon. Dry cleaning has not gained much favor in hospitals (primarily because they use so much cotton, cotton mixtures, and so on).

New types of linens on the market will affect the design of facilities and the equipment used in laundry services. Among the forerunners to challenge the traditional cotton are disposable linens and polyester-cotton blends.

Many hotels and motels are now using only disposable linens in their rooms and a complete line of disposable hospital linens will be available soon. Ecology, cost, storage, and disposal are important problems of this approach. Predominant advantages are easily identifiable patient costs, less need for laundry space and equipment, and lower capital investment. Disadvantages are inpatient and personnel reactions to the quality of disposable linens, increased storage space, and increased load (smoke producing) on the compactor and incinerator. Disposables may be recommended in doctors' offices, treatment rooms, outpatient services, and for some uses in surgery and delivery.

Polyester-cotton blends are new and continuously improving. They have had a considerable impact on laundry-linen services. While somewhat more expensive initially, they tend to last longer and equalize costs over a period of time. The advantages of polyester-cotton blends include increased tensile strength, elimination of press work, less weight, easier to process, colorfast, better appearance, and increased comfort for patients and personnel. Disadvantages, to date, are fluff-dried cotton items such as towels and bath blankets.

Functions. The functions of a laundry-linen service, then, are to:

—receive linen
—process it through laundry equipment
—examine and mend or replace linen
—distribute linen to service areas
—control processed linens not in immediate use
—maintain records for administrative informational systems

In the past, functions also included employee uniform supply, processing, and distribution. Many hospitals continue to supply this service, but there appears to be a trend toward minimizing it.

Laundry-Linen, Interdepartmental Relationships

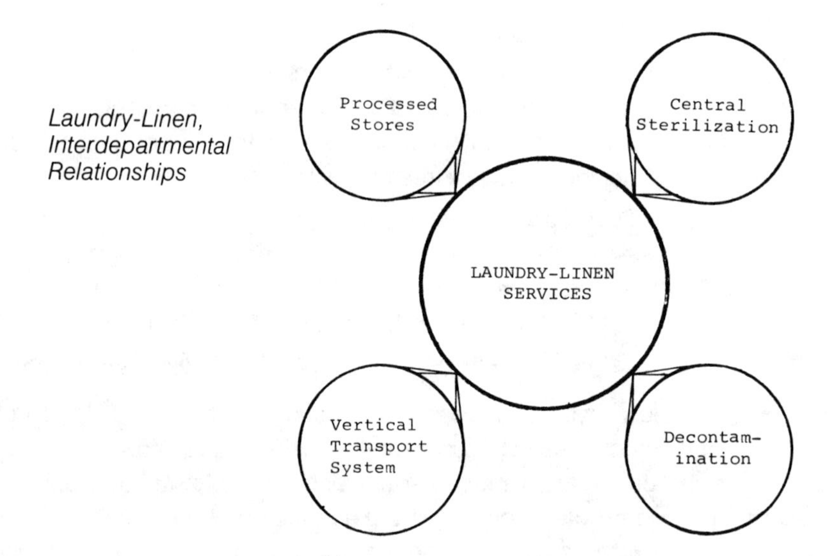

Location. The linen service department should be centrally located on the ground level at an outside wall for future expansion, but it need not be in a prime area. It should be convenient to service elevators or vertical transport systems for delivery of linens and pickup of laundry from patient care units and service departments. Processed stores, central sterilization, and decontamination should be contiguous with this department.

Design. For operational efficiency and control of infection, no cross traffic of soiled laundry and clean linens should be tolerated.

The hospital will have patient and clinical linen requirements ranging from ten to twenty pounds per patient day. A working average of fifteen pounds is reasonable. A linen inventory equaling roughly six times the daily linen requirement should be available to allow the laundry and linen room to work efficiently. This standard will vary if linen services operate on more than a five-day week. The inventory will be in either service, process, repair, transit, or weekend use and no additional linen sets should be stored in the patient's room if good control is achieved. New linens not assigned to immediate use should be held in processed stores until requisitioned by linen services.

All patient linens should be provided on a linen cart exchange system. Delivery may be made to nurse-server units, patient rooms, and so on, depending on operational choice, but the planned quota of backup should remain on the cart in the clean linen room until the time of exchange. Linen standards and quotas to meet patient needs should be established for each nursing unit or department. These quotas should be reevaluated periodically.

Facilities must include space for a cart system; that is, for storing clean, decontaminated carts and for loading and storing loaded carts. Laundry systems and equipment must meet existing building code requirements for construction, utilities, and so forth.

Intradepartmental Relationships. The basic areas of laundry-linen services should be so designed that there is no cross traffic. Linen services is basically an open area, except for the manager's office, storage rooms, and the soiled receiving-sorting area (an element of decontamination). This allows for maximum light and for temperature and humidity control. Equipment should be placed to allow for maximum automation of laundry and mechanized handling of containers to reduce personnel handling time.

The soiled receiving area should be designed as an element of decontamination. It receives laundry by cart, chute, or other mechanical conveyance. Space should be allowed for sorting and weighing prior to processing to maximize the efficiency of processing. After being sorted in decontamination, the laundry is loaded into pass-through washer-extractors (or continuous flow equipment). The carts used to transport laundry to decontamination shall be taken to the cartwashing area for cleaning and preparation for re-entry into system. Linen removed in the laundry processing area is clean. Conditioning and drying are done in a processing area. The placement of equipment, utility requirements, and movement of processed linen between functions are extremely important. Flow should always be away from washer-extractors (or continuous flow equipment).

The shake-out area includes a work area and equipment for folding fluff-dried linens such as thermal blankets, towels, patient gowns, pajamas, wash cloths, and receiving blankets. It should be adjacent to laundry processing and in the line of flow. The flatwork-ironing area requires a spreader, mangle, and folder for efficient processing of flatwork, such as sheets, pillow cases, bath blankets, bedspreads, and so on. This area may also include presses for ironing uniforms and lab coats. It should be contiguous with laundry processing. Lighting throughout should be fifty to seventy foot candles.

Mending and selected linen manufacturing services for the hospital take place here in a separate room. Marking machines, patching machines, and sewing machines are utilized. The sewing room should be convenient to the shake-out and flatwork-ironing areas, since linens needing repair are usually identified in those areas. It should be a closed area to one side of the production line and close to the linen storage and loading area. Lighting required is 100 foot candles.

The linen storage and loading area is the end of the production line. It contains movable shelves to hold processed linens and space for loading linen carts. It should be adjacent to the flatwork-ironing area, shake-out, sewing room, and external hallway convenient to the vertical transport system. Part of the area should be a closed room for storing processed linen above and beyond cart needs. This room should be locked when linen services is closed.

The uniform room is a closed controlled room for holding processed uniforms pending distribution or pickup by personnel. It should be on an external hallway, with one opening into the hall and one into the processing area in order to keep unauthorized personnel out of the area. A suggested location is near employees' facilities.

The laundry manager's office should be enclosed in glass and located for observation of the production line, yet allowing privacy for interviews, record keeping, planning, and so on. Observation of persons entering the department is necessary. The best location is at the end of the laundry processing area, near linen storage and loading.

MEDICAL RECORDS

The medical records department exists primarily to support optimum patient care and must be organized to serve the patient, medical staff, hospital administration, and community. In the interests of economy, accuracy of data, and good communication, all information about a patient should be concentrated in his or her medical record, indexed and filed in the main medical records department.

The medical records program is based upon centralization of all records, utilizing Social Security numbers or a unit record-filing system. Outpatient, inpatient, and all treatment records will be filed within one folder. If the unit record-filing system is used, all record numbers will be issued by the medical records department. The department will maintain cross-referenced indexes of all patient records, including both inpatients and outpatients, and the necessary operations and diagnoses' indexes.

The records area must have adequate space for storage of active and inactive records, for personnel, and for equipment. Design must be functional, with logical placement of work area, good intra- and interdepartmental communication systems, and the best possible means for transporting individual medical records. Special consideration must be given to the types of equipment or systems to be used (for example, files, dictation systems, record storage, distribution systems, and statistical and research systems). It is recommended that automated systems be used as much as possible, including those for storage, record retrieval, card systems, and microfilming.

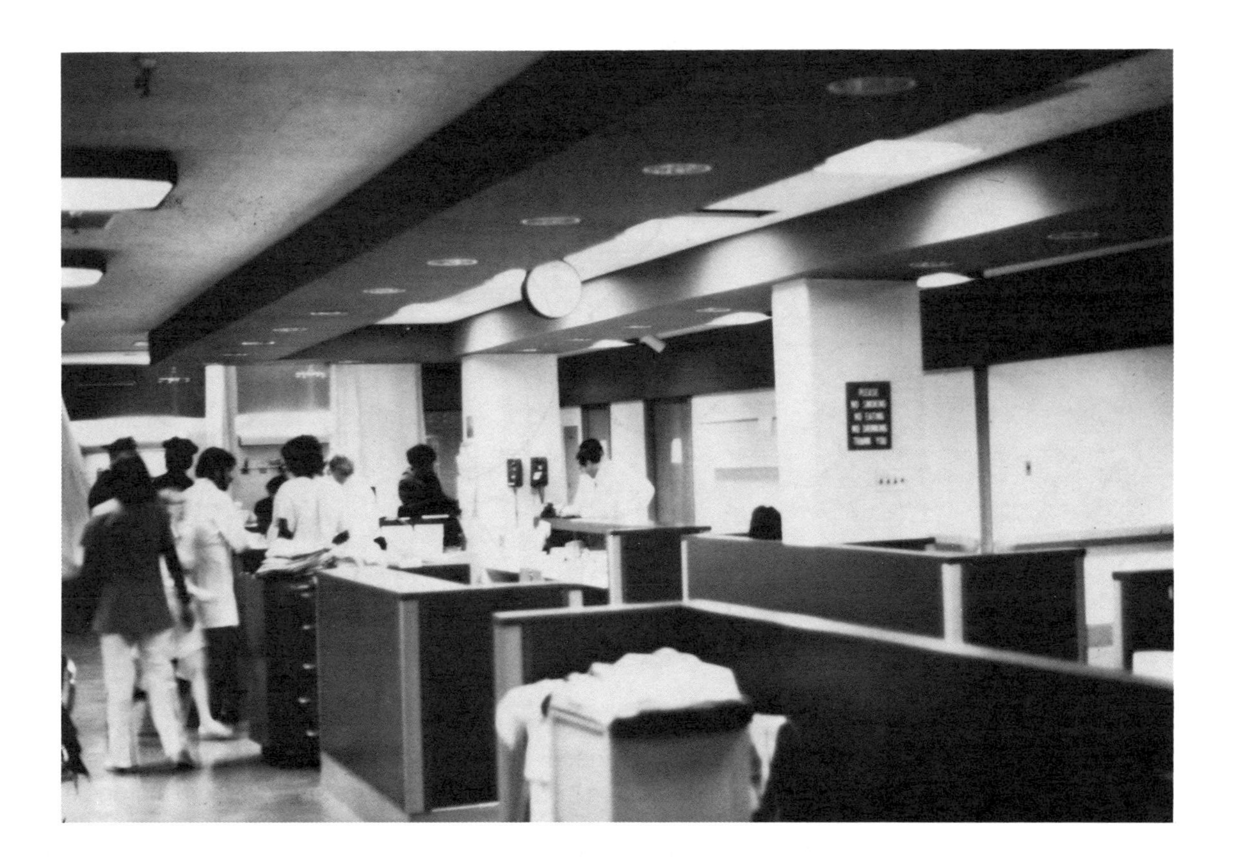

Functions. The medical records department is responsible for several functions.

Maintaining appropriate facilities and services for accurate and timely completion, processing, checking, indexing, filing, and retrieval of the medical record of each inpatient and ambulatory patient admitted to the hospital is the department's primary task. Safeguarding the information in the medical record against loss, defacement, tampering, or use by unauthorized persons is also essential.

The department also provides periodic statistical reports for administration, medical staff committees, medical education, and research departments. These reports should include the number of admissions and discharges by major clinical services, discharge diagnoses and length of stay by diagnosis, types and numbers of operations performed, and age distribution of patients.

Location. The medical records department should be placed where it can provide prompt medical services for the care of all patients (ambulatory as well as inpatients) at all hours. It must be convenient and have adequate accommodations for busy physicians to complete their records or study cases of special interest and also be easily available for research, educational, or administrative purposes. It should be adjacent to the admissions office, the outpatient department, social services, emergency service, the physicians' lounge, hospital administration, and the business office. Because medical records, administration, and the business office are not likely to be adjacent to each other, highly effective communication and distribu-

Medical Records, Interdepartmental Relationships

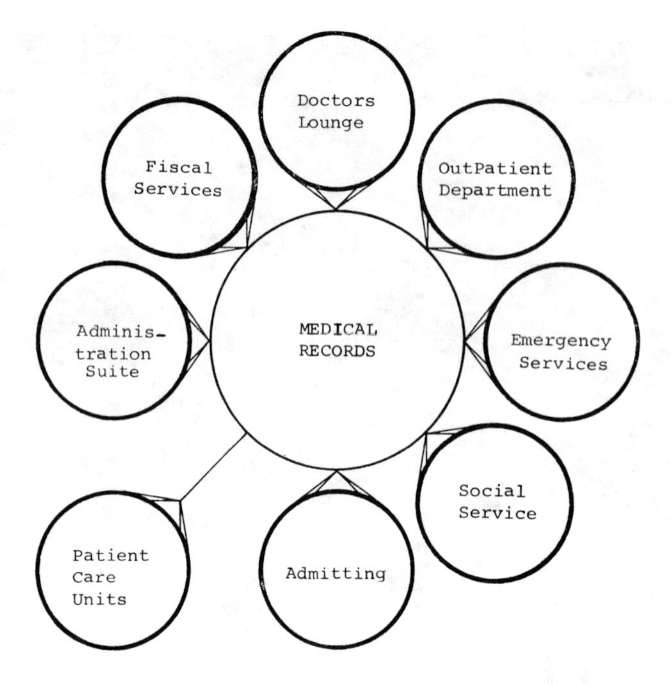

tion systems are recommended. Inactive records, as determined by administration and legal policies, should be microfilmed and stored in the record storage area.

Design. It is recommended that automated systems be used for storage, retrieval, card filing, and microfilming. Record storage files are programmed as open-shelf filing. Dictating and transcribing areas should be planned acoustically to reduce noise.

Intradepartmental relationships. The reception–control area should be located at the main entrance to the medical records department to direct and control persons and material entering and leaving the department. The chief librarian's office should be near reception–control and the doctor's dictation-conference room. The assistant librarian's office could be located near the chief librarian's office, but a decentralized location near record storage and microfilming is recommended.

The doctor's dictation-conference room should be near reception–control, the chief librarian's office, and the central transcription pool. If questions should arise pertaining to transcription of medical records in general, or if additional records are required by the physicians, appropriate personnel are thereby available for assistance. The central transcription pool should be adjacent to the doctor's dictation-conference area to expedite accurate completion of all medical records.

The registry area should be located adjacent to reception–control and record storage. The record storage area will include space for holding charts approximately three years before microfilming. One remote portion of record storage should be designated for microfilming and photostating activities. The microfilm storage area should be located adjacent to the microfilming area of record storage.

Medical Records, Intradepartmental Relationships

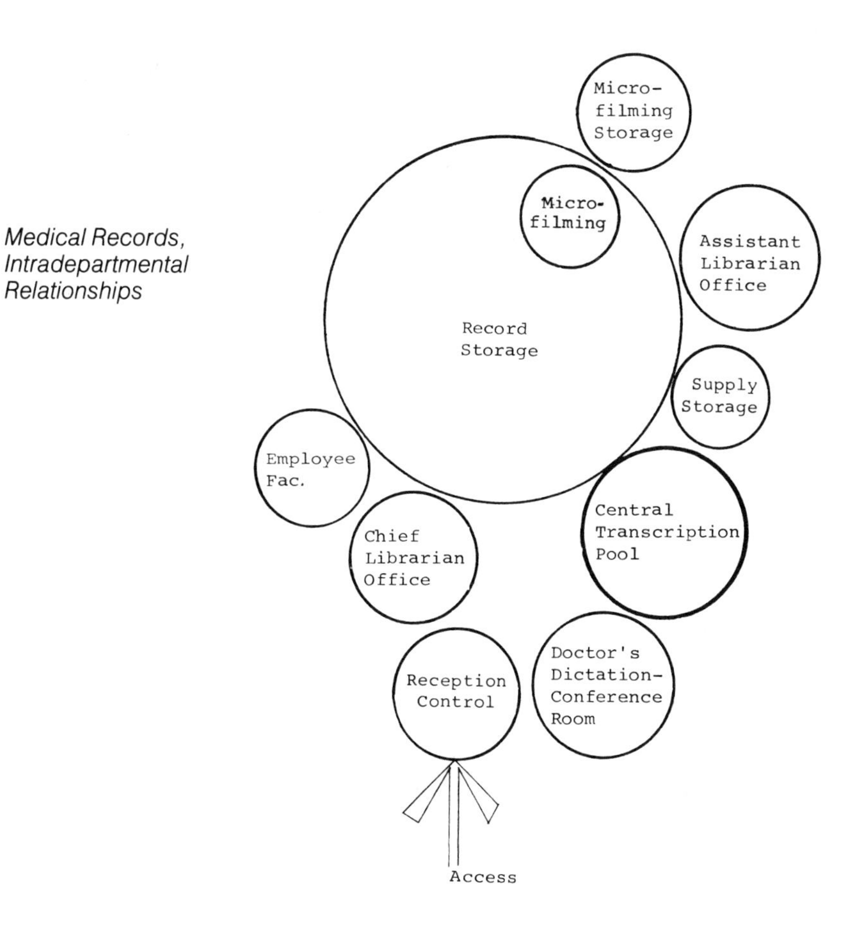

The supplies area should be adjacent to both administrative and filing-storage functions. Employee facilities shall be centrally located, ideally next to the entrance and administrative areas of the department.

ENGINEERING AND MAINTENANCE

The specific needs of the hospital's central plant include all aspects of the design and space requirements for the generation, storage, and distribution of steam; of hot and of cold water; for refrigeration; for ventilation and air conditioning; and for electricity. They are highly specialized and will be finally determined by the consulting engineers and architects on the planning team. Energy use, storage, conservation, recovery, and new sources are the current elements of goal-setting within the hospital.

There is frequently a tendency to minimize problems when making basic decisions about the overall scope of various hospital programs. More often than not, the space needs of the mechanical plant are underestimated. Thus, engineers are forced to fit equipment into inadequate spaces. Thereafter, the operation and maintenance of equipment is handicapped.

The construction contracts should include provisions for color-coding all pipe and duct systems; thus, supply and return conduits are easily identified. This is relatively inexpensive if done at the time of installation and it is invaluable to the engineering-maintenance staff later.

The needs of the engineering and maintenance space have increased proportionately with the development of far more complex equipment. Also, the energy issue is finally coming of age. Consequently, planning must provide space for skilled personnel, equipment, and tools to provide technical support of the physical plant and its equipment, including space for a complete, twenty-four hour monitoring system of the increasingly complex systems and equipment necessary to a modern, efficient hospital.

Concepts of preventive maintenance should be part of each department's functions. However, equipment will still need repair and replacement. Serious thought must be given to planning and providing routine services, but the design must also allow for expansion dictated by the quantity and quality of equipment used by the other services in the hospital. A good example is electronic equipment: if a minimum is planned, it may not justify a specialist and an electronic shop for repair. Future needs, however, may. The possibility must be considered now if such a section is to be operational in the future.

Functions included in the engineering and maintenance department are preventive maintenance, repair, and operation of all equipment, machinery, and distribution lines concerned with the following:

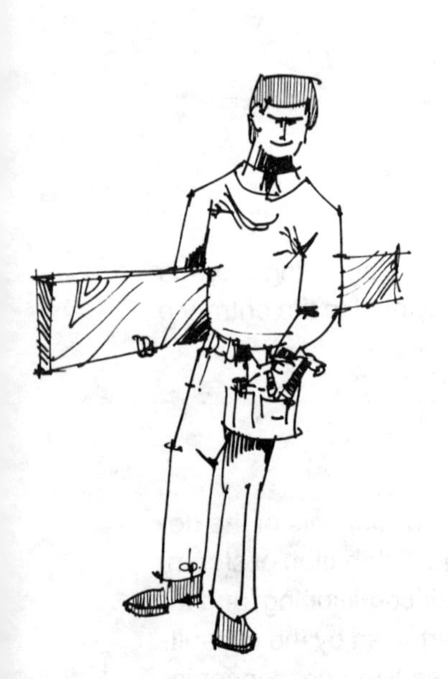

—steam and hot water

—plumbing (including waste disposal)

—electrical systems (equipment, power, and lighting systems, including emergency systems)

—fire detection, prevention and fighting methods and devices

—carpentry

—painting and decorating

—vertical transportation equipment

—communication and mechanical systems

—minor plant alterations and renovations

—grounds maintenance and landscaping

—safety

Location. The best location for engineering-maintenance is on ground level in a nonprime area. Access to service elevators, the boiler plant, mechanical areas, and a loading dock are essential. The main shop areas should be on an outside wall for ventilation and for future expansion. Normal telephone and internal communications systems should be considered. In addition, a pneumatic tube station could be provided for receipt of written job orders.

Engineering and Maintenance,
Intradepartmental
Relationships

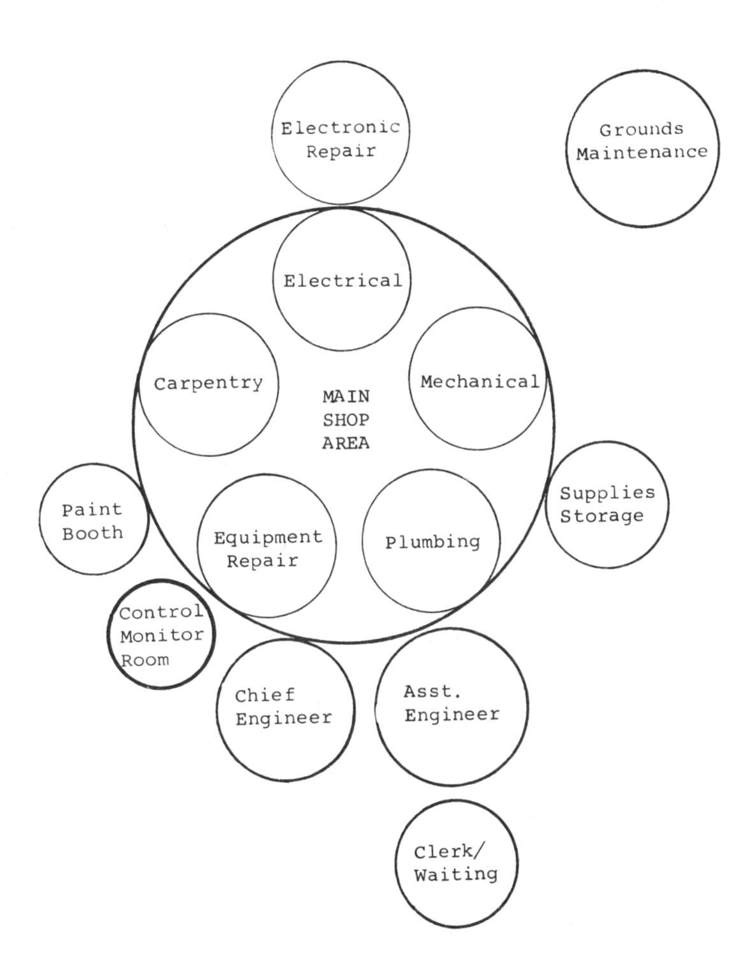

A storage area for grounds maintenance equipment should be provided (outside the entrance) and contiguity with the engineering shop areas is desirable, but not essential.

Design. Basically, the engineering and maintenance department consists of three main elements: an administrative area, the shop areas, and mechanical equipment space. The administrative areas should be compatible in decor, lighting, and general finishes to the other administrative areas of the hospital. The shop areas should be separate and distinct from the office areas and of sufficient size to carry on the following activities: mechanical, electrical, plumbing, carpentry, and equipment repairs. A large open space is recommended with an average lighting level of 100 foot candles. The major area can be divided by movable partitions to allow flexibility of use. Finally, the entire work area should be soundproofed.

Intradepartmental Relationships. The chief engineer's office should be located between the entrance to the suite and the main shop area. The assistant engineer's office should be adjacent to the clerk's office, with an adjacent plan file and drafting room (which may later become office for security). The clerk's office is separate from, but adjoining, a small waiting area, which should be located so as to control access to the offices.

The main shops are large, open work areas divided into major work disciplines and planned as a unified complex. They include: mechanical and plumbing, which should be close together or combined; carpentry, which should be somewhat isolated from other repair areas because it creates so much dust; equipment repair, adjacent to mechanical and carpentry; electrical, adjacent to electronic repair and equipment repair; and electronic repair, which should be well ventilated and as isolated as possible, to eliminate problems caused by dust. The paint booth is an enclosed space, directly adjacent to main shops, for the repainting of equipment. It must be vented according to all pertinent fire regulations. The activity of painting beds and so on will be in housekeeping. The supplies storage room is for all material required by the various work areas.

The control monitor room houses staff, equipment, and panels for complete twenty-four hour monitoring of mechanical and electrical systems. It should be adjacent to the chief engineer's office. This installation will locate and correct potential breakdowns. It is not, however, a substitute for an effective preventive maintenance program and related scheduled inspections and servicing.

Grounds maintenance equipment can be stored near an outside entrance. The relationship of this area to the main areas of engineering-maintenance is not particularly important.

PHARMACY

Factors that affect other areas of the health field also affect pharmacy; for example, population growth; discoveries of drugs, drug preparation, and automated equipment; new distribution techniques; and increased use of drugs in the treatment of disease. Drugs dispensed by a pharmacy have been steadily increasing, and we can assume a continued increase. This will call for a closer look at current methods and practices in pharmacy operation for the present and the future.

A good pharmacy program blends qualified personnel, a modern and efficient facility, sound budgeting, and the support and cooperation of the medical, nursing, and administrative staff of the hospital. In this era, when roles within the health care system are changing, it seems logical that the pharmacy will evolve new roles vis-a-vis the other segments of the health care industry. In addition, the emphasis on reduced cost, and on productivity and efficiency in department operations, will demand new methods (automation), new production approaches (prepackaging and unit doses), and new distribution techniques (automation, decentralization, par-level cart interchange, and so on). Highly automated dispensing is technically feasible at this time. It requires a computer-based ordering system, a computer-activated remote dispensing machine, and a linkage of these components into a coordinated system. The role of the pharmacist in the automated dispensing of the future will be primarily as a consultant on drugs and drug therapy for medical, dental, nursing, and other staff members.

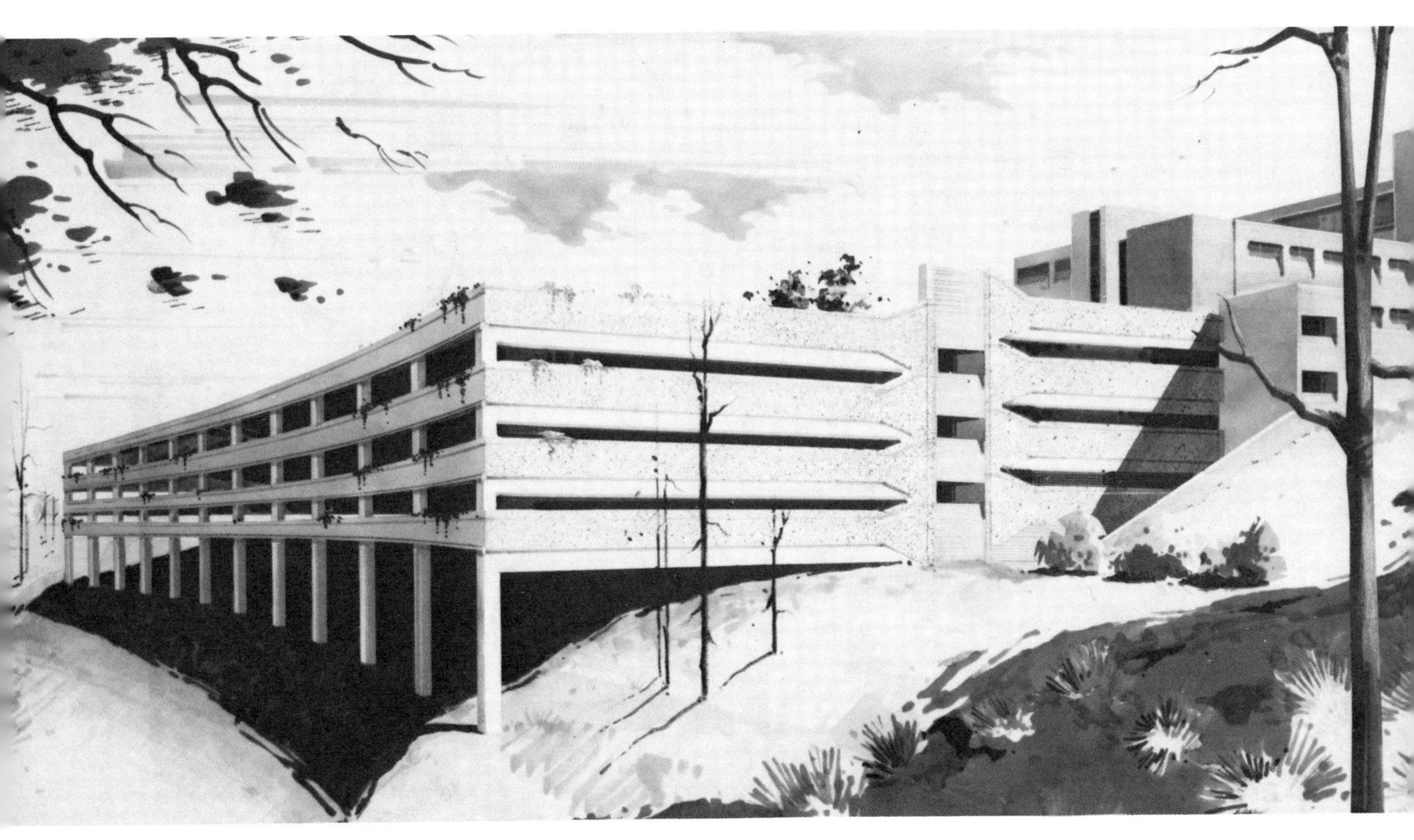

Parking structure. St. Luke Hospital, Fort Thomas, Kentucky

A hospital that is building for the future must include enough flexibility and expansion potential in its initial planning to allow for future revisions in pharmacy service with a minimum disruption to the physical location or assigned space. A guide of 40–100 medication orders per gross square foot of space may be used.

Functions. The basic functions of pharmacy are to:

—requisition, store, compound, package, label, and dispense pharmaceutical items

—make information concerning drugs readily available to pharmacists, physicians, nurses, and other health care personnel

—participate in educational programs approved by the hospital

—plan, organize, and direct pharmacy policies and procedures in accordance with established hospital policies

—implement the decisions of the pharmacy and therapeutic committee

—maintain a satisfactory system of recorded bookkeeping in accordance with the policies of the hospital

Pharmacy, Interdepartmental Relationships

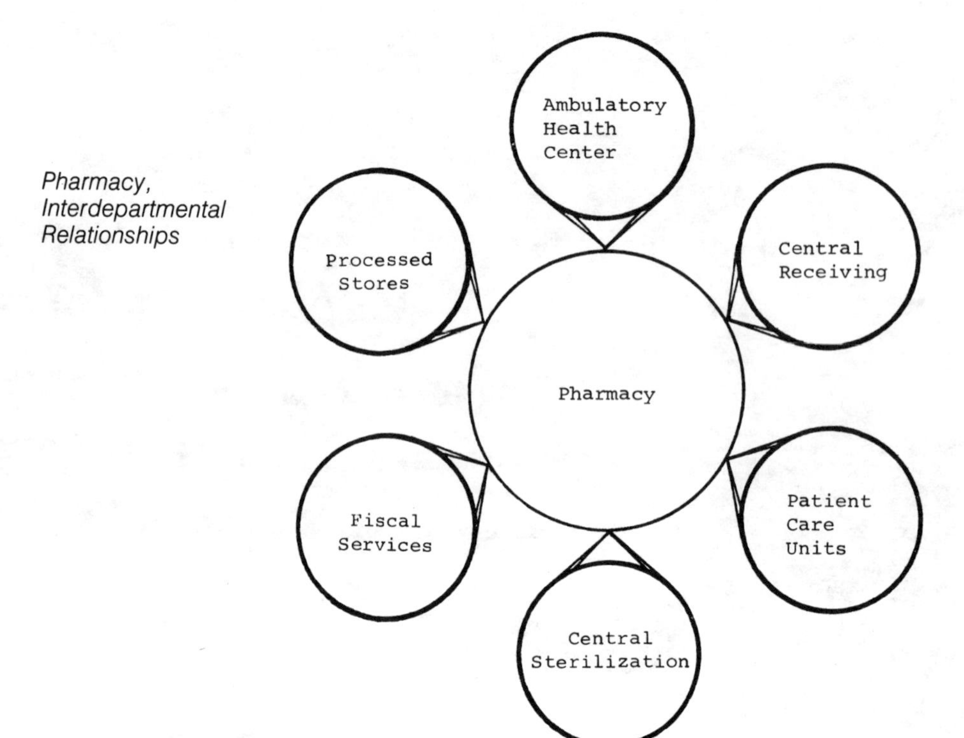

Location. The pharmacy must be convenient to central receiving, the ambulatory health center, central stores, patient care units, and central supply. To accomplish this, a ground floor location close to an elevator servicing nursing units is necessary.

Design. Several mechanical systems will be needed for this department to function efficiently: telephones, terminal transmitters to the computer room for inventory and billing, pneumatic tube for rapid receiving of requisitions and distribution of orders in small quantities, and a cart system to distribute quantities of drugs to designated areas.

Very broadly, the pharmacy is divided into four main areas: administration, worker's production, storage, and an admixture room.

Pharmaceutical supplies may or may not be held in central receiving and storage, but all drugs and other agents of a similar nature (hypodermic syringes, needles, parenteral fluid, alcohol) should be delivered directly to and checked in by the pharmacy. Storage facilities should include routine shelf space laid out efficiently, but must also include locked areas (vault) for safety and accountability of specified drugs. A refrigerated area is also necessary and should be larger than previously thought necessary because of the increased use of materials requiring refrigeration and the storage of admixture parenteral fluids.

The production area should include an admixture area for preparation of parenteral fluids under specific conditions, such as laminar flow and temperature and humidity control. The work area will require dispensers, sinks, a still, work counter space, cart space, and floor and wall-mounted cabinets.

Special attention should be given by the architect to floor, wall, and ceiling requirements, as well as to structural, plumbing, and mechanical requirements.

Pharmacy, Intradepartmental Relationships

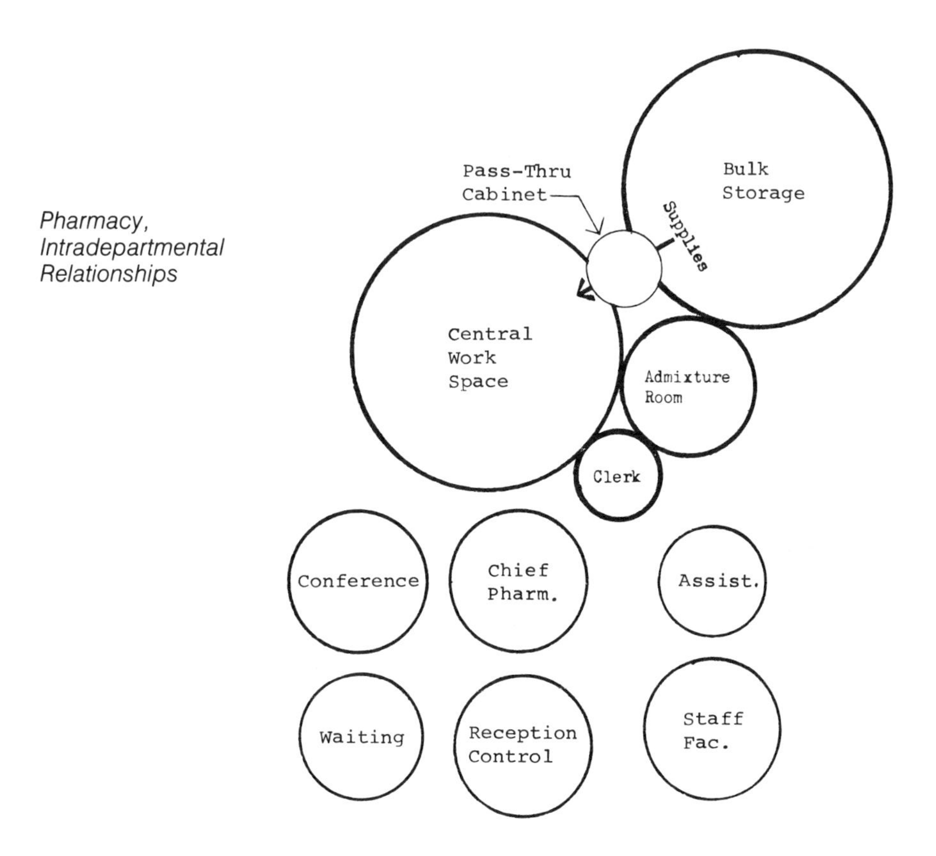

Intradepartmental Relationships. The basic intradepartmental setup follows a natural operational flow of activities.

The administrative area consists of the following:

—control–reception, for receipt of requisitions, visitors to the department, and control of waiting area (the pneumatic tube should be near this area)

—waiting area, designed for employees waiting for drugs and for salesmen or visitors, who should wait outside the administrative area proper

—chief pharmacist's office, away from the stream of activity but within sight of the production area (the assistant's and secretary's offices, or both, should be adjacent)

—conference-library area, for staff meetings, sales conferences, and educational functions

—employee lounge and toilet facilities located adjacent to the conference-library area

The production, or work, area should be designed to allow a free flow of receiving, preparing, labeling, recording, and distributing of required orders or prescriptions. An open corridor around the periphery of an open room is desirable. This corridor should be wide enough for carts to move (par level) and a pharmacist to work. The central portion of the room should be for counters, cabinets, desks, Diebold dispenser, and so on that, in effect, form a sub-storage area. The last work station area in the production line should be for required materials and parenteral fluids. The clerk's office and terminal transmitter should be adjacent to the work station and have easy access to the pneumatic tube system.

The storage area should be large enough to accommodate pharmaceuticals in a volume that is economical to buy and dispense within a given period of time. It should open directly into the work area and contain:

—A walk-in refrigerator with storage and drawers for inside loading. The drawers should be accessible to workers in the production area, and the refrigerator should be used to store required materials and admixture fluids. One large refrigerator would increase efficiency and would eliminate the need for small ones throughout the area.

—Large bulk storage composed of stacked shelves with enough space between stacks to allow for loading directly to a cart. It is suggested that a plan for pharmacy relate the storage areas and the work stations in such a way that the worker's access to the storage area is through a cabinet containing supplies broken down into daily or weekly needs.

—A vault for narcotics and other controlled substances.

The admixture room should be connected with storage (refrigerator) and the work area. It should be large enough to accommodate two people working, include laminar flow candling apparatus, sinks, cabinets for intravenous fluids, drugs, and so on.

EMPLOYEE FACILITIES

Many hospitals contain grouped employee locker and lounge areas that are separate from the individual departments. This space may also exist within each department, but it must be accounted for in the total facility. This area includes toilet facilities with showers, full twelve-inch lockers or convenient double seven-and-a half-inch lockers, and lounge spaces. A layout method to size the total space for these functions is ten square feet per locker required.

PUBLIC AREAS

The public spaces of a hospital are a reference point in the overall traffic and space concept of the entire facility. The hospital lobby should be a spacious one, and the traffic and confusion should be minimal, since good planning diverts much of the traffic to other entrances. The purpose of the lobby will be solely to accommodate visitors. Patient admissions and discharges will be directed away from the lob-

Public Area, Intradepartmental Relationships

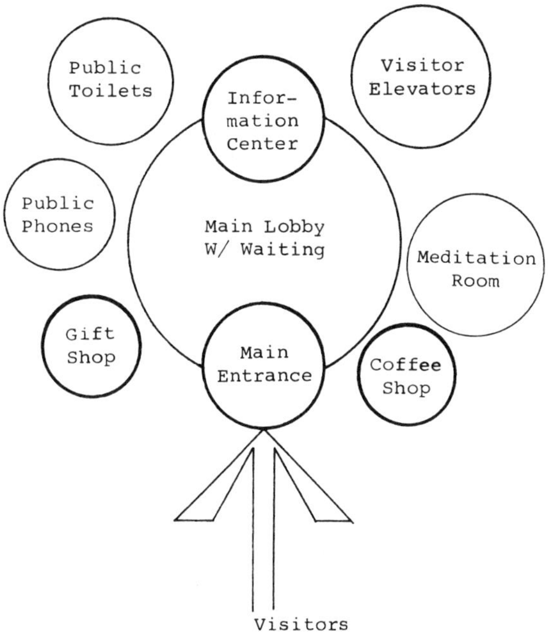

Public Toilets
Information Center
Visitor Elevators
Public Phones
Main Lobby W/ Waiting
Meditation Room
Gift Shop
Main Entrance
Coffee Shop
Visitors

by, and outpatients are provided with waiting areas in the respective departments (see Chapter VIII). Physicians and employees should have their own entrances and exits.

The family member who enters the lobby should be considered an adjunct to the patient within the hospital. Every attempt to properly care for and please the family, as well as the patient, falls within the overall objective of providing for total patient care.

Design. The traditional hospital lobby has given way in some hospitals to a newer concept in design, such as a concourse or expanded central public street, that allows for multiple entrances to the desired hospital areas. The concourse centralizes and controls each type of traffic flow, yet through a series of short hallways allows traffic to flow to all areas of the hospital. This design permits more flexibility in developing interdepartmental plans and should be given serious consideration when planning the design.

Most visitors have the greatest difficulty locating public toilets and the coffee shop. These areas should be easily accessible to lobby guests and not hidden from view. The information center should be located near or facing the entrance doors and main elevators. A program board announcing conferences, seminars, and so on, with proper room locations, should be visible to guests immediately upon entering the lobby.

Visitors' elevators to patient units need surveillance and control. Stairwells should not be visible from the lobby or concourse, and they should be difficult for visitors to find. A desk area near the elevators for volunteer control might be considered. The hospital auxiliary office, gift shop, coffee shop, and meditation room should be adjacent to the lobby or concourse.

Exterior courts and placement of a fine arts program should be integrated into these important public spaces.

CIRCULATION

Circulation is the space within the hospital administrative and support services that is not common to a specific department. This includes corridors between departments, stairwells, public toilets, courts, elevators and lobbies, and material-handling system space. This space must be considered in determining the total square footage of a building concept design.

ADDITIONAL SPACES

Additional space must be designed for functions which are not specifically in administering, supporting, or providing patient services, but are required of any technological institution in modern society. Examples of such services are education-in-service, public relations, security, and warehousing or archives.

Considering the continuous changes in health care service philosophy and its ever-more technologically sophisticated methods, the uses for conference and classroom spaces within a hospital are endless. Most departments will contain some areas for their particular use, but general meeting rooms with attendant administrative offices are also needed. The location of this space is not critical in a primary or a secondary facility.

Public relations, which is dealt with in Chapter VI, deals in both public and patient information. The area must include space for the director and assistant's offices, secretarial services, and production facilities, which might include such elements as layout and darkrooms. The location of this space, beyond providing for easy public access, is not critical.

The security department is divided between administrative personnel and storage spaces, and entrance and site control stations. Given the current usage of centralized electronic security monitoring and communications devices, a central monitoring and administrative area should be located convenient to the major public entrance. Entrance and site control station can be located as needed.

Any service institution as technologically complex as the modern health care facility will need storage space for currently unused equipment and materials. For ease of access and transport this area should be located in the base complex.

X

department planning: medical services

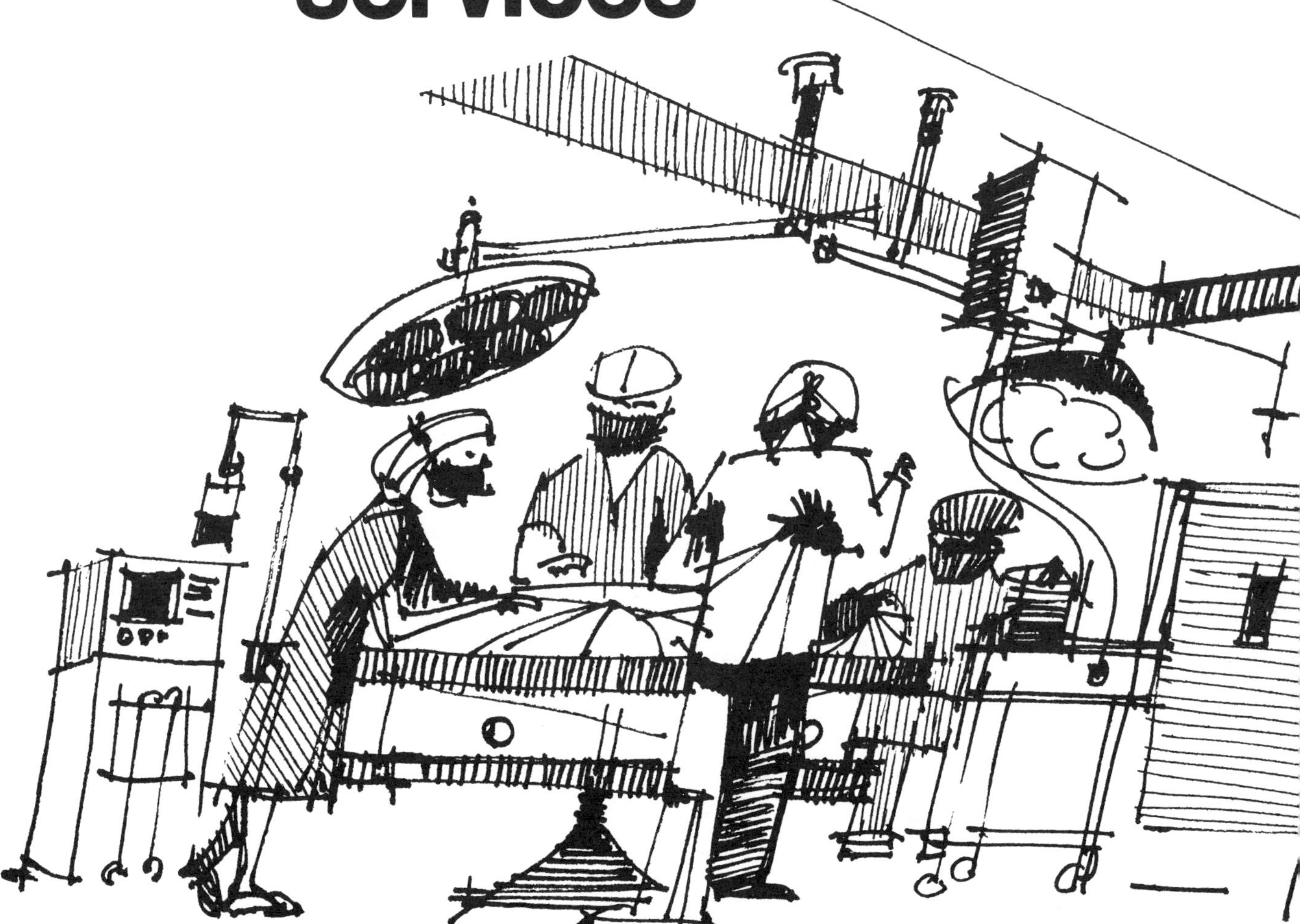

The medical service areas of a health care facility are those areas dedicated to specific diagnostic and treatment procedures. Many of these procedures are not only specialized as such but require equipment with extraordinary utility hook-ups and structural housing requirements. Because of these requirements, the individual areas categorized within medical services are physically the most varied and least interchangeable in the health care facility and careful attention must be paid to their design and construction.

AMBULATORY HEALTH

The concept of ambulatory care is not new, but it has been associated in the past with bargain basement care that is offered to supply clinical cases for medical education programs from the indigent segment of the community. Traditionally, this care has been offered in older sections of hospitals under less than ideal physical surroundings. Modern hospitals must change this stereotype. The number of ambulatory patients is increasing for many reasons, among them the notion that expensive in-house beds should be reserved for acutely ill patients and for as short a period of time as possible. It is becoming obvious that in the future many conditions formerly requiring in-house care can, should, and will be treated on an outpatient basis.

Primary health care centers and neighborhood clinics have made their appearance in various sections of the community; more recently, health maintenance organizations and other prepaid health insurance plans through affiliation

Department	Gross Square Feet per Bed
Ambulatory health center	
Emergency services	10-15
Outpatient services	10
Laboratory substation	2
Social services	1
Admissions and discharge	2
Clinical laboratory and pathology	35
Delivery Suite	13
Nurseries	7
Diagnostic radiology	40
Radiation therapy	10-14
Nuclear medicine	4-6
Human functions	
Inhalation therapy	2
Electrocardiography (EKG)	2
Electroencephalography (EEG)	1-2
Speech and hearing therapy	1
Rehabilitative medicine	
Physical therapy	12
Occupational & recreational therapy	2
Surgery	40-50
Medical staff facilities	3-4

with the local community hospital are being built in the community which offer a wide range of health services. All of these approaches attempt to coordinate the services of the private physician, the hospital, and the existing community health agencies.

The ambulatory care section of the hospital is designed to be a hospital-based ambulatory health center devoted to meeting the changing demands of the community it serves in a facility that offers excellence in patient care. The emphasis is on patient care rather than research or education.

Ambulatory care is defined, broadly, as all health services rendered to patients who need not be hospitalized and who can actively participate in meeting most of their own health needs. Heavy emphasis is placed on preventive services, rehabilitation and long-term care, patient education, and post-acute care after an early discharge from the in-house services. It will offer specialty clinics and diagnostic and treatment services to community physicians, related health agencies, and its own hospitalized patients.

The ambulatory health center should have as its nucleus the emergency services for acute care and the outpatient services for preventive, long-term health maintenance, patient education, and specialty clinics. It is also recommended that admission and discharge, social services, X-ray facilities, a laboratory substation, and a pharmacy dispatch center be part of this nucleus or as close to it as possible. Direct communication is necessary with rehabilitative services, medical records, radiology, nuclear medicine, radiation therapy, mental health, and the business

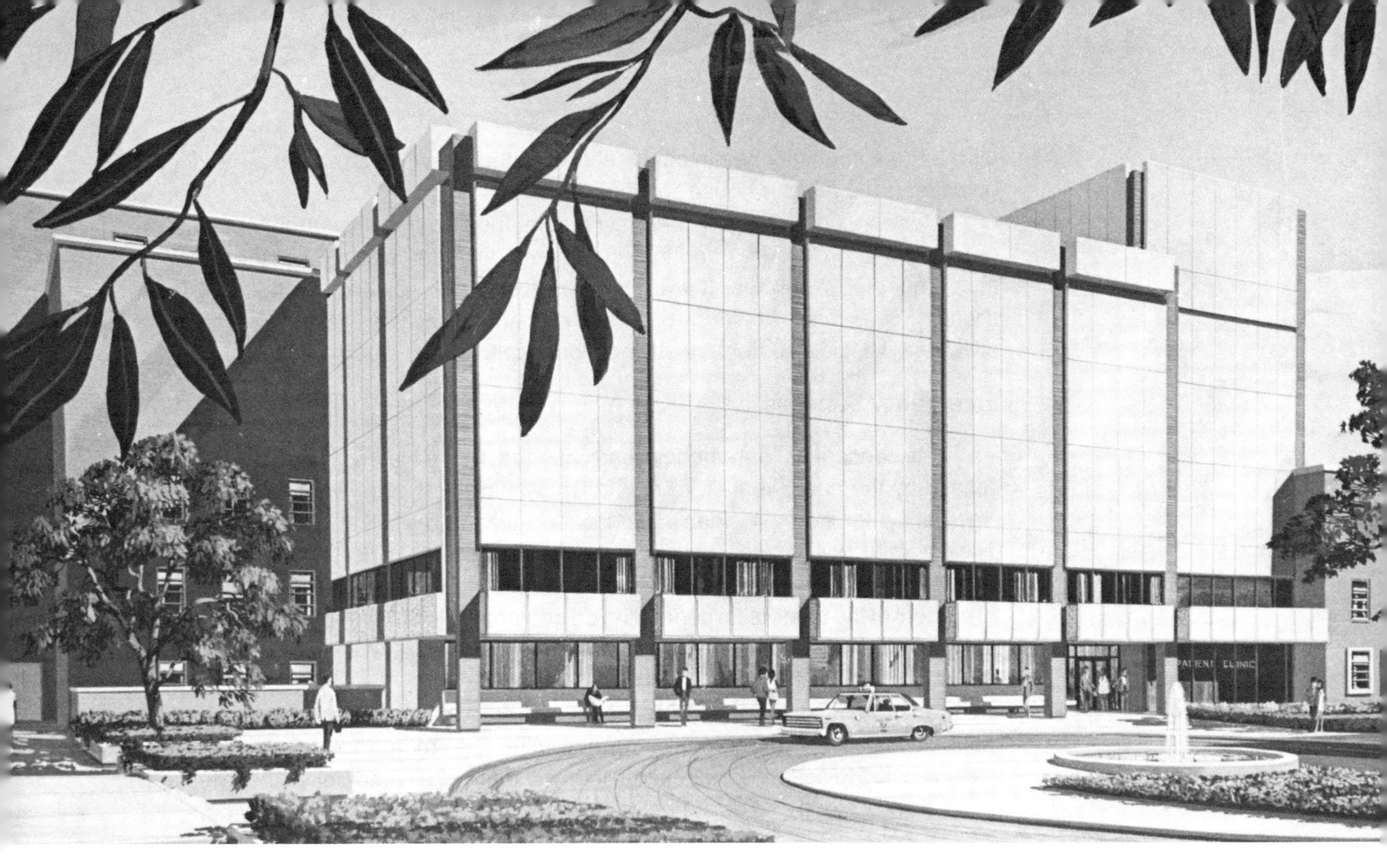

Ambulatory care unit. Washington Hospital Center, Washington, D.C.

Ambulatory Health Center, Interdepartmental Relationships

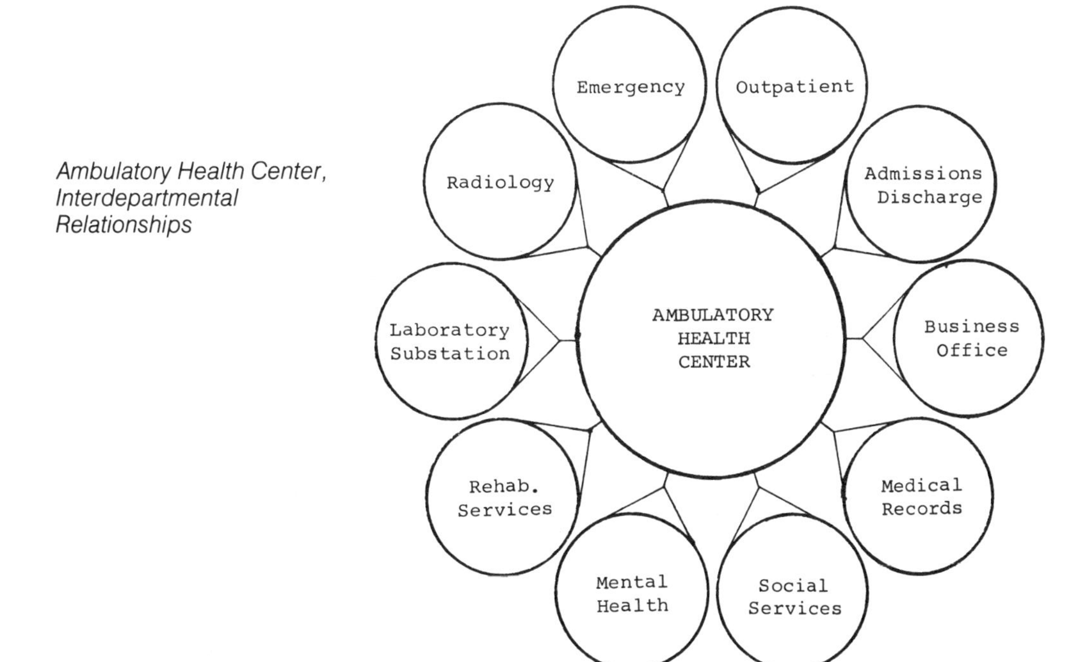

office. The ambulatory health center should further serve as a referral center for all outpatients requiring in-house services.

This concept of patient care may require modifications in current operational concepts and procedures and in departmental attitudes and relationships, and it may require new policies. It will offer, however, more flexibility to meet the fast-changing concepts in health care, greater efficiency in the use of acute-care hospital space and specialized personnel, and more health care for more people.

Emergency Services

The concept of "emergency" has changed from a life and death situation, as defined by the hospital staff, to the patient's interpretation of what constitutes an emergency: for example, inability to locate a private physician, a closed doctor's office, a visitor with no local physician, or a patient who does not feel he can afford a physician. Severe emergencies requiring hospital admission will constitute only 5–20 percent of the total visits, depending on geographic location. The remaining visits can best be described as outpatient visits occurring twenty-four hours rather than the usual eight.

Emergency rooms tend to act as primary care, minor surgery, and outpatient areas when separate programs are not available. The emergency room may also be oversized due to seasonal recreation or tourist traffic in a community. These factors must be understood and documented because they affect the space required.

Planners for emergency services facilities must recognize these changes in function, concept, and demand from the community. They must incorporate flexibility and organize facilities to handle all extremes of emergencies in the most economical and efficient use of space, equipment, personnel, and supplies. Clearly defined policies and procedures are imperative for protection of the patients and the hospital. The emergency program should also fit into a regional or statewide concept for trauma treatment.

Location. Receiving patients and families for primary, or trauma, emergency care and for observation, treatment, discharge, referral, or admission after treatment are functions of emergency services. Parking needs for emergency vehicles, rescue squads, ambulance services, private cars and public transportation must be met adjacent to this department. This department becomes the main entrance during night hours and, thus, must relate to the public and vehicle transportation.

Traffic control within the suite is also critical as the emotions surrounding trauma run very high. A direct relationship to radiology is necessary for timing and movement. The emergency room does not, however, have to be adjacent to the laboratory. Admission, records, and payment for emergency can be entirely in the department or, better, combined with admissions and cashier. Access to patient-staff elevators in order to proceed to surgery is vital in the placement of emergency.

A covered entrance at minimum slope on ground level is the preferred design. Separate waiting facilities for the family, convenient to vending machines or public service, should also be considered.

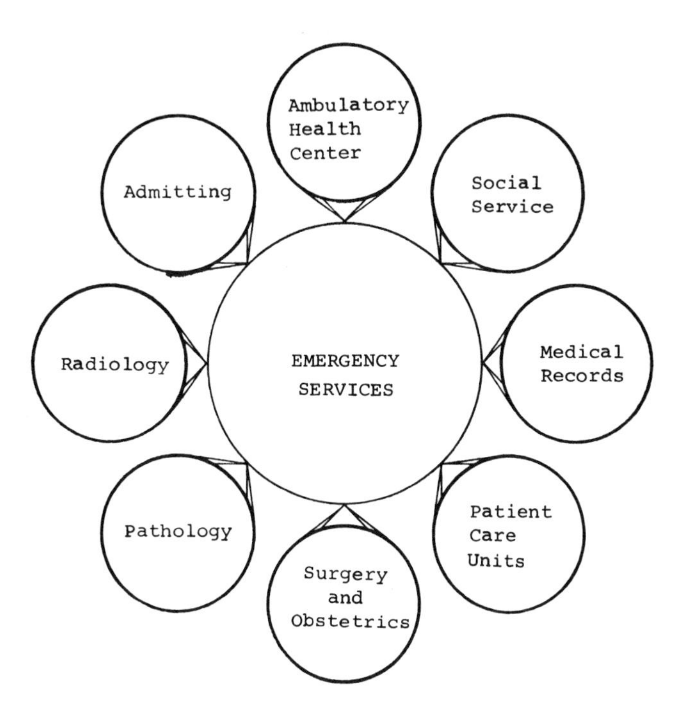

Emergency Services, Interdepartmental Relationships

Design. Size of the department is based upon the ratio of yearly number of visits divided by a factor of visits per gross square feet; four visits per gross square foot is recommended. Emergency service size can also be calculated by setting up a model of the annual number of hours in operation and then determining the average number of visits per hour:

$$\frac{\text{projected visits}}{\text{hours open per year}} = \text{average visits per hour}$$

Suite design should be based upon quick access to the patient by staff and supplies. Holding areas for observation and separate containment areas are often required. Excellent mechanical systems must be designed for procedure requirements and comfort control. The size of treatment rooms is based upon procedures performed. Minor surgery, casts, and multiple trauma must all be considered in the design.

By estimating peak loads and assigning thirty minutes per visit, the number of treatment rooms can be calculated:

$$\frac{\text{visits per hour}}{\text{thirty minutes}} = \text{rooms needed}$$

Intradepartmental Relationships. The administrative area is made up of a reception–control area and a visitor waiting room. The reception–control area is in the entrance lobby to receive patients and relatives. After the data necessary to initiate chart and treatment are secured, patients are sent to triage and visitors and relatives

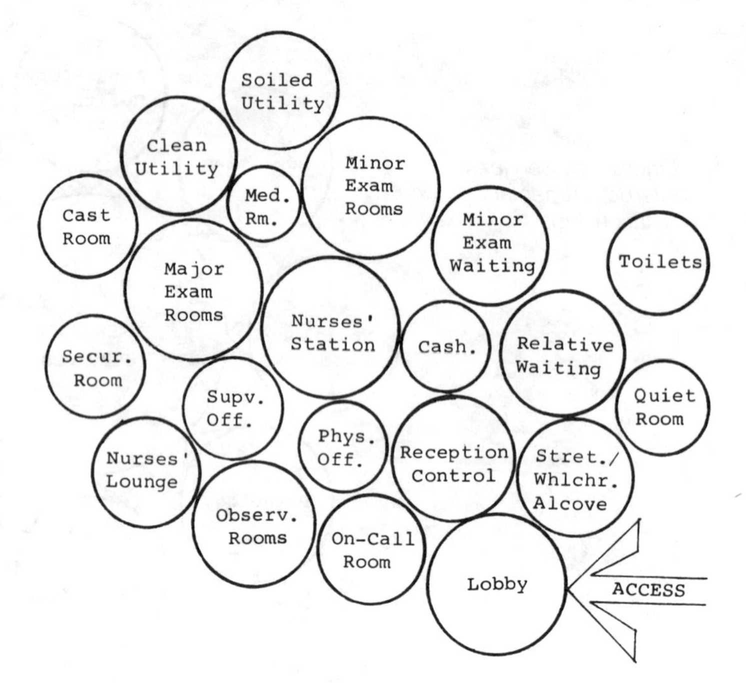

Emergency Services, Intradepartmental Relationships

are directed to an adjacent waiting area. This is a main center of communication and should include equipment for contact within the service and to other areas.

The waiting room is off the reception–control area but under its observation. Waiting visitors and relatives should not be able to see into or hear activities in reception–control or the treatment area, or be able to observe major emergencies entering emergency. Furnishings should create the best possible image of the hospital and there should be a nourishment center in the room plus wall-mounted public telephones. The area should, however, be arranged so that parents can accompany children into treatment areas for minor care and observation, and a children's playroom should be either adjacent to the waiting room or part of the larger waiting room. Separate toilets for men and women should be provided adjacent to the waiting rooms.

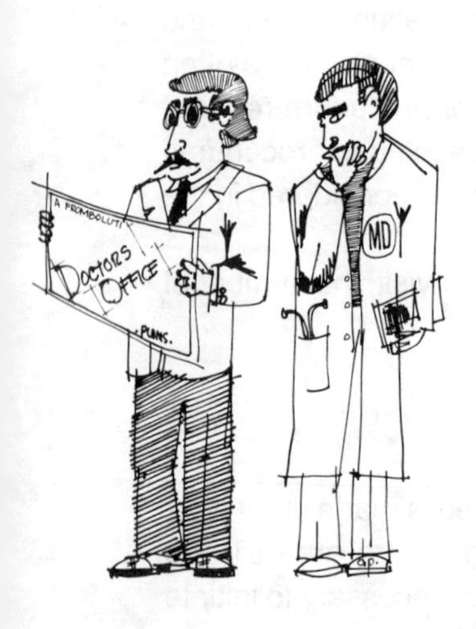

The physician's office should be off the triage reception area for private discussion with relatives. It should contain dictation equipment, as well as regular office equipment, and it may be used by private physicians or emergency service physicians. A quiet room should be adjacent to reception, but separate from waiting rooms. It is used by press and police for interviews and by physicians to control upset relatives and to give consultations.

The on-call room should be located in the administrative area as far away from the reception and activity center as possible. It should be large enough for sleeping accommodations and office equipment for the use of emergency service physicians.

Cashiering and billing should be off the reception desk near the exit from the treatment area. Insurance is checked and the bill prepared, explained, and collected after patients receive treatment and before they leave the service.

The treatment area is enclosed and separated from the waiting area and reception–control. This separation is designed to control which relatives and visitors may enter the treatment area and is necessary to eliminate misinterpretation of activities and the overhearing of privileged conversations. Major examination rooms should be close to the entrance and the physicians' and nurses' stations. They should be connected to one another and should contain oxygen, suction, air, monitoring equipment, surgical lighting, equipment storage area, sink, and a desk. In general, these rooms are similar to intensive care rooms with the addition of a surgical light. They should have direct access to radiology.

The nursing station is adjacent to the physician office and close to the entrance. It must have access to both major and minor examination rooms with a minimum of travel plus easy access to the medicine room (under nursing station control) and the clean and soiled utility rooms (equipped similarly to those designed for the nursing units). A nourishment station (for coffee, soups, and so on) should be in the clean utility room. Both should be close to the major and minor examination rooms.

Minor examination rooms are grouped together away from the traffic flow of major examination rooms. They should be close to the entrance (for ambulatory patients) and equipped as general treatment rooms with the addition of items such as oxygen, suction, air, good lighting, wall-mounted otoscopes. They should be close to outpatient services so facilities such as the eye room, the cast room, and the ear, nose, and throat room can be shared. They should have easy access to the nursing station and to utility rooms. There should be a small waiting room for patients waiting for minor treatment rooms. This allows for removal of minor cases from the waiting area and expedites treatment of patients. Patient toilets should be located for easy access by patients in minor examination rooms. They should contain support bars, a call system, and barrier free design.

Observation rooms are designed primarily to hold patients and clear major rooms as soon as possible. They should be similar to a patient room in equipment and facilities. They should be located away from the entrance and used for emergency care, not as an admission ward. The security room is designed to hold psychiatric patients. It should be a self-contained unit with a toilet. Operational procedures should allow these patients to be admitted directly to the mental health unit.

The supervisor's office should be centrally located and adjacent to the nurses' lounge. There should be a connection at the extreme end of the emergency room to the outpatient department for access to specific facilities in that area. The nurses' lounge should be away from the main traffic flow, but close enough for nurses to be available in the treatment area at a minute's notice. It should contain toilets, couch, chairs, table, and small lockers.

Outpatient Services

Most hospitals have been experiencing tremendous growth in number of visits to and types of services demanded of the outpatient department. Planning must, therefore, provide flexibility and expansion potential and design must consider maximum utilization of space, equipment, and personnel. Control of patient, personnel, and supply traffic is imperative.

Emphasis at this time is on multipurpose examination rooms or broad clinics, such as health maintenance, general medical, and surgical, as well as on specific clinics, such as eye, surgery, dental, and ear, nose, and throat. There is a growing emphasis on multiphasic screening for new patients, health maintenance, prevention, and educational programs. Planning provides for all ambulatory patients, whether referred to the outpatient clinics and services or to ancillary areas of ambulatory care (such as laboratory, admissions, radiology, human functions, and physical therapy), to be scheduled and processed through the outpatient department.

Outpatient Department, Interdepartmental Relationships

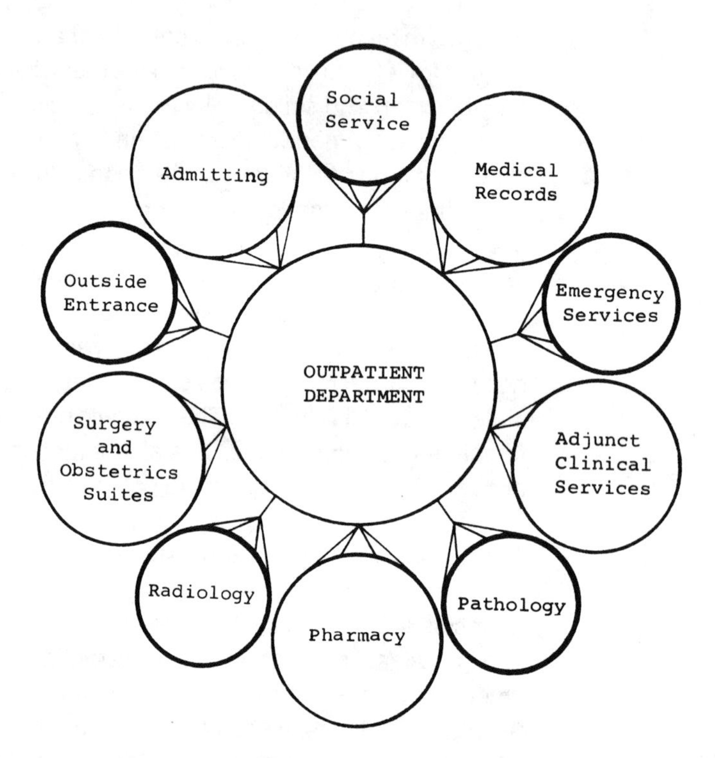

Location. Outpatient services should be adjacent to emergency services, social services, admissions, a laboratory substation, and medical records. There should be rapid access to radiology, human functions, physical therapy, nuclear medicine, and radiation therapy. Rapid service should be available from the pharmacy also. Outpatient services should be on the ground level with its own entrance from its own parking lot and must be able to handle wheelchair and stretcher patients without hazard to walking patients.

Design. The outpatient department is basically a separate entity. It is recommended, however, that doors be installed between emergency services and outpatient services to allow certain specialty areas to be available to emergency services after outpatient hours. For security reasons, the major portion of outpatient services should be locked at a specific time. Every effort should be made to supply necessary services in a manner that approximates a visit to a private physician and to retain the patient's self-esteem while receiving care in this facility. The patient is visualized as moving from the special entrance to the receptionist, the specific clinic, the appointments clerk, the cashier and billing, and then out until the next appointment. The total number of visits per year divided by the factor of visits per gross square feet of space equal the department size. A factor of eight to ten visits per gross square foot is recommended. The following calculations are made in determining size of examination rooms:

2 visits per room per hour × 4 clinic hours per day =
8 visits per room per clinic day × 220 clinic days per year =
1760 visits per room per year

The total number of visits to the clinics (that is, to general clinics, specialty clinics, primary care clinics, and private clinics) is divided by the number of visits per examination room per year to get the number of square feet per examination room. Space must be added for support services.

A central appointments area channels all inside and outside calls for appointments to clinics and ancillary services. The use of private offices allows additional services to be developed (for example, psychology, nutrition, nurse clinicians). This concept increases the use of space and the flexibility of the service. Rooms are to be equipped for multiple uses and given enough flexibility to be used as specialty clinics when the need arises. Changes of equipment should be the only changes necessary to transform the rooms into specialty rooms. Examination rooms also serve as preparation and recovery rooms for ambulatory surgery.

A patient education room provides preventive care through planned lectures for patients waiting for physicians. Such classes might include orientation of inpatients to outpatient services facilities and functions, prenatal care, and Medicare and Medicaid benefits.

Intradepartmental Relationships. Outpatient services is divided into two major areas: administration and treatment. Administration includes the following areas:

—lobby-waiting
—cashier-billing
—reception–control
—central appointments
—registrar-interview
—manager secretary
—nurse supervisor

The lobby-waiting area is at the entrance to the department and is under the observation and control of the receptionist. Cashier-billing is off the waiting area, with the same control as the receptionist over patients entering and leaving the department, allowing them to control billing and collection.

Outpatient Services, Intradepartmental Relationships

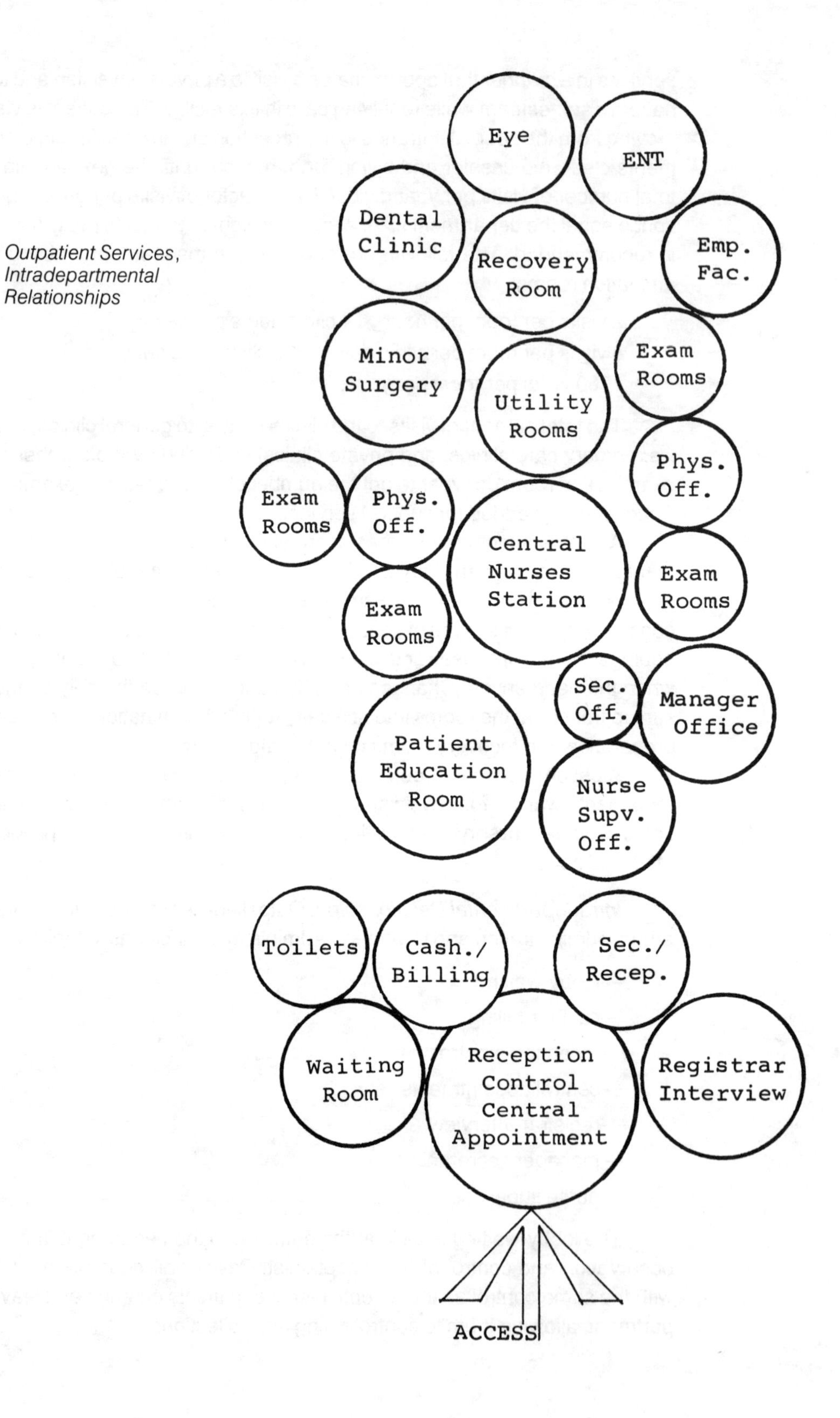

Reception–control and central appointments areas are located off the lobby-waiting area to receive and direct patients. The department should be designed so that, at the end of a visit, the patient must pass this area on his way out. Future tests or visits, as ordered by the physician, will be scheduled here. The registrar-interview area is for interviewing new patients, determining their eligibility for a clinic, and beginning their charts. It should be located off the lobby-waiting area.

The manager secretary and nurse supervisor should have adjoining offices forming an administrative suite. I recommend that they coordinate ambulatory care services from this location.

The patient education room is a classroom and a conference-library area for the department. It should be located close to the administrative offices and the treatment areas.

The treatment area is divided into three unequal parts: diagnostic and screening clinic, general clinics, and specialty clinics. The size of each facility depends on administrative decisions defining the extent of care to be offered to ambulatory patients.

The diagnostic and screening clinic should be located to one side of the treatment area and close to the administrative offices. This clinic serves as a health maintenance clinic, gives initial physical examinations, and should be equipped for multiphasic screening procedures. The physician's office is located between two examination rooms equipped for special purposes. The examination rooms might also serve as a pediatric clinic or as a preparation room for ambulatory surgery. The general clinics are in a multipurpose area and form the center of the treatment area. Screening and specialty areas should be on the periphery of this area, within easy access. The examination rooms are visualized as rooms with good overhead lighting, a sink, wall-mounted scopes, manometer, and X-ray view screens. The physician's office is placed between two examination rooms. Intra-communication allows the physician to call his own next patient and schedule the next patient visit or diagnostic test with the appointments clerk. The central nursing station is at the entry to the treatment area and contains medicine closet, charting area, and communications equipment. It is adjacent to utility rooms and has quick access to examination rooms, surgery, and so on. The clean and soiled utility rooms are adjacent to the nursing station and central to treatment areas. They should contain storage space, a work counter, and storage for backup carts.

The specialty clinics are designed for diagnostic and treatment procedures requiring specialized, fixed and movable equipment. They should be planned with as much flexibility and utilization as possible (for example, cyctoscopies and proctoscopies should be scheduled in minor surgery). These clinics should be at the distal end of the outpatient department and connected to emergency services. Design should allow for the specialty clinics to become part of emergency services when the rest of the outpatient department is closed. The dental clinic should be equipped for routine dental work, X-ray, and emergency work. There should be a small area for laboratory work, film developing (ninety-second), and film storage. Ophthalmology and otorhinolaryngology clinics should be equipped to handle emergencies, routine examinations and treatments, and procedures not available in the specialist's office.

Rooms should be equipped for minor surgeries not requiring general anesthesia and for general diagnostic procedures. They should function as a surgical center and be available to area physicians for ambulatory cases not requiring overnight care. Cases should be scheduled but allowing some flexibility to handle emergencies. A recovery room to hold patients for observation after surgery or treatment should be within easy access of minor surgery, dental, eye, and ear, nose, and throat clinics. It is suggested that this area be visible from the nurses' station for supervision and observation. There should also be a toilet off the recovery room. Other specialty clinics might be available, including high risk obstetrics, neurology, orthopedics, diabetes, arthritis, kidney, gastrointestinal, thoracic, plastic surgery, dermatology, and endocrinology.

Home Care

The trend toward providing out-of-hospital health services has accelerated sharply since 1966. All segments of the health care delivery system have had to reorient themselves to new obligations and, in many instances, new opportunities for service. Home health services have been established in various agencies as well as hospitals. The services offered include all or part of the following: home nursing care, physical therapy, occupational therapy, nutrition, speech therapy, social service, and home health aids. Perhaps the greatest contribution of home health services to their patients would be to coordinate existing services in the community and in the hospital. Home care for discharged patients, patient visits to selected hospital services, and assistance on admission to the hospital would certainly be proper responsibilities of the hospital home health services. Once actual community needs are determined, some consideration should be given to extending home health services beyond planning and coordination.

Location. This service should be located in the ambulatory health center, if possible, near admissions and discharge, social services, physical therapy, outpatient services, emergency services, and outside entrances. It should include a coordinator's office, secretary and file space, and a waiting area.

Laboratory Substation

The advantages of a centralized clinical laboratory are well known and documented. The disadvantages tend to be minimized in discussion, but they create some of the major problems in the efficient functioning of the laboratory.

Centralization means that the ambulatory patients from outpatient services, admissions, emergency services, and private physician offices, in addition to inpatients, must be handled in the laboratory facilities designed primarily to handle specimens. The tendency in such a situation has been to regard the needs of the ambulatory patients as an interruption to the established daily workload necessary to meet in-house patient needs. The increased use of automation in the laboratory has compounded this problem. The ambulatory patient must now wait for a "run" to be completed before his test can be programmed. This means that the patient must wait in an area where he can misinterpret many of the personnel's actions and comments and overhear data that should be confidential.

The admissions departments of modern hospitals have encouraged pre-admissions procedures to shorten the time between the patient's arrival at the hospital door and his being established in his room. The tendency has been to set up procedures whereby laboratory personnel are sent throughout the hospital to collect the specimens. This is costly in both personnel and time.

Emergency service requests are usually for simple, routine tests to speed the physician in establishing his treatment plan or sending the patient home. These orders interfere with routine laboratory work and are costly in personnel and time. Requests from outpatient services are usually not urgent. Problems arise when attempting to schedule the patient for testing at the convenience of the laboratory. The patient often has to make a separate visit for testing or wait until the laboratory is free. More often the former prevails, with an unhappy patient facing problems of transportation, babysitting, even time off the job to obtain these diagnostic services. This is difficult for the patient to understand and leads to poor hospital image.

Functions. A laboratory substation would improve laboratory service to ambulatory patients and would have major advantages. New procedures could be implemented for pre-admission workup in the substation; this would place patients from admissions in their rooms shortly after arrival. Urgent admissions and emergency service cases could be served more rapidly in the emergency area, with a minimum of disruption to the central laboratory. Laboratory needs of private and regular ambulatory patients could be handled at the time of visit. Procedures involving patients and specimens would be in separate areas, thus improving the quality and delivery of service and care. Inpatient stat requests could be handled in this facility to eliminate interruptions of routine operational procedures.

Location. The laboratory substation should be adjacent to emergency services, outpatient services, and admissions. Proximity to medical records and the business office would also be an advantage. A minimum of personnel, space, and equipment would be necessary to establish this substation. It would require the same utilities and basic module considered necessary for the laboratory area and would include a work area, toilets for patients, and venipuncture booths.

Social Services

The concept of total health care has resulted in an increased use of social services. The department goal is to contribute to the total medical care provided by the health team and is directed toward achieving the optimum state of patient health.

Functions. The function of the department is to aid the physician and the community in rendering quality care to the patient. Department objectives are achieved in collaboration with physician, nurse, administrative staff, and other personnel involved in the patient's care. These objectives are to:

—give the entire health team a better understanding of the patient in relation to his social and emotional environment

—help the patient and family accept the illness and any residual physical disability

—assist the patient and family with problems precipitated by the illness

—encourage optimum utilization of medical care

—encourage more effective use of hospital beds for the acutely ill through utilization of other community resources for the chronically ill

—encourage development of new resources for unmet social service needs

—participate in studies that will contribute to improved patient care and health programs in the community

The specific purpose of the department is to enable the patient to make full use of medical care, both preventive and therapeutic, and to achieve the fullest possible physical, emotional and social adjustment.

Location. Since the department is involved with both inpatients and outpatients, it is desirable that the director of social services be located in an area that facilitates communication with other department heads. Two approaches are currently prevalent:

—a dispersed department with offices located in the inpatient area for easy access to patients and staff

—a centralized department with offices in one area and workers scattered about as needed.

Ideally, the department should be centrally located, near the ambulatory care area, medical records, physical therapy, and admissions (and discharge) and should have easy access to physicians' lounge, finance, and administration.

Intradepartmental Relationships. Basically, the department is a suite of offices with privacy for interviews, conferences, telephone calls, and dictation. It would include a director's office, receptionist-secretary, waiting room, workers' offices, supply storage, conference room-library, and toilets.

CLINICAL PATHOLOGY LABORATORIES

The clinical pathology laboratory is very complex and is best described by dividing it according to function.

Functions. The hematology division is dedicated to performing those laboratory procedures which pertain to diseases of the blood and blood-forming organs. The blood bank and blood transfusion division is involved in typing and crossmatching bloods; blood fractioning, processing, and stocking; and blood donor programs.

The clinical chemistry division performs quantitative and qualitative analyses of substances found in many tissues, body fluids, and secretions. Clinical chemistry may be further subdivided for functional and organizational purposes into automated, routine, special, and radioisotope. Radioisotope studies (wet) measure the

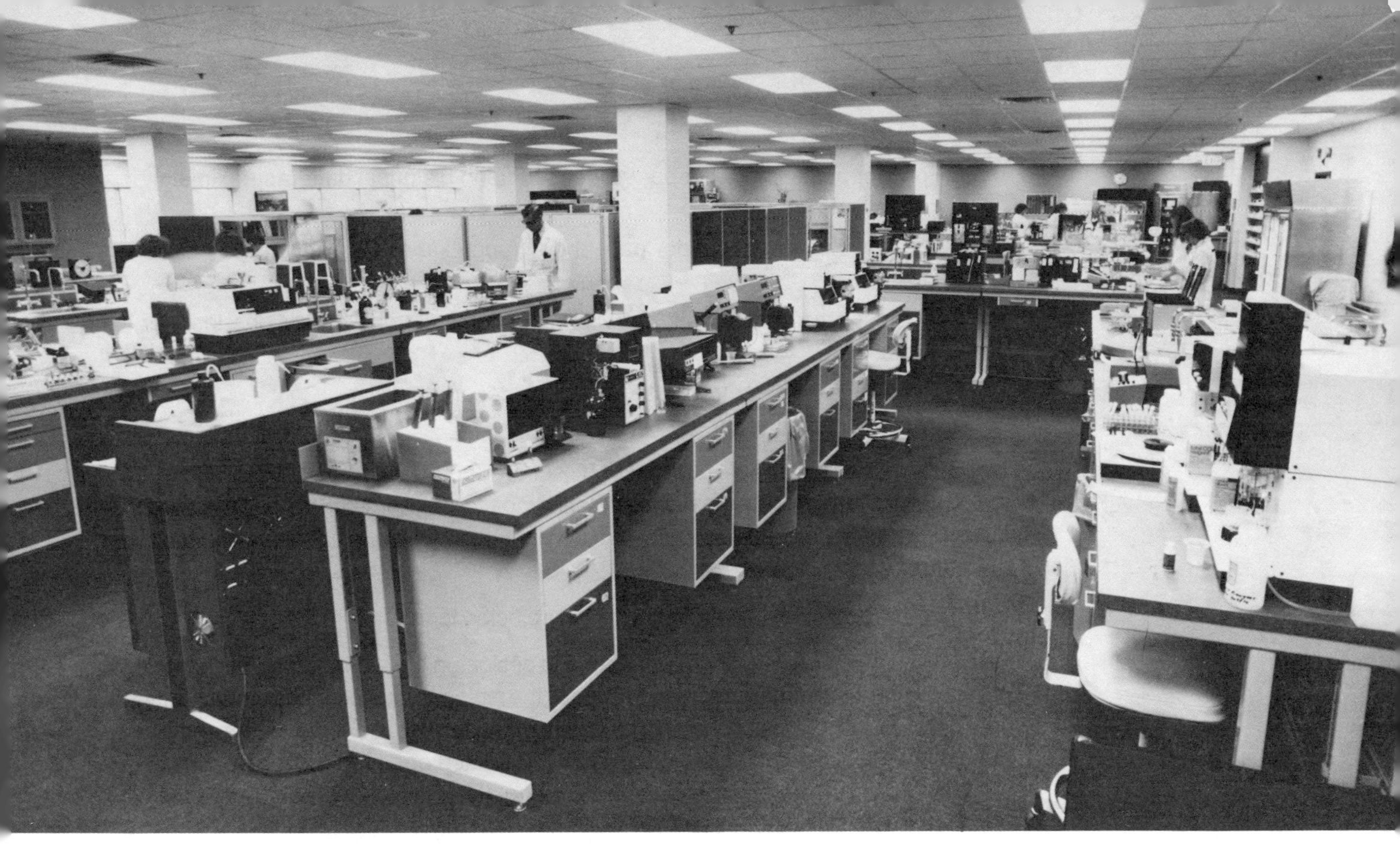

Pathology Laboratory. St. Luke's Medical Center, Sioux City, Iowa

utilization of radioactive chemicals (radioisotopes) in the diagnosis and treatment of disease. Special chemistry studies may include endocrinology and toxicology determinations.

The clinical microscopy division performs a variety of studies that really do not fit into any one given area of the laboratory. These include urinalysis, semen analysis, and gastric analysis.

Microbiology and parasitology study microorganisms, bacteria, fungi, viruses, and pathogenic protozoas.

Serology, or immunology, is the division that monitors immunologic disease through laboratory testing.

Cytopathology examines and interprets cells from body fluids and secretions for diagnosis of malignancy, effects of hormones, and so on.

Location. The laboratory should serve and be convenient to the ambulatory care units of emergency and outpatient, surgery and obstetrics, radiology, and intensive care.

The autopsy area should be included in a pathology department, with an easy access to emergency and the patient units through nonpublic corridors. The morgue should have access to an outside mortuary-ambulance dock in a nonpublic space.

Design. The amount of space needed by this department can be calculated as follows:

—project outpatient tests per visit based upon historical data (approximately three tests per visit)

—project inpatient tests per patient day (approximately twenty tests per patient day)

—project emergency tests per visit (approximately one-half to one test per visit)

$$\frac{\text{total tests per year (projected)}}{\text{tests per square foot}} = \text{gross department size}$$

Use 50–70 (custom up to 100) tests per square foot, based upon automation of the lab. An alternative means of calculating space is to project tests per patient discharge (same as admissions; that is, approximately three tests per patient discharge).

$$\text{admissions} \times \text{tests per discharge} = \text{projected tests}$$

The use of modules is recommended in designing the laboratory. This applies not only to the work station design, but also to the piping layout for the essential utility services. For the work stations, ten feet by twenty feet will give room at one end for equipment and casework used jointly between related open modules. The dimensions desired are workbenches twelve feet long, thirty inches high, with a working depth of twenty-three inches to offer maximum flexibility.

Modules should be open within subdivisions and closed between subdivisions. The open concept can be landscaped with movable partitions for flexibility. Open areas include hematology, urinalysis, biochemistry, chemistry, automated analyzer center, and secretarial-clerical areas. Closed areas include bacteriology, parasitology, serology, pathology-histology, sterilization and glass washing, blood bank, and offices.

The laboratory needs hot, cold, distilled and ionized water. Not all laboratory subdivisions require all kinds of water; however, flexibility is enhanced if each unit can be converted easily by adding or deleting portable equipment. Because distilled water will meet or exceed every requirement for water in the laboratory, it should be piped to all points where water is used.

Air conditioning, with a well-defined pattern of air movement, is necessary to provide an acceptable environment in the laboratory. Chemical fumes, vapors, heat from equipment, and the undesirability of open windows contribute to this need. A slightly negative air pressure, relative to other hospital areas, should be maintained in the laboratory because of contaminants and odors that originate there. Strict attention must be given to the effect of the various hoods required in certain of the laboratories on the problem of maintaining a smooth and controlled flow of conditioned air.

Intradepartmental Relationships. The following areas are needed: space for the major subdivisions, reception and waiting, blood donors, blood bank, automated equipment and computer room, glass washing, storage, administrative offices and

Clinical Pathology Laboratory, Intradepartmental Relationships

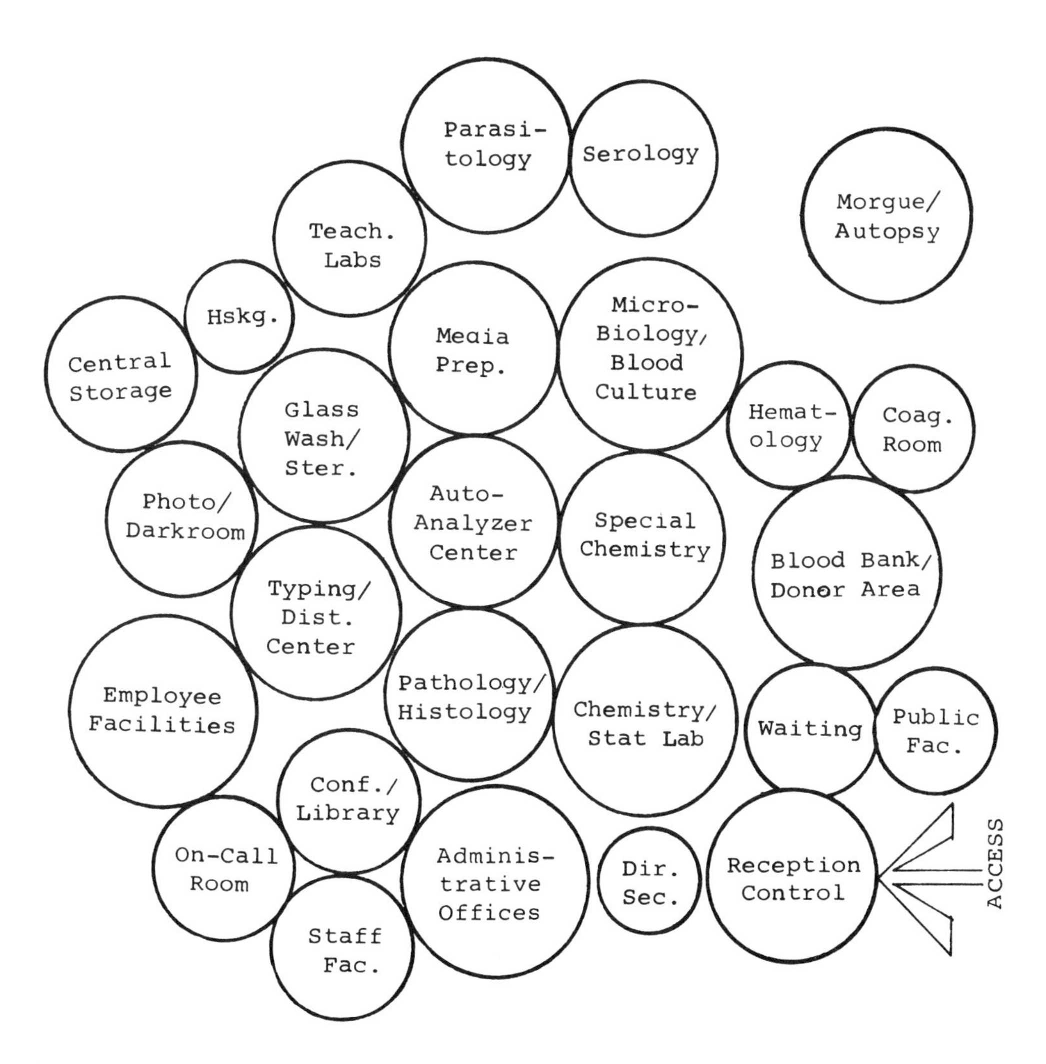

typing and distribution center, conference room-library, staff facilities, morgue, autopsy, specimen storage, and housekeeping.

Layout should reflect support relationships and incompatibilities: hematology should be adjacent to the blood bank, urinalysis adjacent to biochemistry. Pathology and histology units should be near access and support units (such as the cutting room, frozen section, cytology and the autopsy room). Bacteriology should be adjacent to serology and both should be located farthest away from other laboratories to minimize cross-contamination. A stat station should be located in the emergency portion of the laboratory near the entrance. A soiled glass collection and a flash specimen sterilization area must be accessible to all laboratory units, but closely related to microbiology, serology, and chemistry. The laboratory director's office should be adjacent to pathology and the secretarial–clerical areas should be central to the laboratories and the automated analysis center. Personnel facilities should be located for easy access by the whole staff.

DELIVERY SUITE

The delivery suite is basically a self-sufficient aseptic area that must be as remote as practicable from the entrance to the obstetrical service to reduce traffic and air turbulence and to provide privacy for the patient. It should be close to a vertical transport, to the nursery, and to the obstetrical nursing unit.

The delivery suite includes four areas of activity: labor, delivery, recovery, and support services. These areas should be located and related to facilitate movement of patients between them and observation of patients by the unit personnel.

Design. Estimate .22–.45 delivery per gross square foot and fifty deliveries per year per obstetrics bed. Labor rooms should be close to delivery rooms, but not so close that the two areas are intermixed or that patients can overhear or view delivery room procedures. They should provide maximum comfort and relaxation for the patient and should have facilities for examination, preparation, and observation.

Single rooms are recommended, as they eliminate the necessity for a patient preparation room and an observation room for questionable or infectious patients. Single rooms provide greater privacy for the patient and permit the father to visit during labor. Each labor room should have a lavatory with gooseneck-type spout and foot- or wrist-operated controls, soap dispensers, and paper towel dispensers for hand washing by the patient, the nurse, and the physician.

Doors should be four feet wide to allow passage of bed or stretcher. Each bed should be furnished with oxygen and suction outlets, nurse call system, and lighting controls. A toilet and lavatory for each labor room is desirable, although patient needs can be met with a toilet room, shower, and dressing cubicle facility convenient to all labor rooms. The patient's personal belongings can be put in her labor room or in a central locker room convenient to all labor rooms. Air conditioning, controlled humidity, and "piped in" music are desirable for this area. A nurse charting desk or area is also desirable.

Design of the delivery room should consider the welfare and safety of the mother and newborn. These include availability of equipment and supplies, built-in protection against anesthetic explosions, auxiliary electrical systems, adequate air conditioning, and finishes that promote aseptic conditions. Minimum size of a delivery room should be eighteen feet by eighteen feet. It is suggested that one delivery room in the suite be equipped for caesarean section. Serious consideration should be given to installing a fetal monitoring system. These systems are increasingly being considered necessary to good obstetrical care. Flooring should be conductive and installed in compliance with recommendations of the National Fire Protection Association. Ceilings should be made of a smooth, waterproof material for ease of cleaning.

An emergency call system, foot- or elbow-operated, must be installed in each delivery room; a dome light and buzzer must be in the corridor over each delivery room, in locker rooms, in the lounge, and at the nurses' station. A nurses' intercom system must be provided among these same areas as well as in the delivery room with connections to the fathers' waiting room to allow communication from the mother and physician to the prospective father.

Recovery rooms should be designed for close observation and special care of the mother by the labor-delivery nursing staff. Recovery can be in a delivery room, a labor room, a bed in the maternity nursing unit, or a room used exclusively for this purpose.

It is recommended that the hospital study the labor-recovery room concept, whereby the patient is placed in a labor room, is moved to delivery, and then returned to the same labor room for recovery care. This requires more labor rooms, but it minimizes square feet needed for the total suite, allows more patient privacy, minimizes utility outlets (such as suction and nurse call) and minimizes cleanup procedures for staff. Placed close to the entrance of the delivery suite, they allow the fathers to visit during labor and recovery with a minimum of penetration into the delivery suite. A labor-recovery room needs no more equipment than does a routine labor room.

A birthing room, set up for natural childbirth, has a home-like atmosphere and delivery support.

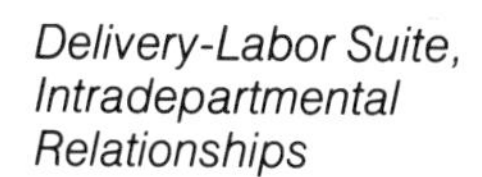

Delivery-Labor Suite, Intradepartmental Relationships

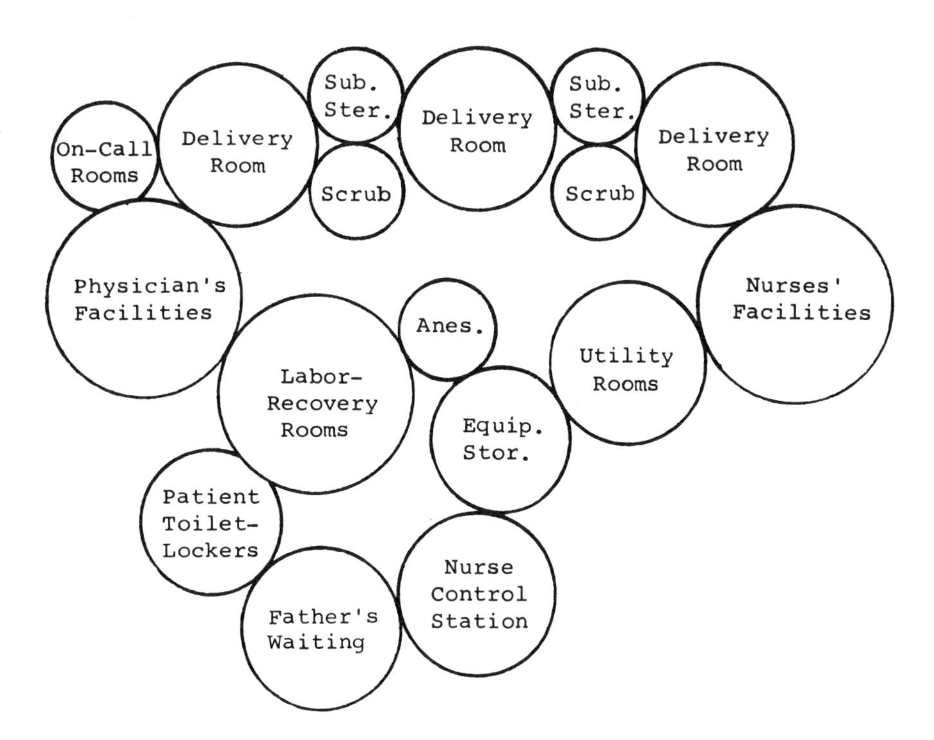

Intradepartmental Relationships. The nurses' station is the administrative control center of the suite. It should be located to control who enters the suite and have easy access to all areas of the suite and contain an intercom to all areas in the suite as well as telephone communications to all other areas of the hospital.

The physicians' facilities should contain a locker room, toilets, shower, and lounge. The locker room should hold lockers and benches and provide an area for clean scrub suits and an area for soiled linen. Adjacent to the locker room should be

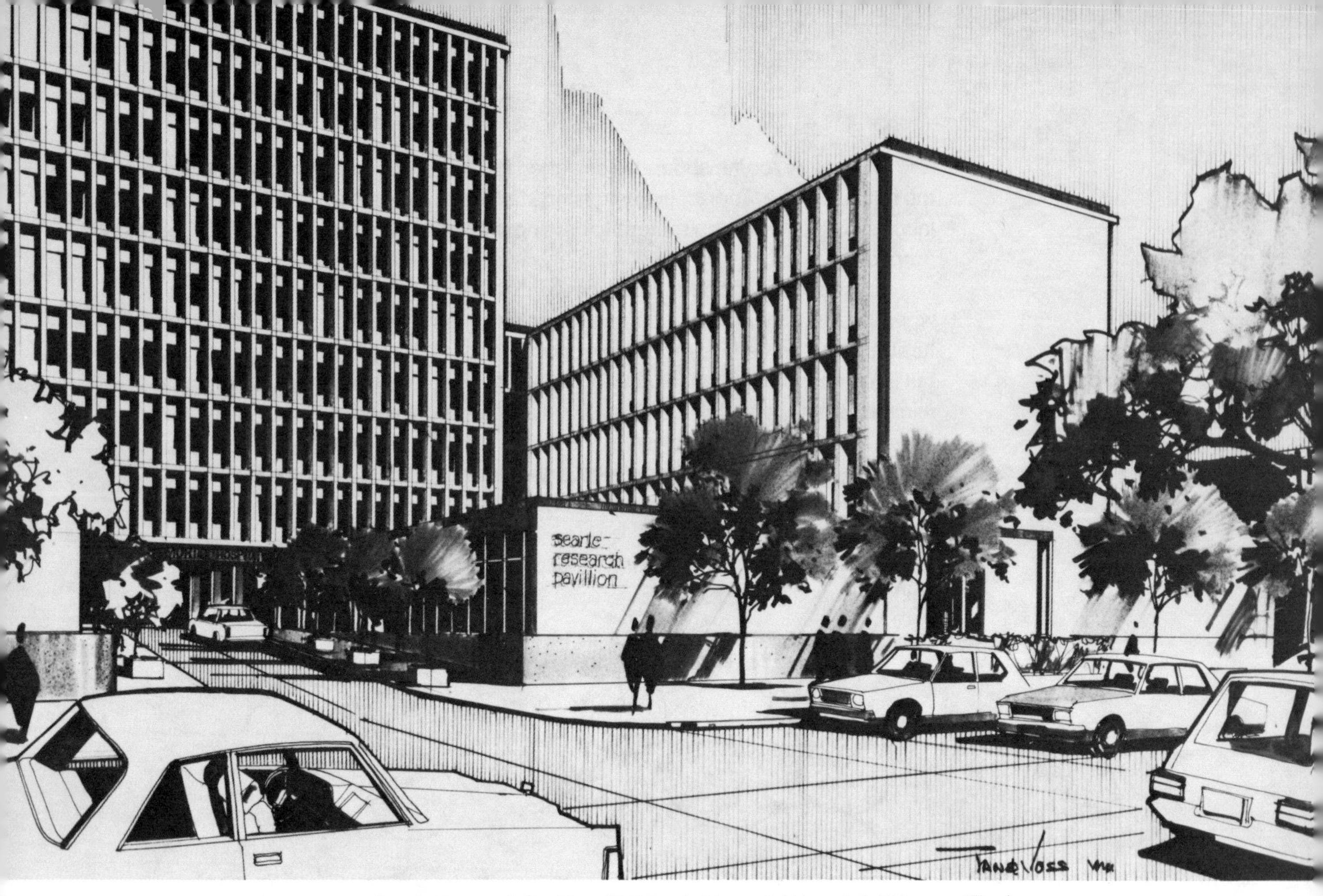

Searle Research Pavilion, Children's Memorial Hospital, Chicago, Illinois

toilets, lavatories, and showers with dressing cubicles. Movement into the suite should be from the outside, through the locker area, and then directly into the substerile area of delivery. The lounge should accommodate a couch, chairs, bookcase, and magazine table. A recessed film illuminator should be provided, as well as a desk and chair for chart work. Cubicles for dictation are also desirable. Nurses should have separate locker, toilet, and lounge facilities. Location and space requirements are similar to those of the physicians' facilities. It is recommended that a nourishment center be adjacent to both the nurses' and physicians' facilities. On-call rooms should have single sleeping accommodations so that they can be used by men and women.

Scrub and substerilization areas should be adjacent to the delivery rooms. One area including three scrub sinks should be available for every two rooms. The sinks should be equipped with gooseneck spouts, foot-operated controls, thermostatically controlled temperature valves, space for nail brushes, sterile caps, and masks, and an easily visible clock. Access from recessed scrub area to either delivery room should be easy. The substerilization area may also be shared between two delivery rooms and should include space for supply storage, a sink, and a high-speed washer-sterilizer for emergency sterilization.

The soiled-materials holding room should be centrally located for easy access from delivery rooms and labor-recovery rooms. It should be large enough to accommodate a sink, carts for soiled linen and trash, and storage space for germicidal solutions and utensils. The clean utility room should also be centrally located for easy access from delivery and labor-recovery rooms. Space should be allowed for clean linen carts, sink, and storage space for supplies. Medications may be centralized in this room, but locating them in the nurses' station may be preferred.

Requirements for anesthesia facilities can best be determined by the anesthesiologist: however, a room should be provided for storing gas cylinders and equipment. Space for storing a forty-eight-hour supply of gases is considered adequate. Gas storage rooms should not connect directly with delivery rooms, should have a conductive floor, and should be individually vented to the exterior of the building. Special attention must be given to electrical wiring and fixtures in this area.

The fathers' waiting room is a vital support area. It needs to be considered as part of the delivery-labor suite, although it does not necessarily have to be within the suite. It should be a comfortable waiting room, supplied with nourishment, and have easy access to the suite and the obstetrical nursing unit.

Space must be allocated, away from the stream of traffic, for storage of large pieces of equipment not frequently used but necessary to the unit.

NURSERIES

Concepts and principles of care in this area have evolved rapidly, with conflicting reports on the results obtained under any one design, location, or guiding concepts and principles. The traditional nursery has given way to the concept of nurseries: full-term newborns, observation, premature, isolation, high risk, and intensive care. Their physical location is decided by the chiefs of obstetrics and pediatrics and by the director of nursing, since availability of staff and professional philosophies influence their choice. This is especially true of isolation and premature nurseries. The tendency has increasingly been to locate these on the pediatric service, with the premature nursery as part of the neonatal intensive care unit.

Functions. In general, the nurseries should be planned to provide for the best means of care for the safety and the welfare of the infants, with space, facilities, and equipment designed to minimize the possibility of infections.

Location. The nurseries should be located in the obstetrical nursing unit as close to the mothers as possible. It is also desirable to locate the nurseries as close as possible to the labor-delivery suite in order to minimize travel distance and exposure of newborn.

Design. The number of infants in each nursery should be limited and may be regulated by state code. There should be wide spacing of bassinets within each nursery, separation of bassinets by cubicle partitions, and limits on the number of bassinets served by one nurses' station. There should be separate facilities for premature infants and for observation of infants suspected of having infectious conditions. All nurseries must provide optimum conditions of temperature, relative humidity, and ventilation. Space requirement standards vary from 30–60 square feet per bassinet.

Intradepartmental Relationships. Many hospitals plan a maximum of twelve bassinets in a full-term newborn nursery. Since normal staffing requirements indicate a need for one person to care for every six infants, larger nurseries do little to conserve staff. Smaller nurseries provide better conditions for care for infants, since cleaning the units is easier, and the possibility of one infant's incubating an infectious disease and subjecting all other infants to the same disease is minimized. The full-term newborn nursery should also contain the following facilities: clean area, camera room or area, examination room, physician's area, soiled holding area, formula room (breakout area), and locker-dressing and wash area for personnel, as well as a common lounge.

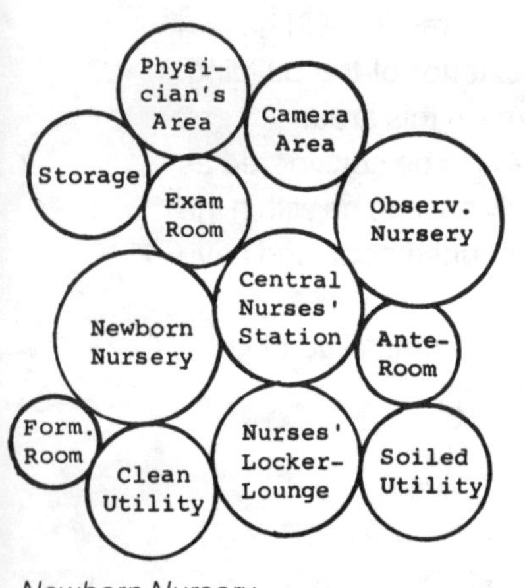

Newborn Nursery, Intradepartmental Relationships

The nurses' station is a control point. It also provides work space for the nurses and an area for treating infants. The desk should be placed so that the entrances from the corridor and from the station to the nurseries can be supervised. The nurseries should be visible through observation windows in the partitions. A rack for charts, a waste receptacle with foot-controlled cover, and two chairs will be needed.

Observation Nursery. An observation nursery should be provided for infants suspected of infection. When a positive diagnosis is made, the infant is transferred elsewhere in the hospital and placed on isolation precautions. If diagnosis is not positive, however, the infant may be returned to the regular nursery provided he has not been exposed to an infected infant in the observation nursery. The observation nursery should be a completely separate unit, but it should be located adjacent to a full-term nursery, with a glazed partition between to permit observation by the nursery staff. A minimum of forty square feet per bassinet is recommended to provide adequate space for bedside care and treatment of the infant.

An anteroom should be provided between the nursery and the corridor. This area should contain the same facilities as the work and treatment areas for full-term nurseries. Such facilities include a work counter for the nurse, a sink with gooseneck spout and knee or foot controls, a hook strip, and shelves or cabinet for clean gowns for the physician and nurse.

Premature Nursery. The premature nursery requires forty square feet of space per incubator or bassinet and is used for the care of infants with a low birth weight. This nursery, if located in pediatrics, may accept premature infants born outside the hospital; if the nursery is located in a postpartum unit, it is recommended that infants born outside the hospital not be admitted to this nursery.

In a premature nursery, where suitable environmnetal temperature and humidity are maintained, only 50–75 percent of the infants may require incubators. Aside from the incubators, furnishings for premature nurseries will be similar to those in full-term nurseries. A utility table, infant scales, and a rocking chair should be available for tending the premature babies who do not require incubators. One double oxygen outlet should be provided for every two bassinets or incubators, and each premature nursery should contain a centralized suction bulb or a mechanical suction device with a soft rubber tip and individual catheters for individual infants and a regulator to limit suction. The same work area facilities are needed for premature care as for full-term newborns. If the premature nurseries are to be located in postpartum, then locker rooms can be shared with the staff of the full-term newborn nursery. If it is to be located in pediatrics, an adjoining locker, dress, and wash area must be provided.

Isolation Nursery. An isolation nursery requires 50–60 square feet of space per bassinet and is designed for the care of infants who have an infectious disease. Infants requiring care in an isolation nursery have not usually been transferred from the hospital's other newborn nurseries, but rather have acquired the disease after having been discharged from the hospital.

Cubicles could be used to separate infants from each other, but research has shown that they are not very useful in preventing the spread of disease. An open room is, therefore, acceptable. Strict isolation techniques must be practiced by the staff in caring for these infants. The same elements for care of the infants are required in the isolation nursery as in the premature nursery. A clean utility area, examination room and work area, and soiled holding room are also required, as are facilities for staff to change and scrub.

DIAGNOSTIC RADIOLOGY

Functions. Diagnostic radiology is an ancillary department for the entire hospital facility. It serves both inpatient and outpatient needs and is critical in determining what treatment or surgical procedure is necessary. Nuclear medicine and scanning are likewise diagnostic tools. Radiation therapy is a treatment facility. Advances in technology and treatment within the fields of radiology and oncology will vary the space needs of the future. Improvement of image intensification, reduction exposure, radio and color scanning, new radioactive element selection, thermography (scanning with infrared light), sonography-ultrasonic visualization, wound sound scanning and echoencephalography, laser radiation, field emission X-ray tubes, xerography, and computer adaptions are all recent advances.

Location. Radiology should be adjacent to emergency, convenient to surgery, and accessible to inpatient travel from the bed units. A mix of both inpatient and outpatient services, this department and the department of radiation therapy should be located on ground level.

Design. Department of Health and Human Services guidelines suggest 3.4–4.5 procedures per gross square foot (g.s.f.). Department size can then be calculated as follows:

$$\frac{\text{projected procedures}}{\text{4 procedures per g.s.f.}} = \text{basic department size (g.s.f.)}$$

A method of computing examinations per discharge or admission will result in an average number of procedures per admission (2.5–3.5), adding the average of examinations per emergency visit (.10–.50), the total number of procedures can be calculated as follows:

inpatient admissions projected ×
(av. exams per admission) +
(emergency and outpatient visits projected ×
(av. exams per visit) =
total exams projected

Based upon a range of 5,000–6,000 procedures per room per year (4,000 inpatient and 7,000 outpatient), the number of radiology rooms required can be calculated:

$$\frac{\text{total procedures projected}}{\text{5,000-6,000 per room}} = \text{number of rooms}$$

The number of rooms multiplied by a gross square footage of 1,500 per room (includes entire X-ray space) yields the gross square footage needed for the entire department. Space for new technology such as linear accelerators and scanning must be added to the ratios and calculations above.

The combination cancer oncology–radiation therapy is a custom outpatient and inpatient program located with the ambulatory care, the clinic, or adjacent to radiology. A primary cancer center is designed to handle 300 new cases per year while a tertiary facility is designed for 500.

Intradepartmental Relationships. The reception–control area under direct observation should be located at the entrance to the department, adjacent to cashier-billing and the waiting room. The area should include a desk, pneumatic tube, and storage cabinets. The billing clerk might share the same area to handle insurance and payments by outpatients. Toilets, lockers, and dressing area should be part of the patient waiting area. A wheelchair and stretcher storage area should be located within the control area.

The administrative area is on one side of the department, away from the traffic of patients, physicians, salesmen, and visitors, and is controlled by the receptionist. The chief technician may be located in this area but is better located central to the treatment area to allow supervision of activities and personnel. A film-viewing area should be close to the radiologist's office and the conference room.

The diagnostic-treatment area is complicated. The flow of patients is visualized as proceeding from waiting areas to radiography or fluoroscopy rooms. These rooms should be designed around a central core that includes the chief technician's office, equipment storage, a housekeeping closet, supply storage, and a barium room (which must be adjacent to the fluoroscopy rooms). There should be a control-monitoring generator room between each two diagnostic or fluoroscopy rooms. A holding area where stretcher patients are observed until films are checked is recommended for radiography rooms, and a toilet room for each fluoroscopy room should

Radiology, Intradepartmental Relationships

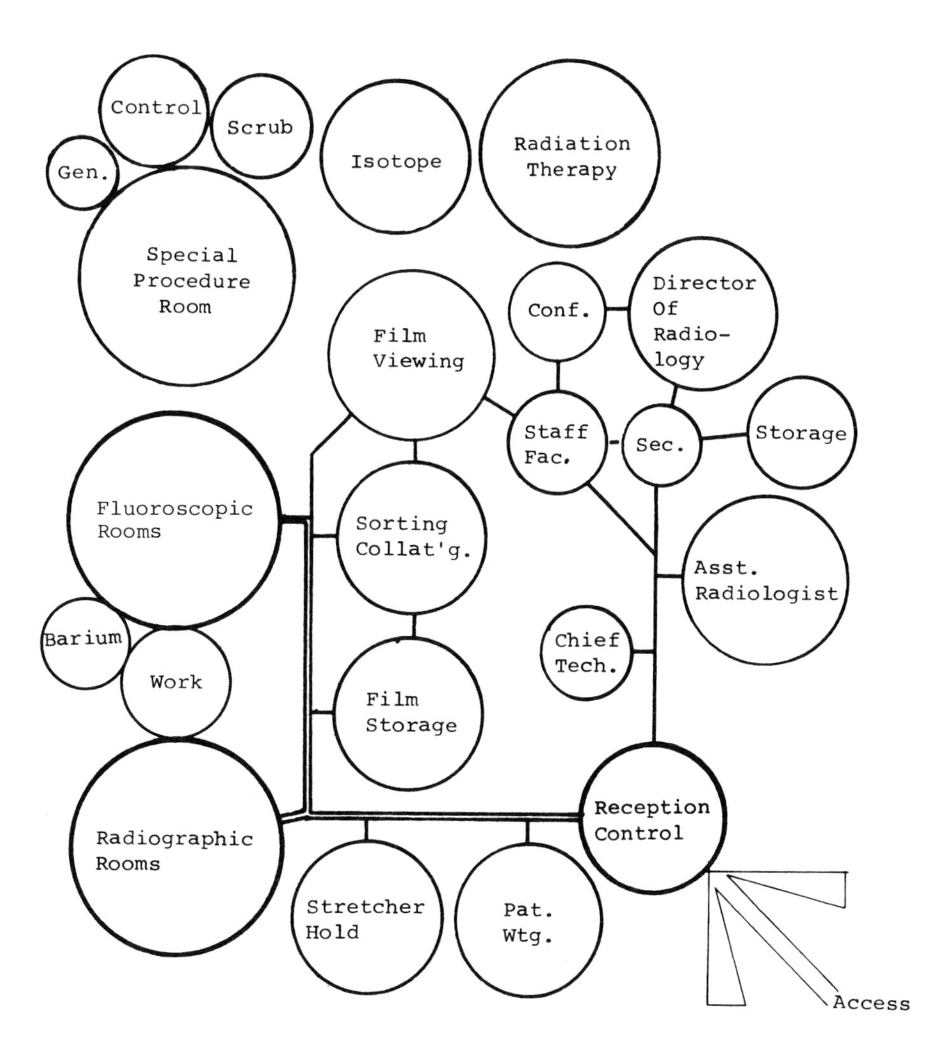

form the work core between examination rooms. Further, one room close to the entrance should be designated as a chest X-ray room and one general diagnostic room should be connected with the emergency-outpatient area. One darkroom is recommended for each four general diagnostic rooms, while daylight processing may be done in a control location within the suite.

The work area is designed to remove the flow of films from general department activities and to include several smaller areas. A film-viewing area should be adjacent to the radiologist's area and contain dictation equipment. There should be a sorting and collating secretarial pool for typing and distributing reports to appropriate areas and attaching a copy of each report to the X-ray film prior to forwarding it to storage. Film storage should be adjacent to the secretarial pool and accessible only to administrative staff for conferences and viewing films with the appropriate physician. Space should be allocated in this area for a film copier. Current film storage must be within the suite; past films may be in a large storeroom elsewhere in the hospital. There should be an area for small group meetings, study, and demonstrations.

Special Procedure Rooms

The planning of a diagnostic radiology department requires that separate consideration be given to rooms used for special diagnostic procedures. This poses design problems not encountered in conventional radiography and fluoroscopy rooms. Hospital policies will determine the range of these procedures and, therefore, design specifications. These procedures can include cardiovascular radiology and angiography, neuroradiology, tomography, urography, and operating room procedures. When the latter is planned, consideration must be given to National Fire Prevention Association code requirements for areas in which an anesthetic agent is used.

Ideally, the special procedure rooms are located close to or within the operating room suite, intensive care units, emergency, and diagnostic radiology, either on the same level or with an exclusive elevator or hallway to connect them. These adjacencies are necessary for maximum efficiency of technical staffing, maximum utilization of space and equipment, and centralization of film processing. It is essential that special procedure rooms be manned and operated by personnel under the administrative control and direction of the director of the department of radiology.

Cardiovascular and neuroradiology can include such procedures as pneumoencephalography, ventriculography, cerebral angiography, venography, peripheral arteriography, selective arteriography, cardiac catheterization, and sphenophotography. One room should be devoted to these procedures and should handle three or four per day. There should be a control room, a monitoring room, and a scrub room between each set of rooms. Space must be provided for such things as automatic biplane equipment, a sliding-top table with image recording system, X-ray tube support, support stand for lateral X-ray tube, a television monitor, a stand, storage cabinets, a sink, and a portable operating light. A room for tomography and urography should be adjacent to the cardiology room and should share controls, monitor scrub area, and so forth. Procedures carried out here will depend upon the equipment selected.

Special attention should be given to walls, floors, and ceilings, as well as to shielding, electrical and water requirements. Should direct adjacencies with diagnostic radiology be impossible, serious thought should be given to automatic systems distribution of films and records and to patient traffic flow.

RADIATION THERAPY

Functions. Radiation therapy is basically a tissue-destroying procedure. This department varies in size according to the type of services and program offered. A primary center may contain an older cobalt unit or a mega-electron volt linear accelerator. A larger facility may contain equipment ranging from orthovoltage to a 20–MEV accelerator. Future considerations for neutron equipment may affect both space and program.

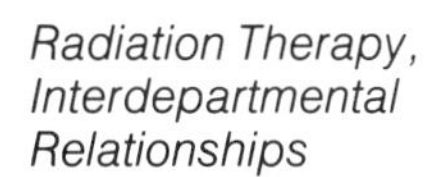
Radiation Therapy, Interdepartmental Relationships

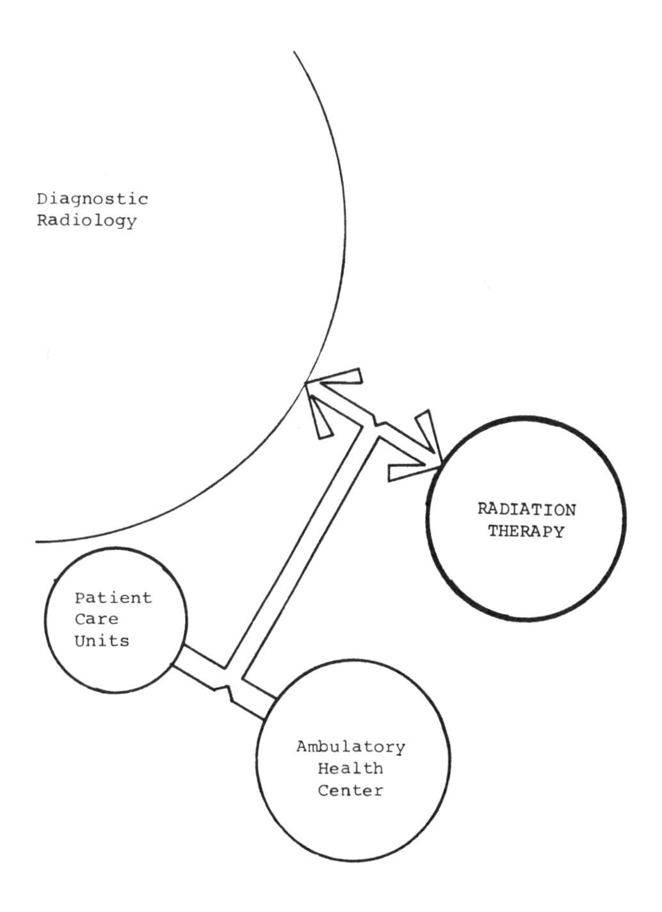

Location. Because of the dense shielding required by radiation therapy and national standards for design, this department must be carefully located so that it does not block future planning and expansion. Three-foot-thick walls and ceilings with required access for the placement or removal of the equipment are a major design element. Radiation therapy is used to treat both inpatients and outpatients and should, therefore, be adjacent to radiology and ambulatory care. Most patients will be ambulatory; hence, the radiation-therapy unit requires easy access from the ambulatory care center, diagnostic X-ray, and vertical transport facilities.

Radiation therapy should be put where it will adjoin the earth on several sides and have no neighbors directly below. It is also desirable to have this department adjoining the diagnostic X-ray facilities, but the two units are not dependent on one another and can be separated.

Design. Many outpatient cancer treatment programs are combined with the radiation therapy department; thus, the specific design is based upon projected use. Because of the seriousness of the diseases treated here this space must present a pleasant atmosphere concentrating on patient and visitor comfort. A computer tie-in is desirable.

The use of cobalt 60, 400–kilovolt X-rays, and Cesium 137 requires concrete walls thirty-six to fifty-four inches thick for shielding; up to twenty-four inches is needed for protection against secondary radiation. Equipment itself requires special shielding. Large cables will carry voltage from large transformers to the suspended apparatus necessary to provide precise positioning of the accelerator. Tube operation is controlled from a console that determines length and intensity of X-ray discharges. An adjustable table is required to position the patient and to hold the X-ray cassette. This entire assembly is usually enclosed in lead to protect personnel. When linear accelerators are used, X-ray personnel must be able to observe the patient's treatment from outside the room, by window, television, a mirror arrangement in the adjacent hallway, or any combination of these.

Radiation Therapy, Intradepartmental Relationships

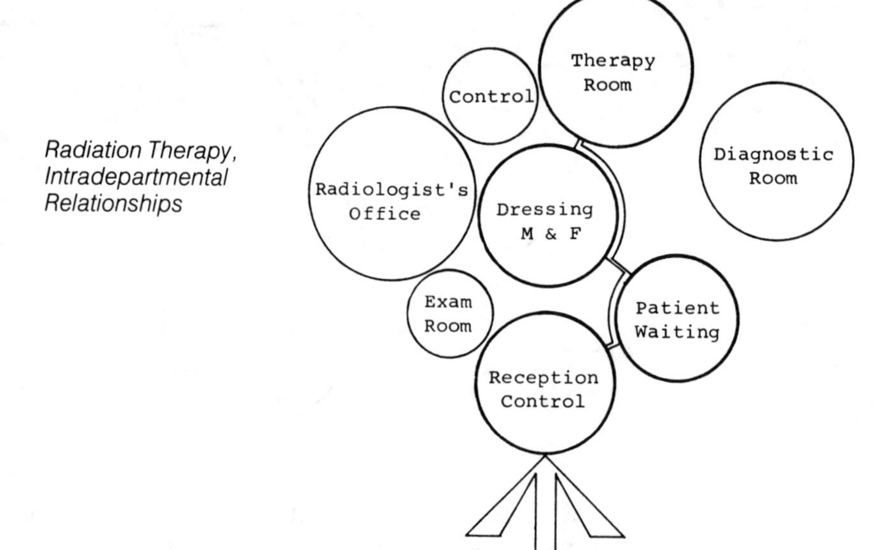

Intradepartmental Relationships. Reception-control receives patients, directs them to other elements in the department, and makes appointments for future visits. The waiting area is close to reception-control, the dressing area, and the diagnostic room and should be observable from reception-control. Waiting patients and relatives should be unable to view the rest of the department. The dressing room should be next to the waiting area.

The diagnostic room can be within the suite or not. It can be put in diagnostic radiology if facilities are not available in the radiation therapy suite. Its basic purpose is for procedures necessary before radiation therapy or evaluation of treatment programs or both.

The radiologist's office should be close to the radiation therapy room and should have an adjacent examination room for pre- or post-treatment examinations and for examination of new patients.

The therapy room is designed with proper shielding and protection. Space required will vary with the choice of equipment. The control room is adjacent to the therapy room; from it, radiation personnel control treatment and observe the patient during treatment.

NUCLEAR MEDICINE

Nuclear medicine is the internal administration of radiopharmaceuticals to diagnose or to treat disease. Close cooperation among chemists, physicists, biomedical electronic engineers, and physicians has helped make this department one of the most rapidly growing areas of the hospital. In 1934 only one radioactive substance was in use—deuterium oxide (heavy water). Today, more than 100 radiopharmaceuticals are on the market.

Functions. The functions of the department are to provide:

—safe, reliable, and accurate screening tests

—information otherwise unavailable to the physician on the structure and function of an organ or system

—information to support the probable diagnosis

Location. The department should be adjacent to:

Nuclear Medicine, Interdepartmental Relationships

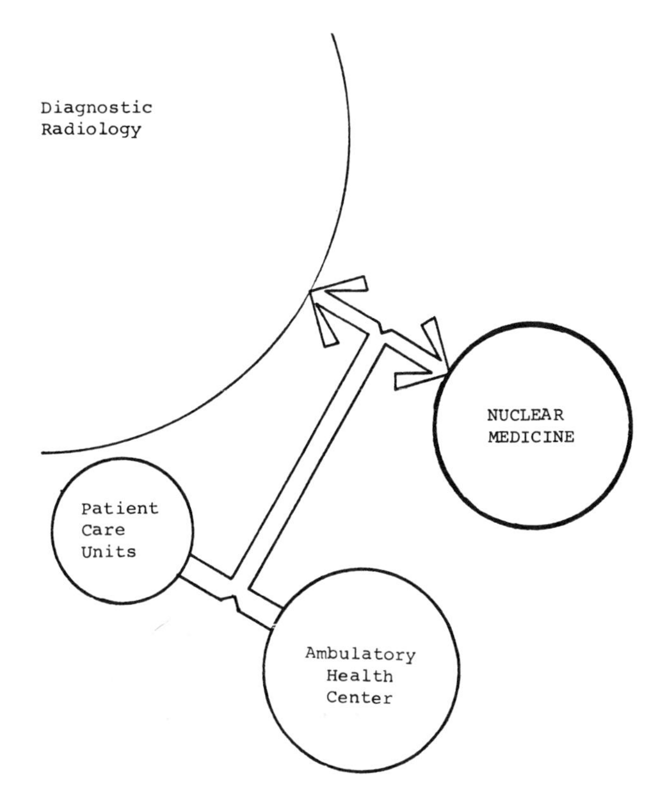

—diagnostic radiology, and use the same receptionists, waiting area, and stretcher-wheelchair holding area
—outpatient services and entrance, because many of the patients will be ambulatory
—social services, laboratory, and medical records (these are desirable adjacencies but can be located within a short walk, with good interdepartmental communications

Design. The following basic types of recordings are used in nuclear medicine:

—dilution techniques (blood counts)
—concentration (iodine in the thyroid gland)
—dynamic recording (renograms in kidney diseases)
—static organ, or pool, imaging (to determine size, shape, position, architecture, and function of an organ or pool)

Radiation exposure from nuclear medicine procedures is well within the established safety levels.

A computer tie-in will be of increasing importance. Nonetheless, special construction for radiopharmaceutical storage and disposal of wastes is necessary.

Consideration also needs to be given to a design which separates the "in vitro" and "in vivo" procedures.

Utilities for the area must reflect electricity needs for specific equipment selected, adequte lighting, and control of light.

Nuclear Medicine, Intradepartmental Relationships

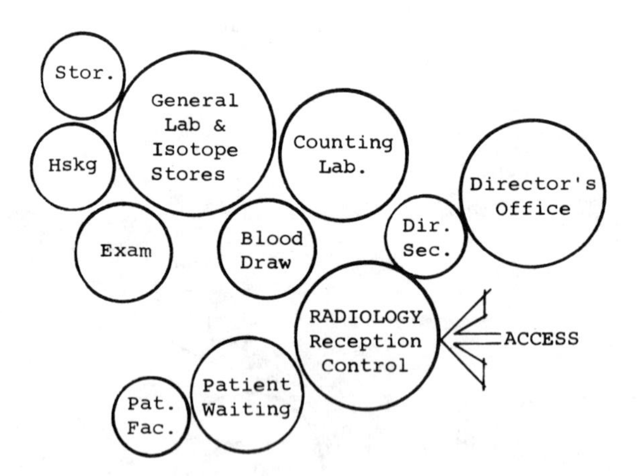

Intradepartmental Elements. The administrative area includes the director's office and the secretary's office. The treatment area is made up of examination rooms, a counting lab, a small room for drawing blood, and a general laboratory and isotope storage area (including waste storage). Supporting areas are equipment storage, ninety-second film developer, and housekeeping.

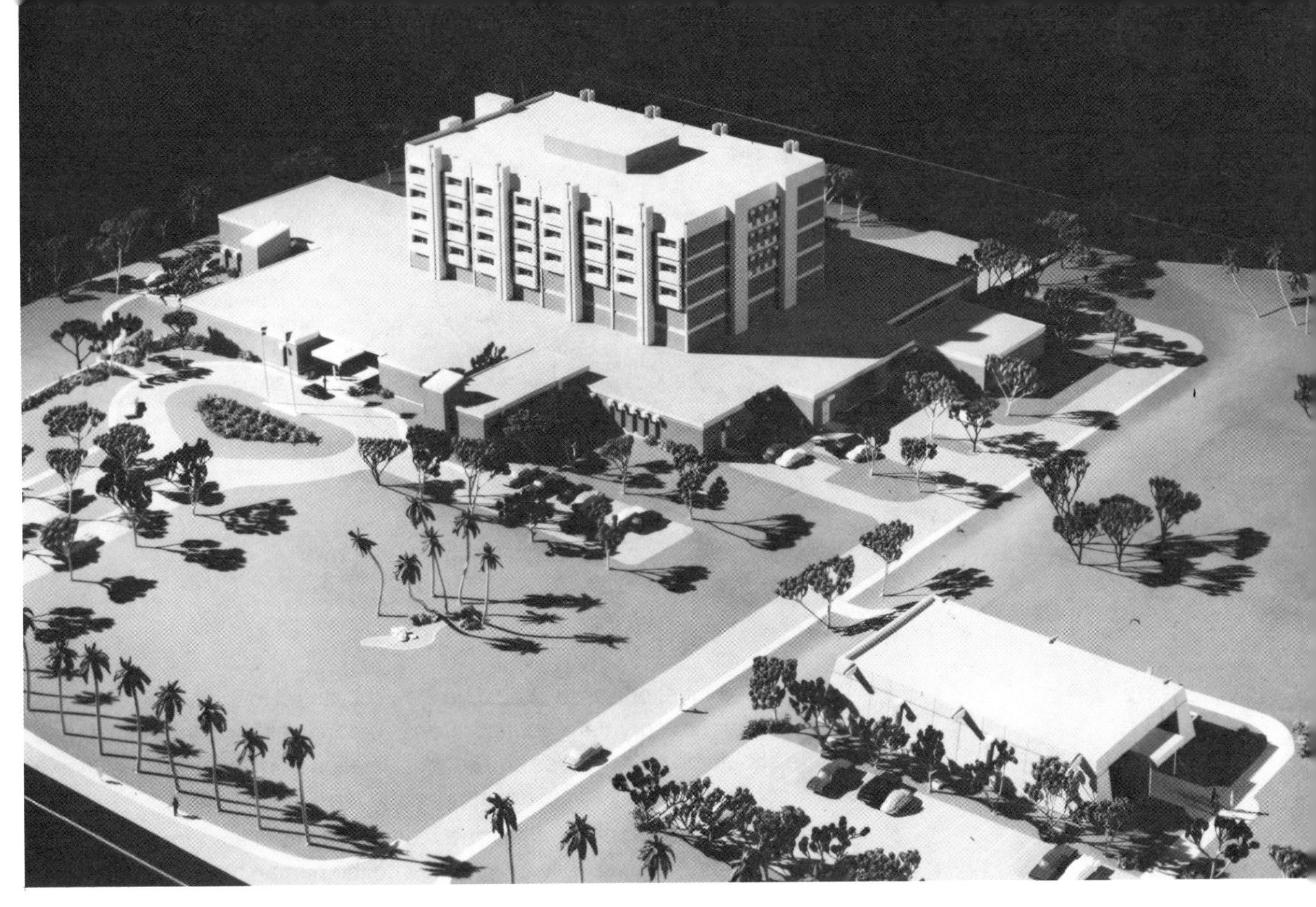

San Pedro Sula Hospital, Honduras

HUMAN FUNCTIONS

Human functions, or special services, are a group of diagnostic and treatment procedures. They function either as isolated services with a minimum of administrative supervision or as services offered by a department that does not view them as one of its primary functions. All too often they occupy reclaimed space not designed for them nor allocated for maximum utilization of their services. The most familiar of these services are electrocardiography, electroencephalography, basal metabolism, inhalation therapy, pulmonary function, kinegrams, electromyelograms, exercise tolerance testing, chest physiotherapy, and echoencephalography.

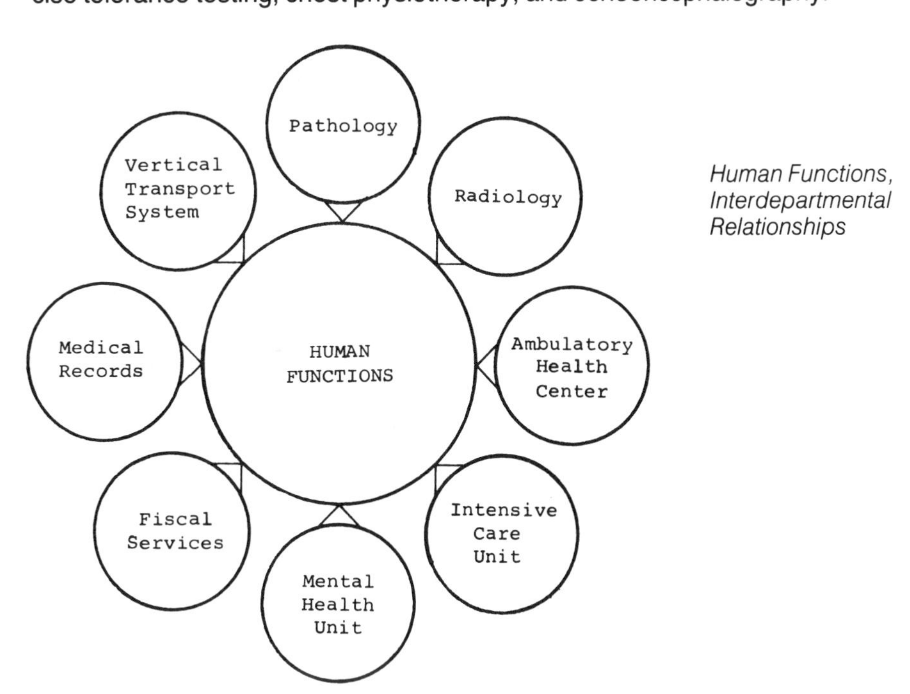

Human Functions, Interdepartmental Relationships

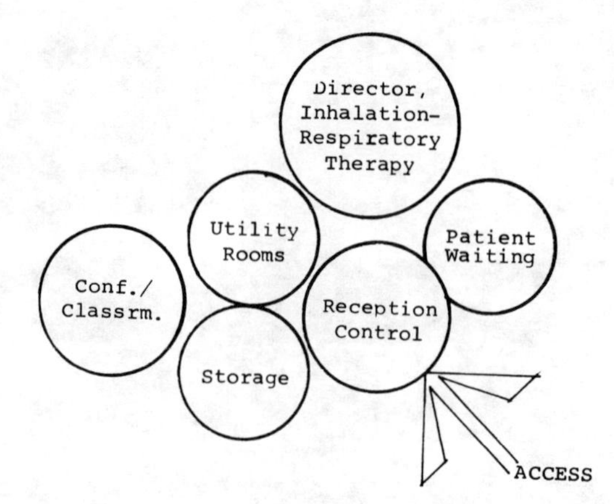

Human Functions: Central Core, Intra-Departmental Relationships

The human functions area should be located central to the clinical laboratory, radiology, the ambulatory care center, intensive care unit, and the mental health unit. There should be easy access and communication with the business office and medical records, and with vertical transport to the other patient units.

The central core should contain one reception-control area for all services; it should be located off a main hallway leading into the human functions department. Reception-control should have easy two-way communication with all services in the department and with outside departments. One common waiting area should be located adjacent to reception-control for observation and additional control before referring the patient to the appropriate service.

A conference-classroom should be designed for conferences by any or all services, instruction classes, patient-staff conferences, and staff-private physician conferences. It should be the farthest away from the entrance and easily accessible to all services.

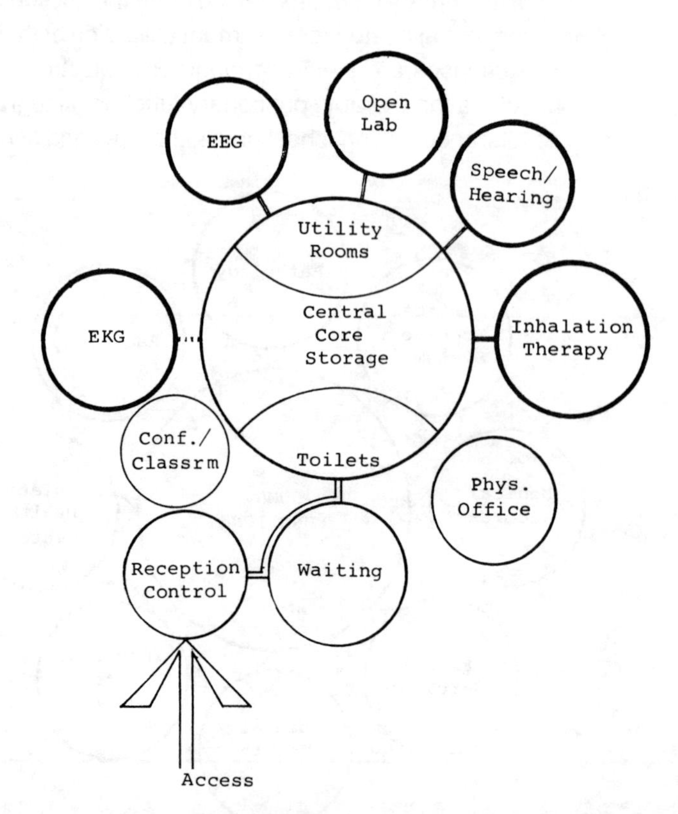

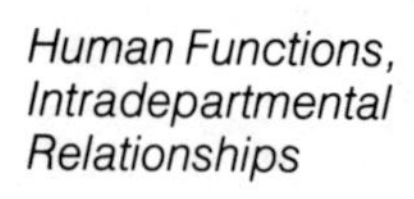
Human Functions, Intradepartmental Relationships

There should be one clean and one soiled utility room located centrally for easy access by all services. A storage-supply room should be centrally located for easy access.

There should be inhalation and respiratory therapy. Office space for physicians assigned to it should be located close to reception–control and the inhalation therapy–open laboratory area of the human functions suite.

Inhalation Therapy

Statistics indicate that twenty-five percent of the patients admitted to a hospital require some sort of inhalation therapy during their hospitalization. Demand for services has been increasing from intensive care units, emergency services, cardiorespiratory arrests throughout the hospital, and other patient care units. In teaching hospitals, this service has been organized into a separate pulmonary, respiratory, or inhalation therapy department.

Assisting the physician, through referral, in the management of patient's respiratory problems is a basic function of inhalation therapy. Specifically, this means handling all respiratory support, including artificial ventilation, tracheostomies, and endotracheal tubes, and treating all patients requiring postural drainage and chest percussion. Inhalation therapy also maintains patient and administrative records on procedures and activities and participates in continuous staff education programs regarding the use of inhalation therapy equipment.

Location. Inhalation therapy should be located to one side of the human functions department, close to reception–control and the waiting area. It should have easy access to intensive care, inpatient areas (via vertical transport), emergency services, operating-recovery room, and outpatient services.

Design. Design of the inhalation therapy area will be affected by an administrative decision on whether ambulatory patients are scheduled for treatment in the area or in the ambulatory facilities.

Every twenty-four hours equipment from patient care units must be disassembled, washed, cleaned, reassembled, serviced, packaged, separated, and sterilized. A good distribution system is necessary for efficient flow of this equipment from patient units to decontamination to inhalation therapy and back to patient units. Area utilities should include oxygen, suction, and air. A good communication system is vital to this service.

Inhalation therapy requires a wide variety of fragile and expensive equipment, including ventilators, flowmeters, humidifiers, nebulizers (mechanical and electronic), oxygen analyzers, and volume meters. These will need a fairly large storage area.

Intradepartmental Relationships. The chief therapist's office should have traditional office furniture and equipment, be close to the entrance to the suite, and have good visibility and access to treatment units. The secretarial clerical area is for maintaining statistics, compiling reports (charting area for technicians) and so on. It should also contain filing space.

The storage area is designed to hold movable equipment, small processed equipment, and supplies. It is recommended that the latter remain on an exchange cart to one side of the room, while movable equipment is stored on the opposite side; this will enable the therapist to respond more quickly to request for services.

In the normal operation of the department, there will be a need for the therapist to adjust and repair inhalation therapy equipment and to break down, clean, and maintain highly specialized equipment above and beyond routine decontamination. Space for this should be provided adjacent to the equipment storage area and should contain utilities, a workbench, and wall-mounted cabinets.

The treatment room itself is partitioned into cubicles for examination and treatment of both inpatients and ambulatory outpatients.

Electrocardiography (EKG)

Functions. Electrocardiography produces hard-copy readouts of heart function to assist the physician in diagnosing disease, establishing a treatment plan, and evaluating the effect of the treatment on the patient. Equally important functions are evolving in preventive care and observation of the patient's heart function during surgery.

Location. Electrocardiography should be located within the human functions area on the opposite side of the central core from inhalation therapy. It should be easily accessible to ambulatory patients and designed to allow personnel to leave rapidly for other areas of the hospital.

Intradepartmental Relationships. The chief technician's office is space for private interviews, administrative functions, and coordination and control of the suite. It should be located close to the entrance to the suite, with easy access to the other rooms. The reading room is an area for cardiologists to interpret and dictate diagnostic findings. It should be adjacent to the work-preparation area and the chief technician's office and should contain a computer terminal.

The work-preparation area is space for cutting, splicing, and preparing recordings for interpretation and filming. It should be adjacent to either the reading room and diagnostic laboratories or the computer-telemetry recording and readout space. In the latter case, the two areas would be combined. The work-preparation area should also include copying equipment.

Laboratories for taking EKGs of ambulatory patients can be located either in the suite or in the outpatient department. Consideration should be given to providing one room, with access to pulmonary functions units, for exercise testing.

There should be space close to the entrance and exit, for housing equipment not currently in use. A supplies storage area would hold supplies germane to EKG only.

Electroencephalography (EEG)

Functions. Electroencephalography measures the electrical potentials of the brain at the scalp or, in surgical procedures, at the surface of the exposed cortex;

electrical response in a contracting muscle; and eye oscillations associated with sound in order to diagnose epilepsy, trauma, tumors, and other brain diseases.

Location. The electroencephalography suite should be located in a quiet section of the human functions area to avoid distraction of the patients during examination. It should also be separated as far as practical from main electrical cooridors or equipment that will affect recordings. There should be easy access to intensive care, mental health, ambulatory services, and vertical transport to other patient areas.

Intradepartmental Relationships. The chief technician's office should be situated so that he can see the laboratory rooms and have privacy in handling other responsibilities. The file-dictation-reading room is an area for physicians to read recordings and dictate findings. It also serves as a filing room. It should be near the chief technician's office.

The preparation and control room is designed for preparing (wiring) the patient for an EEG and contains equipment for recording while observing the patient through a glass wall. It should be large enough to prepare two patients at a time, one on each side of the room, and should have dual controls located central to both EEG laboratories. The EEG laboratories, themselves, will accommodate a patient lying down or in a supine position during the testing procedure.

SPEECH AND HEARING THERAPY

This unit diagnoses speech disorders; diagnoses and treats hearing deficiencies; provides speech correction and development; and prescribes audiological prosthesis. The ideal location for speech and hearing therapy is adjacent to the central core and next to inhalation therapy. Since most patients for testing and treatment will be ambulatory, it should be easily accessible to the ambulatory health center. The department should include:

—reception–control room
—waiting area
—speech pathologist's office
—audiometric screening room
—therapy rooms
—storage room

REHABILITATIVE MEDICINE

The modern hospital, in its efforts to deliver comprehensive care, must consider carefully the contribution of rehabilitative medicine as part of its inpatient and ambulatory patient care. The department should be organized to provide for continued specialized treatment of a variety of prolonged, often reversible, physical and mental disabilities.

Rehabilitation Medicine, Interdepartmental Relationships

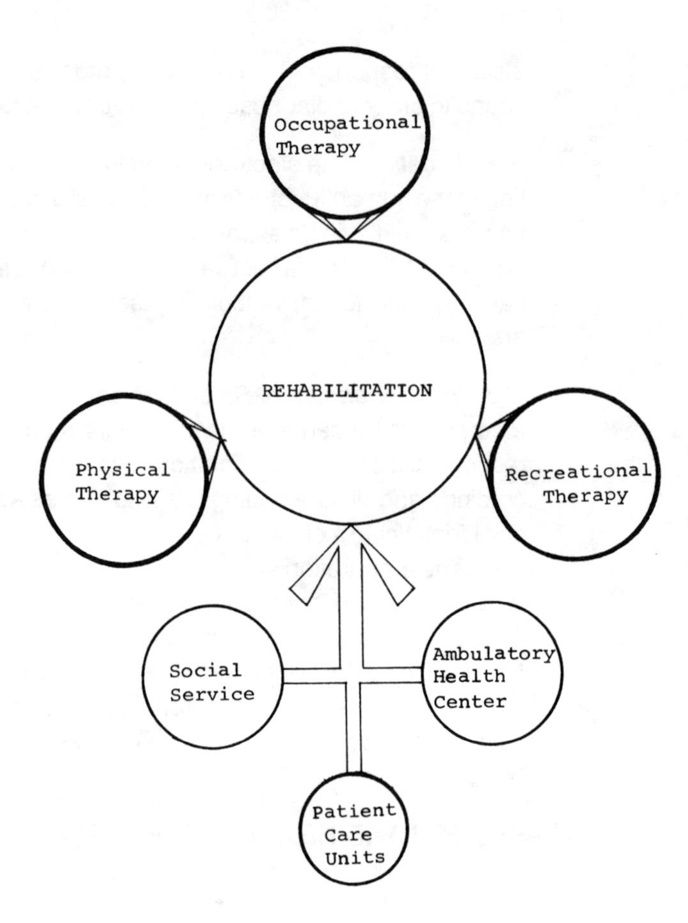

Physical Therapy

Functions. The following are functions of physical therapy:

—to obtain certain kinds of information needed for diagnosis, prescribed therapy, and evaluation of patients

—to prevent or minimize residual physical disabilities

—to return the individual to optimum living

—to accelerate convalescence and reduce the length of hospital stay

Location. The function of the physical therapy department is closely related to its location within the hospital. The area should be centrally located to minimize travel and transportation problems, to accommodate ambulatory patients, and to facilitate bedside treatment. It should also be close to the central elevators if it is to meet the growing demands of the medical team. The department should have easy accessibility to both inpatients and outpatients, with a minimum of heavy doors to manipulate. It should be adjacent to social services, to other rehabilitative services (such as speech therapy and recreational and occupational therapy), and to outpatient services. The orthopedic service should be as close as possible.

Physical Therapy, Interdepartmental Relationships

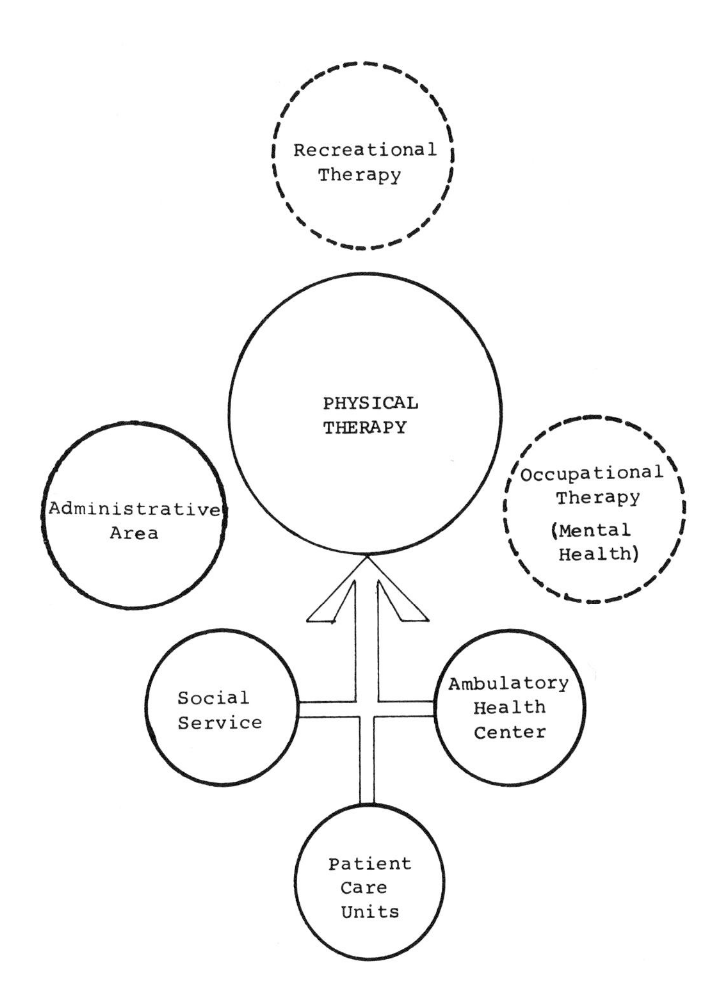

Design. The number of treatments can be projected on the basis of the number of inpatient treatments per patient day plus outpatient treatments per visit. If each treatment requires forty-five minutes to one hour, the number of treatments per station per work day is ten to twelve.

total treatments ÷ days of operation ÷ 10
= number of treatment stations

number of treatment stations × 600 g.s.f.
= department size

Intradepartmental Relationships. Physical therapy is usually divided into three areas, which are designed to meet specific requirements for given types of treatment and the special equipment involved: a treatment booth area, a water treatment area, and an exercise area.

Treatment booths should be large enough to accommodate the therapists working on either side of the table without moving equipment or extending into the hallway or other work space. Ideally, the cubicles should have full walls on three

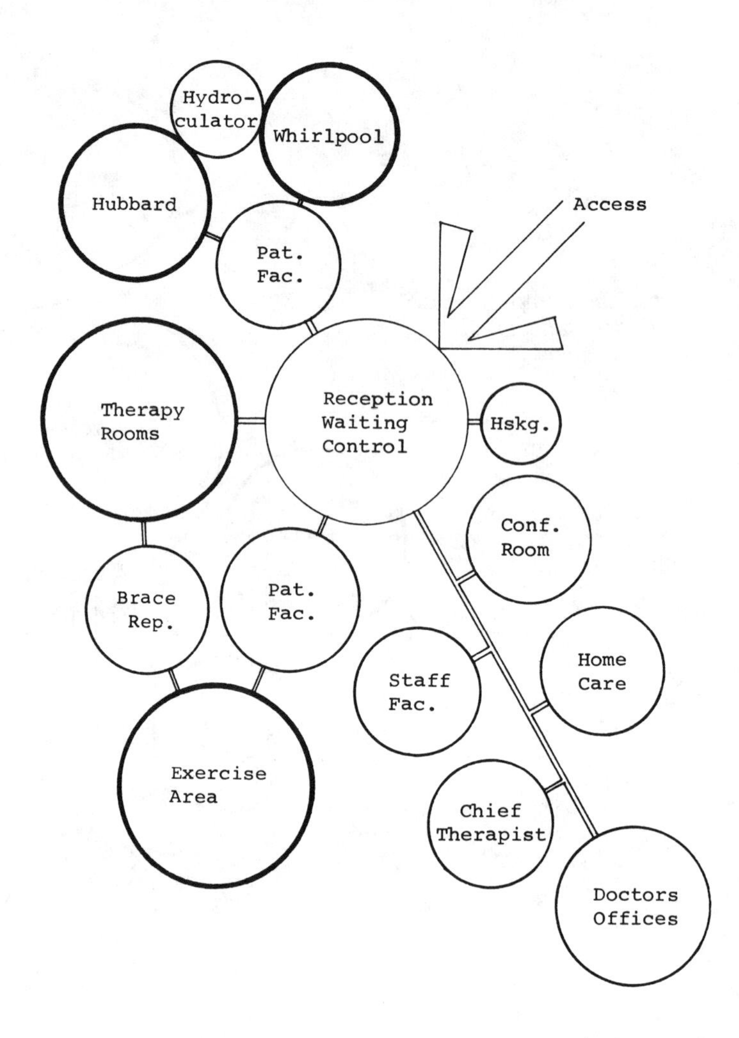

Physical Therapy, Intradepartmental Relationships

sides and a sliding door across the front to allow for privacy and easy access by wheelchair or stretcher. Dressing cubicles should be adjacent to this area and should allow patients to dress and undress in privacy before treatment. Some system of lockers for patients' valuables should be investigated. This area, because it involves most of the treatments given by the department, should be close to the reception area.

All equipment in the water treatment area that requires special plumbing and water supply should be concentrated into a subarea adjacent to the other treatment areas and the reception area. Special care in planning must be given to reinforce ceilings of areas below, to provide special drains, to absorb noise, and to control humidity. The Hubbard tub should have its own room to accommodate the large tub, mixing tanks and filters, and overhead lifts or hydraulic elevator lifts necessary for efficient use. A higher ceiling than normal should be provided. Enough space must be allowed for maneuvering a stretcher in and out of the room. This area must also include space for examination and exercise outside the tub to eliminate moving the patient to another treatment area. Tanks to provide whirlpool treatments for both arms and legs are needed. These tanks should be located to allow accessibility by wheelchairs without interfering with other patients receiving treatments in this subarea. The hydroculator area is a special area for preparation of hot packs and overnight storage of carts. Storage of the large amount of clean linen used in water treatments and disposal of wet linen after treatments must also be considered.

The open exercise area is a large rectangular or square room for individual or group exercises. It should be planned with enough flexibility to accommodate a variety of stationary and movable equipment for patients with limited mobility (those using crutches, wheelchairs, or canes) and steps or mats for floor and weight exercises for fingers, arms, legs, and so on. The equipment should be located to allow maximum circulation through the area and to minimize falls and other hazards to patients with limited mobility. The floor covering should be nonslip vinyl and at least one wall and the ceiling should be designed to allow safe attachment of built-in equipment.

Occupational and Recreational Therapy

These are subdepartments of rehabilitative services whose function is to apply their techniques through processes of demonstration and training. They should have a close relationship to physical therapy for continuity of care and adjacency to the mental health unit.

Occupational Therapy, Intradepartmental Relationships

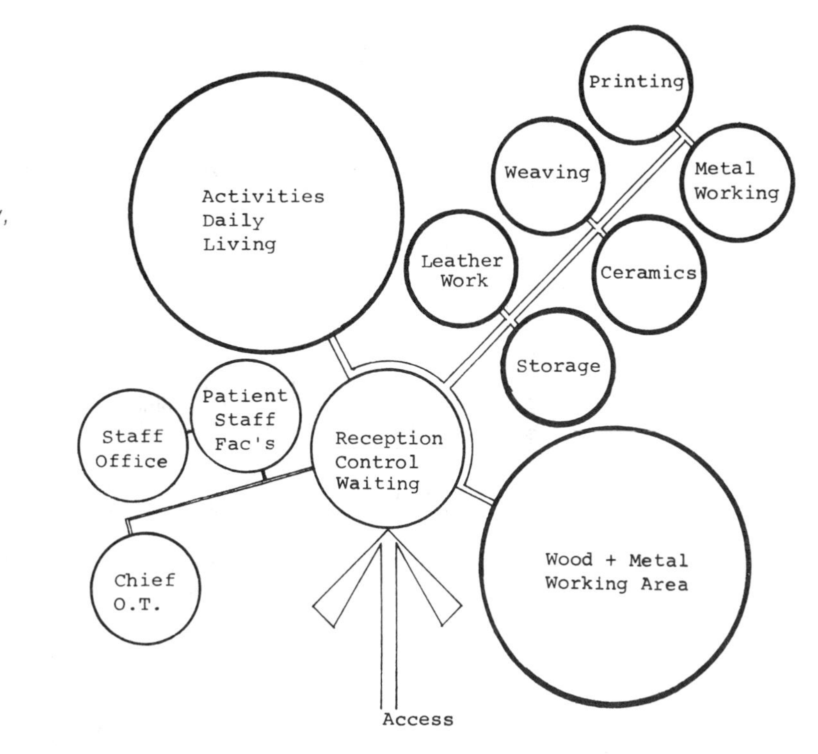

SURGERY

Many programs separate outpatient surgery from the main surgery facilities. As much as one-third of all surgery may be performed on an outpatient basis, thus reducing the space needed for the main operating room. Surgical functions include anesthetization, surgical treatment, and recovery of scheduled as well as emergency trauma patients. Surgical treatment may be major or minor, specialty or ambulatory outpatient procedures.

Location. Ambulatory patient surgery should be accessible to patients from the outside. Surgery receives inpatients via traffic corridors connecting the bed floors through non-public corridors and elevators. Ideal adjacencies would be to emergency, radiology, the clinical laboratory, central supply, intensive care, the physicians' lounge and anesthesiology. The best location allows an uncomplicated flow of patient, staff, and clean supply traffic.

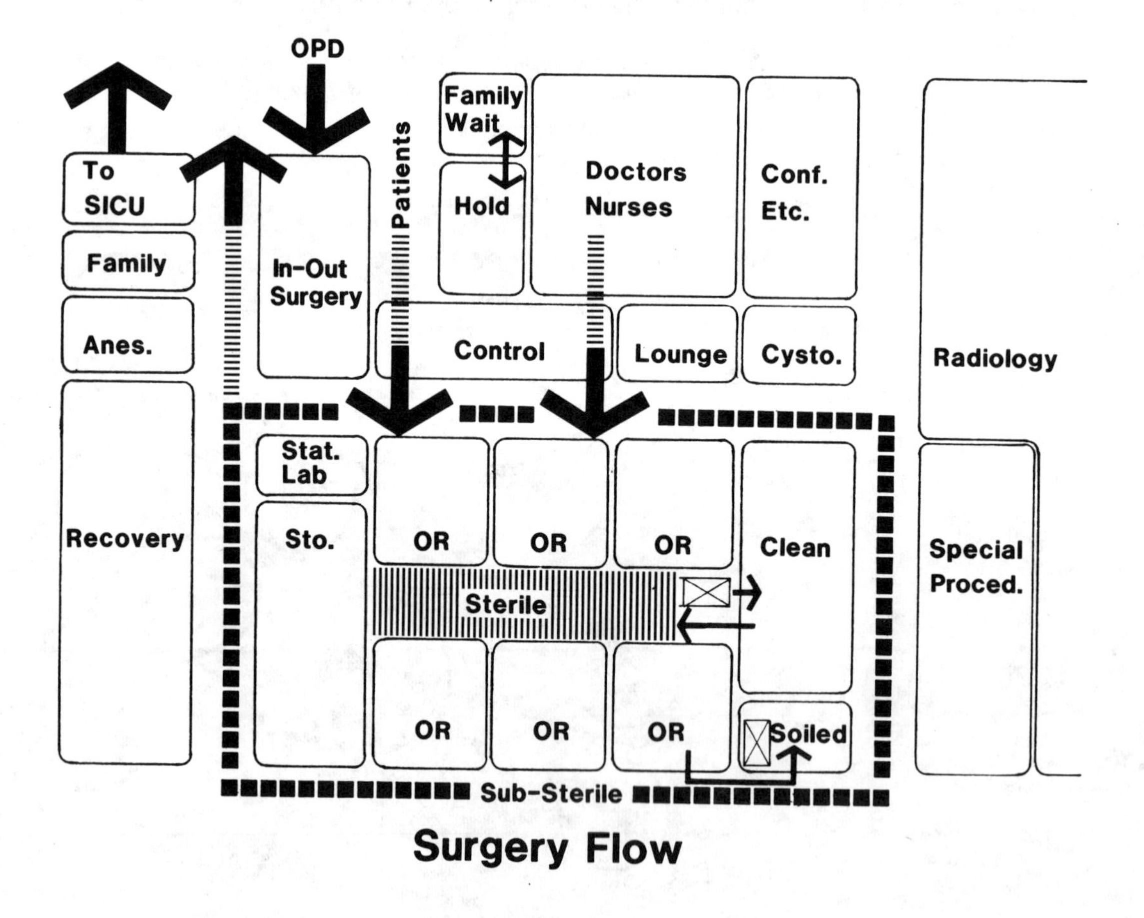

Surgery Flow

Design. Starting with a determination of the yearly total number of procedures to be performed in the hospital, calculations can be made to determine the number of operating rooms and the total surgical space required as follows:

$$\frac{\text{total procedures per year}}{\text{procedures per room per year}} = \text{operating rooms required}$$

gross square feet per room × operating rooms = surgery space required

An operating room requires 1,700–1,900 g.s.f. The average primary and secondary hospital (approximately 400 beds), with a balanced mix of subspecialists, can perform 1,000–1,300 procedures per operating room per year (total of major, minor, and cystology procedures). A major tertiary hospital, however, averages fewer (750–1,000) procedures per room per year because the procedures themselves are more complicated. Thus, if the probable total number of procedures per year equals 10,000 (using a yearly room average of 1,000 and an average of 1,800 g.s.f. per room) the surgical space specifications would be as follows:

$$\frac{\text{10,000 procedures}}{\text{1,000 per room}} = \text{10 rooms required}$$

1,800 g.s.f. per room × 10 rooms required = 18,000 g.s.f. of surgery

When calculated on the basis of the architectural space standard of 40–50 gross feet per bed, the approximate surgical space can be figured as follows:

400 beds × 40 g.s.f. = 16,000 g.s.f.
400 beds × 50 g.s.f. = 20,000 g.s.f.

Using a standard planning ratio (of .30–.50 procedures per g.s.f. of surgery space) simplifies these calculations:

$$\frac{\text{10,000 procedures}}{.50} = \text{20,000 g.s.f. of surgery space}$$

Intradepartmental Elements. Space is needed for the following functions:

—family waiting rooms (with privacy)

—patient holding area

—surgery control station (with pharmaceuticals)

—anesthesia storeroom

—sterile supply space

—major operating rooms (twenty feet by twenty-four feet)

—minor operating rooms

—flash sterilizer space

—substerile corridor

—special procedures rooms (twenty-four feet by thirty feet)

—cystology rooms (and film processing)

—frozen section laboratory

—film processing

—decontamination and soiled materials receiving room

—recovery room (1.5 beds per operating room)

—recovery support room and family quiet room

—supervisor's office

—anesthesia office

—head nurse's office

— consultation-conference room

—doctors' and nurses' lockers

—technicians' lockers

—operating room staff lounge

—stretcher and wheelchair storage

—storage of stock and rolling equipment (this space is usually grossly undersized)

—housekeeping areas

MEDICAL STAFF FACILITIES

Comprehensive health care planning requires that the medical staff of a hospital be involved in overall operations planning as well as in planning the individual course of treatment for the individual patient. This can best be accomplished if the design of the hospital incorporates medical staff facilities within or near the administrative services center. These facilities should include an informal lounge-conference area for discussion of patient care and offices for formal physician-to-physician contacts. The offices of the director of medicine, the directors of services, and the president of the medical staff should also be located in the administrative services center to allow for maximum contribution to planning and operation. The use of centralized medical staff facilities could also provide space for physician activities such as pharmaceutical and professional displays, a check-in register, and an information center for posting announcements of meetings, clinic services, and surgical schedules. It could also be used as a medical staff and professional guest entrance, thus avoiding the main entrance.

Location. Medical staff facilities should be within the administrative services center, with a separate entrance from an adjacent, designated parking area. It should be adjacent to medical records and the medical library, with easy access to vertical transportation, admissions office, ambulatory care center, and social services.

Intradepartmental Relationships. The locker-coat area should be provided with unassigned lockers for the use of medical staff members while in the hospital. Toilet facilities should be adjacent to the lounge and locker-coat area. The lounge should contain several sofas and comfortable chairs and one wall should contain slots for mail and messages. A doctors' registration station should be located at the entrance to the lounge.

Medical Staff Facilities, Intradepartmental Relationships

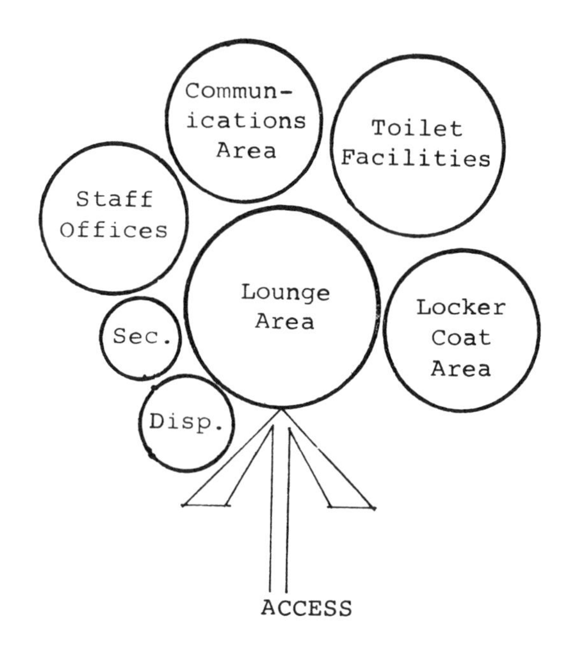

The communications area should be separated from the lounge by an acoustical divider. It should contain no fewer than four soundproof carrels with telephones tied into the dictating system of the medical records department. These telephones also should be used for placing local calls concerning patient care.

A display area should be allocated for salespersons who wish to contact physicians. It should be in the lounge and communications area.

Medical staff offices are provided for designated representatives of the medical staff. They should be easily accessible from the lounge without having to use central hallways. The secretary's office is designed for one secretary to handle the needs of the medical staff offices.

Medical Staff Facilities, Interdepartmental Relationships

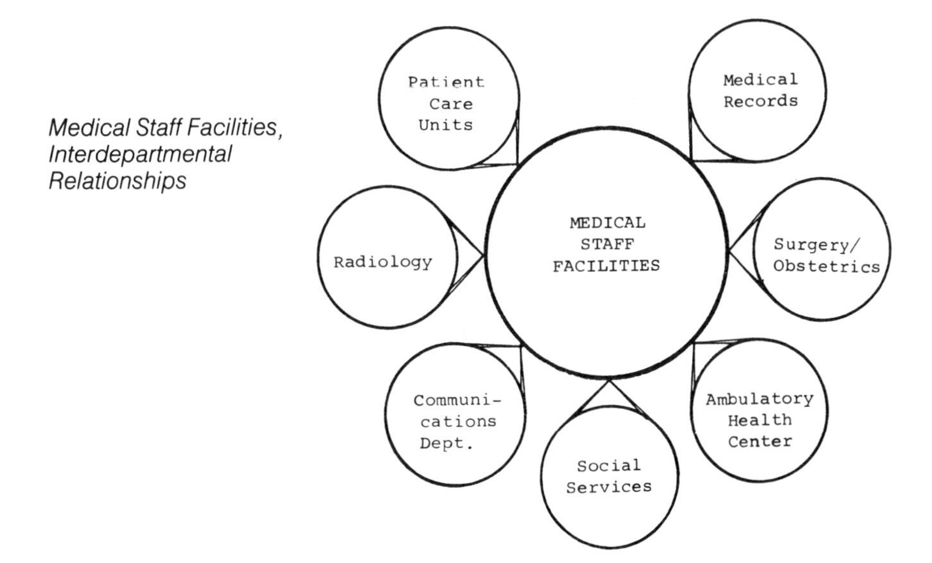

XI

department planning: nursing services

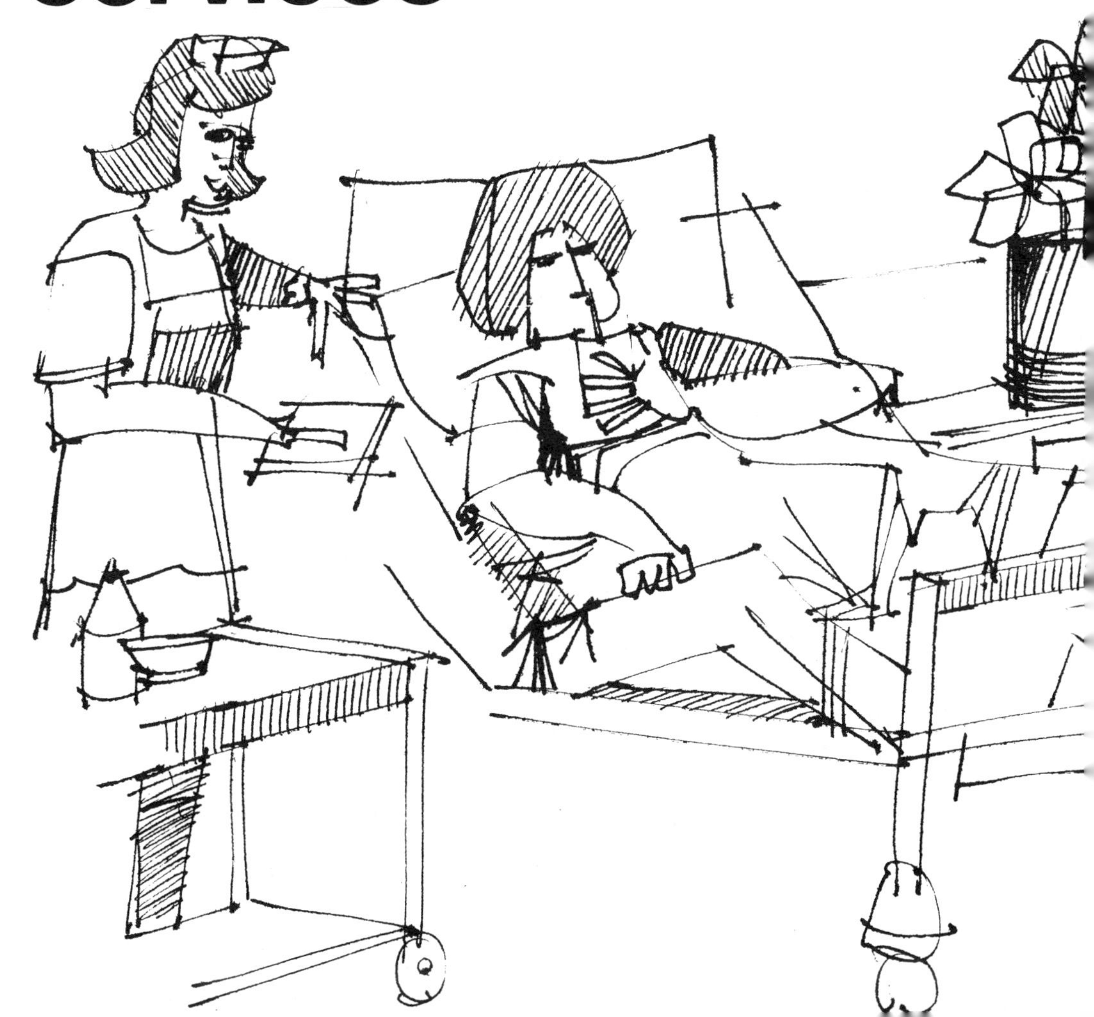

Good nursing services result from and are part of coordinated administrative and clinical planning. The primary purpose of the nursing department is to give comprehensive, safe, effective, and well-organized nursing care to all patients. Furthermore, the department is responsible for teaching programs for nursing and auxiliary personnel.

The nursing department constitutes the largest single group of hospital personnel. Properly administered, it is the mainstay of the organization from the standpoint of supporting administrative requirements, rendering effective patient care, and promoting good community relations. While dependent upon all other hospital departments, it serves as a focal point for much of the administrative coordination necessary among departments.

NURSING SERVICES ADMINISTRATION

The offices of the director of nursing and of the nursing administrative staff should be contained in an administrative suite to improve the coordination of nursing services. Some health facilities are now decentralizing nursing administration by

Department	*Gross Square Feet per Bed*
Nursing services administration	2.5
General nursing units	400–420
Pediatric unit	400
Obstetrical unit	400
Intensive care complex	500–550
Intermediate unit	400–420
Long-term care unit	450–500
Extended care unit	450
Holistic medicine	10
Mental health unit	600–700
Psychiatric inpatient unit	450–500
Rehabilitation unit	500
Cooperative care	500
Psychogeriatric unit	500
Sports medicine unit	10
Hospice unit	550

placing supervisory staff in the patient care areas for which they are responsible. This is designed to improve patient care and administration-staff communications.

Nursing administration is responsible for:

—constantly evaluating and improving the nursing care of patients

—maintaining stable staffing patterns

—selecting, orienting, and assigning nursing personnel

—maintaining adequate nursing records for clinical and administrative use

—keeping nursing service policies, procedures, and functional organization up to date

—maintaining effective relationships between the nursing department, hospital departments, and medical staff

The nursing services administrative suite should contain the following:

—director's office

—supervisors' offices

—secretary's office

—secretarial pool

—conference room–library

—employee facilities and lounge

Nursing Services Administration, Intradepartmental Relationships

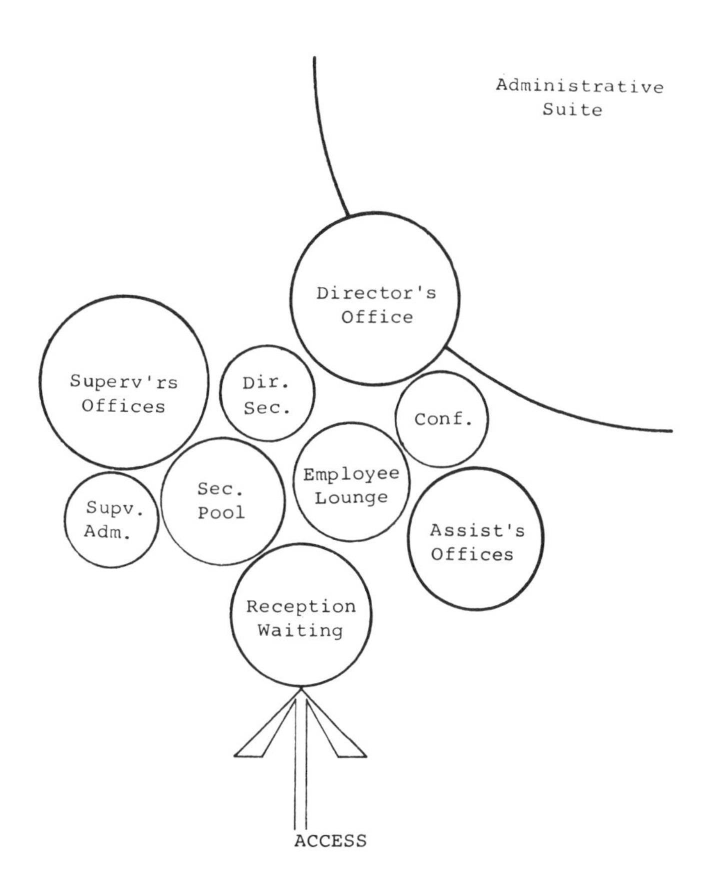

General Nursing Units

A nursing unit is a self-contained, independently operated and controlled group of rooms for patients designed for either special or general care. The size, shape, and components of the nursing units affect the hospital's efficiency.

Traditionally, the size of a nursing unit has been twenty to thirty beds. Recently, the trend has been toward units of thirty to forty, forty to sixty, and sixty or more beds per unit. The floor plan of a unit does have an effect on the efficiency of the unit; nonetheless, beyond twenty to twenty-five beds per unit a breakdown tends to occur with the duplication of utilities, telephones, nursing stations, and so on. The smaller size also permits a higher level of nursing care and lends itself to either individual or team care, when this concept is used. Combined twenty to twenty-five bed units can also produce overall night coverage efficiences in staffing and unit management.

The size of the patient room, or how the beds are distributed, is also undergoing changes. The trend is toward more single-bed rooms and elimination of the four-bed room. A unit design that includes a combination of single and double rooms retains efficiency of operation, keeps construction costs down, and gives the individual hospital flexibility in meeting the needs of its community. The ideal room is the double room with two separate entrances, two doors into the toilet, and a folding partition that separates the beds, for privacy.

The structural shape of units has also undergone innovation and experimentation in an effort to maximize hospital efficiency: the single corridor, the cross, the circular, the triangle within a pentagon, radiating corridors (or snowflake) and so on. These designs achieve varying degrees of success in meeting the following goals:

—low construction cost, consistent with need

—efficient, low-cost operation and use of personnel

—maximum care and supervision of acutely ill patients

—patient privacy and comfort

The size and shape of a unit must, in the long run, be determined by the functions and the operational procedures taking place within the unit, and flexibility in planning must be retained to permit innovation and the introduction of more efficient procedures.

Functions. A nursing unit is made up of three primary components: the patient room, the nurse control station, and the work unit areas.

The patient room is a clearly defined area of space designed to provide a safe, aesthetically pleasing, therapeutic milieu conducive to recuperation, and it must contain space necessary for equipment, staff, and the emergency needs of the patient. The nurse control station provides work space and a view of patient rooms in a manner that facilitates the relationship between work needs and patient care. Its location allows nurses to control and direct traffic entering and leaving the unit, as well as traffic and activities associated with the care and safety of the patients in the unit.

Space must also be allocated for work that takes place outside the patient's room. Work areas serve four purposes: handling materials necessary for patient care, handling and maintaining communications and patient records, meeting the specific needs of the staff, and providing space for either social or physical needs of the patients.

Location. The nursing unit is highly dependent on vertical transportation, communications, and mechanical or pneumatic systems for its relationships with such departments as dietary services, operating rooms, central stores, pharmacy, laboratory, and X-ray. Careful consideration must be given to the choice of these systems in order to produce maximum operational efficiency within financial limitations.

Design: General. Any doorway that may admit a patient in a bed, including classrooms, elevators, treatment rooms, operating rooms, trauma rooms, and radiology rooms, should be four feet wide and at least seven feet high to accommodate traction frames and ciro-electric beds. Handicapped requirements should be consulted for current standards. Handicapped access, for instance, requires 12–18 inches of space at the edge of the door to allow wheelchair patients to open and close it. Corners in corridors that have a projected heavy traffic flow of movable equipment, carts, and beds should have additional protection from bumping. All electrical outlets in the unit should be installed at least three feet above the floor, and all rooms in the nursing unit and within the service should have at least two outlets per wall. Isolated circuitry must be considered; therefore, grounding of all electrical equipment must be provided. Most new hospital equipment today is adapted for low-voltage outlets, including portable X-ray machinery. If food carts will be used to serve patient meals, then 220-volt outlets must be provided in the corridors outside patient rooms.

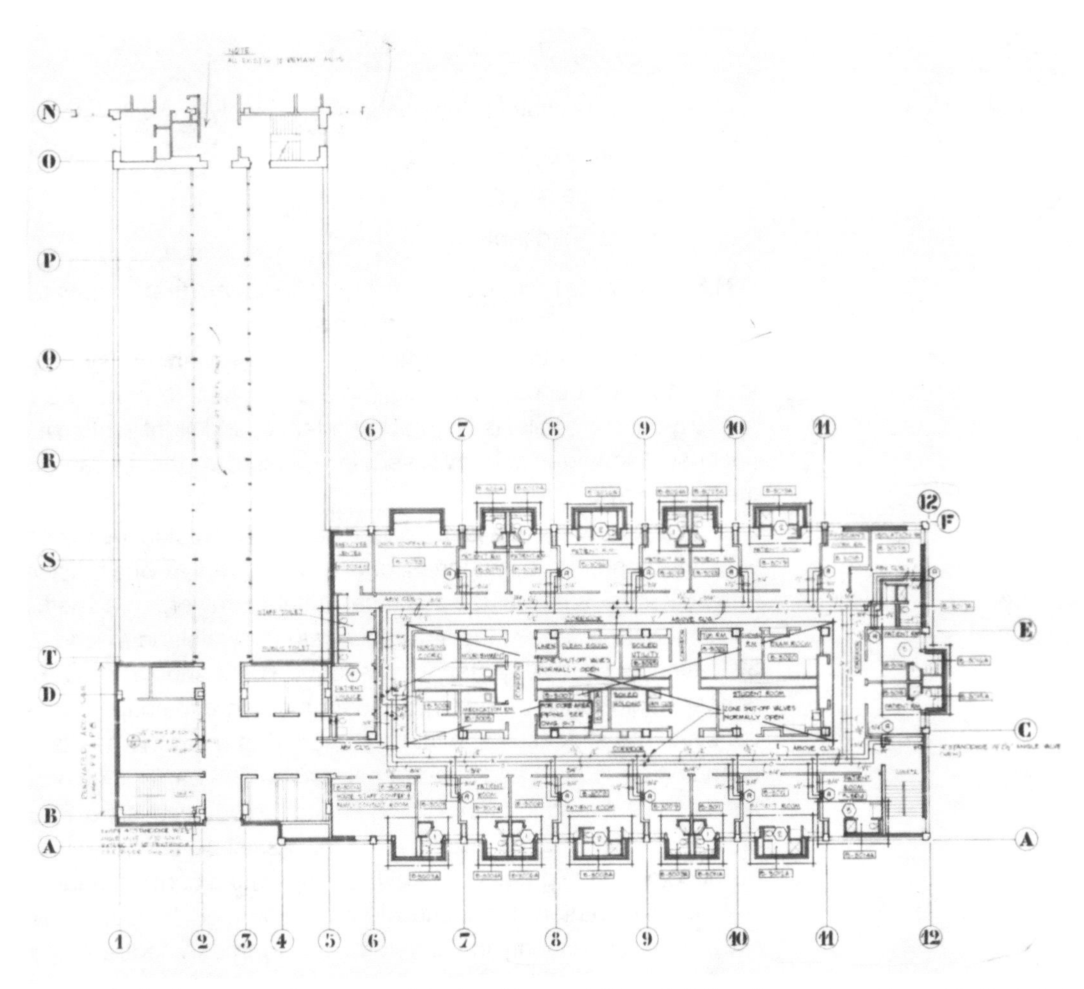

Patient rooms and nursing unit design. Marcus J. Bless Building, Georgetown University Hospital

Design: Patient Rooms. Design of patient rooms must consider the traditional elements of patient care and patient comfort. However, new trends in equipment utilization, treatment procedures, and diagnosis make it imperative that hospital design be flexible enough to encompass not only those ideas that now control patient environment and care, but also new health care delivery concepts. Thus, the general patient room must be designed with enough space and equipment to meet the requirements of today's emergency care procedures and tomorrow's special equipment.

Movable and fixed equipment should fit into 130 square feet of space in a private room and 200 square feet in a semiprivate room, adding an additional 40 square feet per person for toilets and showers. In a double room, sufficient space is required to allow the passage of one bed past the other without moving the other bed. In designing the patient room, careful consideration must be given to accommodating wheelchair and limited mobility patients.

The minimum amount of movable equipment for each private patient room should include the following:

—a bed

—a lounge chair for the patients (preferably one with a footstool)

—a visitor's chair

—a bedside stand

—an over-bed table

H.H.S. standards require a minimum of 100 square feet for private rooms and eighty square feet per patient in semi-private rooms.

The toilet, with an emergency call button within easy reach, should have a flush valve for bedpan cleaning (unless disposable pans are used). Circulation space around the toilet is of great importance, and night lighting must be considered because disoriented or heavily sedated patients frequently cannot remember where the bathroom is.

In a private room a lavatory can be placed outside the water closet; a semiprivate may contain two lavatories, one inside as well as one outside the water closet. The sink area must include electrical outlets, drawers or a shelf, and a mirror. The mirror should be above the sink, flush with the wall, and extend low enough for use by seated as well as by standing patients. There should also be a paper towel dispenser within reach of the sink, and toothbrush and soap holders which drain into the sink. The sink itself should be designed to meet the needs of both the patient (standing or seated) and support personnel. The basin should be deep enough to prevent splash and the faucet high enough to be accessible. Faucet controls must be the wrist-action type, for they not only assist personnel in washing their hands, but accommodate patients incapable of operating conventional valves.

A combination shower-tub is recommended for each private room, with a shower installation only in the semiprivate rooms. A central tub is included in each nursing unit for the use of patients in semiprivate rooms. The shower-tub should be designed to provide multipurpose use of warm water therapy techniques, foot soaks, and bathing without wetting dressed incisions, wounds, or casts. A track-mounted shower nozzle with vertical flexibility is desirable and the shower head should be attached to a hose that can be hand-operated by the patient or by support personnel.

The bedside console should be designed so that it may be placed on either the left or right of the patient's bed or, in case of an emergency, out of the room. It should be convenient to the patient, but not interfere with care. A storage drawer for the patient's personal items should be provided. There should be additional built-in storage to accommodate the patient (bedpan, urinal, emesis basin, toilet tissue, towelettes) and to accommodate the nurse (washbasin, towels, wash cloths, soap). A telephone should be mounted on the console, along with switches for operating the lights at the head of the bed, the reading lights, and the ceiling lights. A ceiling or a wall-hung television should be in the direct line of sight from the bed.

It is recommended that a central communications system for patient control of television, radio, and nurse calls be convenient to the patient. Many different nurse call systems are available. One type utilizes a central station which monitors all patient calls for nursing assistance and relays the call to the nursing station closest to the patient. This system should utilize coaxial cable to allow for future systems innovations.

There should be a built-in wardrobe, with at least two drawers, that will accommodate three suits or dresses, a suitcase, and shoes. A nurse-server or storage closet can be placed on the corridor wall so that it can be stocked via doors in the corridor and used via doors in the room. (This design only accommodates certain supply systems and is therefore optional.) The unit should include two sections, an upper and a lower, both divided into shelves. Its purpose is to feed clean supplies to the patient from the corridor and to hold isolation linen. The bottom section may be used for bagged contaminants or trash and may be removed from the corridor side.

Lighting should be designed to meet the aesthetic and environmental needs of the patient as well as the service needs of the nursing staff. It is recommended that a reading light be fixed at the head of the bed and a night-light on the baseboard near the head of the patient's bed. There should also be ceiling mounted bathroom lighting and vanity lighting for the lavatory area. The patient should be able to control levels of all lighting. A window should provide natural light and a view outside from the bed. Location of the window is important for patients, as it helps them to retain their orientation in time. Regardless of what window design is chosen, it should seek to eliminate the hospital maintenance problem of cleaning or replacing drapes, shades, or blinds upon discharge of the patient: ventilation of smoke from the room through a window is required by the life safety codes.

Design: Nurse Control Station. The nursing control station must be situated on the nursing unit so that it provides optimal visibility of the patient wings. Station design must also include needed communication and record-handling systems. The amount and variety of the traffic and materials that flow past the control station make noise or sound control design of primary importance. Sound control provides a minimum level of noise, a maximum consideration for the patient, and a greatly reduced possibility of staff conversations being overheard by friends and relatives of the patient. Equally important to design considerations is the ability to meet the various needs of the staff.

The patients' need to feel secure can be gratified visually with a well designed nursing control station. Patients are often awake and fearful or anxious during normal sleeping hours. If they require reassurance from the staff, the appearance of the control station should be welcome and comforting. It is imperative that the nursing control station design not project a negative or off limits atmosphere to the patient.

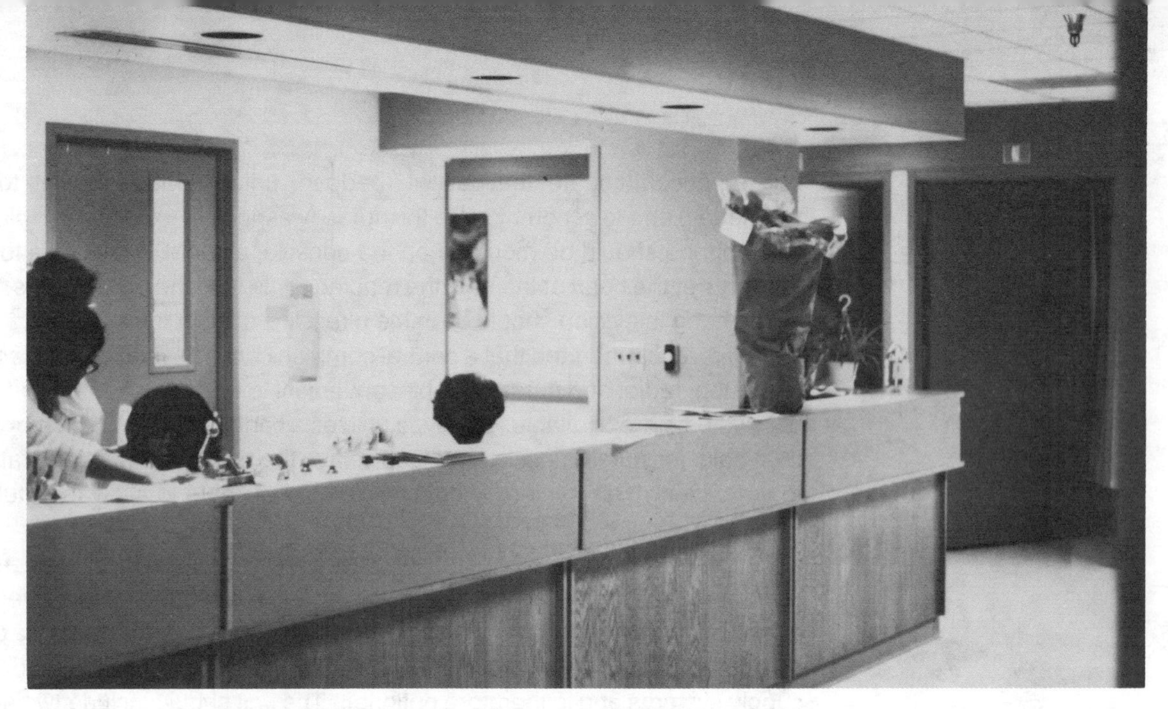

Nursing control station. Capital Hill Hospital, Washington, D.C.

Also, the nursing control station should be designed to prevent the visual effect of a cage around the staff who work in the area. This effect is undesirable for both the staff and the patient.

The nursing control station should provide space for patient chart storage, paper and form storage, chairs in the viewing area, nurses' charting and reporting area, physicians' charting area, and communications requirements. Corridor control should also be kept in mind. The communications bank must be able to accommodate patient communication systems, telephones, addressographs, dataphone, and, in the future, electronic monitors and computer terminals.

Design: Work Areas. Regardless of the managerial method used by the hospital's nursing personnel, nurses' functions encompass patients, visitors, physicians' orders, and general coordination of all individuals and activities directly or indirectly related to the patient. Because of this degree of responsibility, it is recommended that design elements be geared toward providing control from a central point in the unit. Those work areas that are used frequently by personnel on the unit should be placed close to the control station. Further, frequently used work areas should be located directly in front of the viewing area: for example, medical areas; the linen, clean supply, and equipment utility areas; janitor and housekeeping closets; and soiled utility areas.

The medicine room should be large enough to accommodate personnel and teaching needs and be under continual observation. It should include an acid sink, double-locked narcotic boxes, wraparound counters with formica tops, and built-in cabinetry, unless unit close carts are used. If a pneumatic tube system is incorporated, it should be accessible to the medicine room. A small refrigerator for drugs requiring cooler temperatures should be located off the nurse charting area. A unit dose system cart may be programmed in this area.

The soiled utility areas hold used patient items for return to the various processing areas. As a result, they should be as close to the unit's entrance or automated transport junctions as possible. The soiled utility area requires a large splash-proof sink with a foot-operated faucet. Shelving of formica or stainless steel for tray coverage and space for a soiled linen and a trash cart are also recommended.

Regardless of the type of general food service system used by the hospital, the nursing unit requires a nourishment center. It should contain space for an ice-maker, a full-sized refrigerator with freezer, a cabinet area with a toaster, and an automatic tea, soup, and coffee dispenser. The concept of convenience food is fast gaining acceptance in this area. The nourishment center should be designed to provide room for expansion in the future for such items as a microwave oven.

The clean utility room should be large enough to accommodate shelving for patient items such as soap, toilet paper, tissues, mouthwash, toothpaste, paper forms, and requisitions. Prepackaged admission kits may be used, but replacements will be needed. A large splash-proof sink is required, and a deep basin is recommended for hand-washing. Shelving for dressings, intravenous equipment, antiseptics, small kits, and so forth should also be provided. It is anticipated that linen will be distributed to each nurse server cabinet or a linen exchange cart on arrival, nonetheless, space for a linen cart with extra linen should be included in the clean utility room. An exchange cart system does not require the wall storage. Regardless of the delivery system to be used, the distance between the elevator and the clean utility room should be kept to a minimum.

The treatment room should be large enough to accommodate a large, deep sink located adjacent to the treatment table. The examining table should be carefully evaluated to provide the patient with the greatest degree of comfort during examinations. Emergencies do occur in nursing unit treatment rooms, so the table must be versatile enough to provide for emergency patient care. Arm boards for use during the administration of intravenous solutions and rollers with locks are necessary. Since the table will be used for procedures and treatments that cannot be performed comfortably in the patient's bed, lighting is of critical importance. A small ceiling-mounted swivel-operated light, which can be directed toward any part of the body, is recommended. A bathroom should adjoin the treatment room and should include a toilet and bedpan flush valve. A small shelf for urine specimen containers and a lavatory for hand-washing are also required. Hand rails and an emergency call button should be located in the treatment room. This room should be soundproof. The central tub room should be adjacent to the treatment room and contain one high tub, one low tub, and a sitz bath. It should be possible, by using a ceiling-mounted curtain, to afford privacy for all three areas.

The conference classroom should be located near the control station. It is used for in-service and other educational programs and for planning patient discharges.

When selecting the location of the patient dayroom on the nursing unit, its function and its relationship to other areas of the unit should be considered. The dayroom is designed to be, first, an area where the ambulatory patient can relax in a change of environment and visit with relatives or other patients, and, second, an area where the patient's visitors can wait while hospital personnel carry out routine

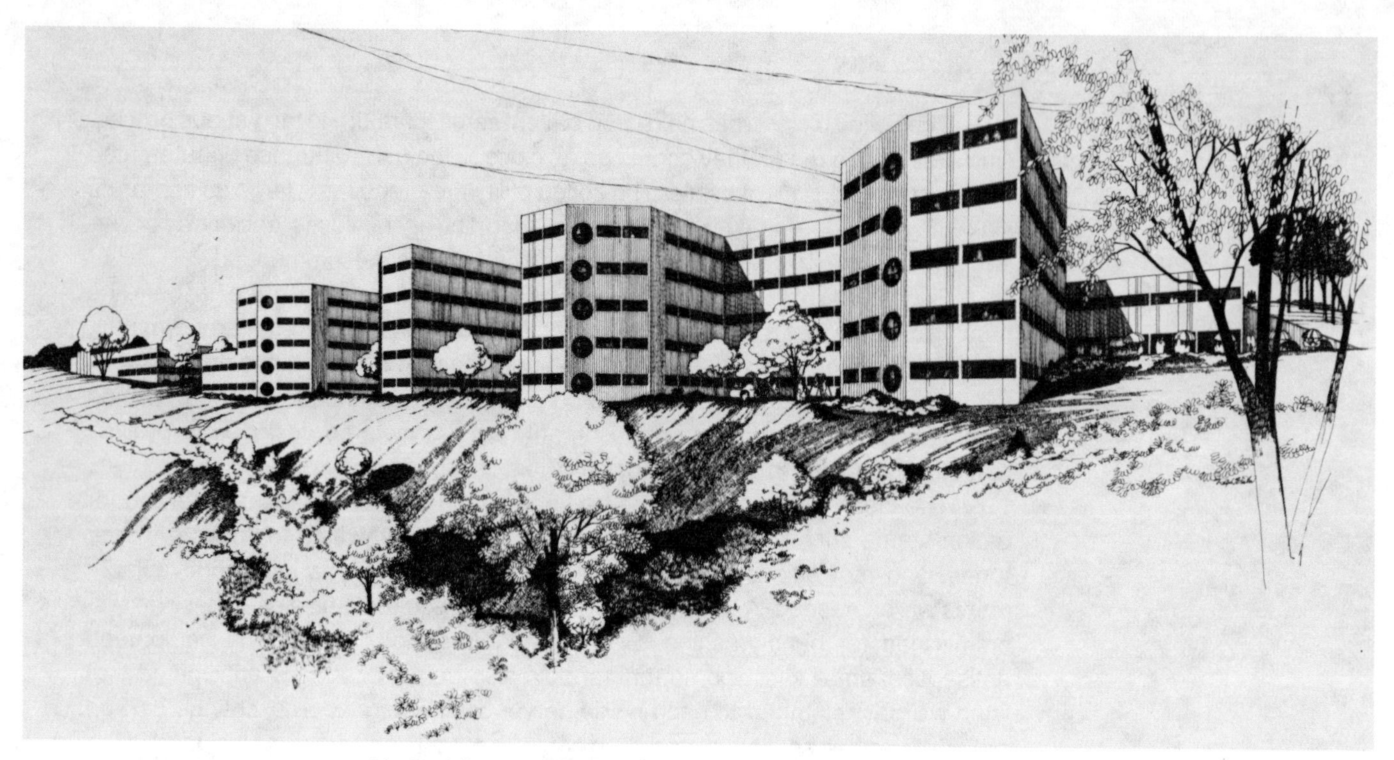

Medical Center of Beaver County, Pennsylvania

or emergency procedures in the patient's room (therefore, it should have a line of sight relationship to the patient's door). A separate visitors' waiting room can also serve this function. The dayroom should not be an area for hospital personnel to congregate, nor should it become a charting room for physicians and nurses.

The dayroom should be located so as to encourage patients to use it, yet it need not be centrally located for access to the nursing control center, the treatment or medicine rooms, the nourishment center, or the linen and storage areas. The ambulatory patient's needs for these are minimal. It should be distant from the entry into the unit and off the main traffic pattern so that ambulatory patients will not impede or accost physicians, nursing personnel, hospital staff, or visitors. Finally, the dayroom should be located so as to facilitate supervision by the nursing staff, while at the same time minimizing the possibility of the patients' misinterpreting professional activities or overhearing private or confidential communication between staff, other patients, and visitors.

The dayroom should be provided with the following:

—one round table (high enough to accommodate patients in wheelchairs, that will seat four persons,

—individual seating, including large chairs with footstools and rocking chairs (construction and material should be selected for ease in cleaning and maintenance, as well as comfort)

—a large television

—two electric outlets per wall

—small tables (for lamps, ashtrays, and so on)

—a magazine and book rack

—outlets for oxygen and suction (hidden behind a wall picture or painting)

—storage cabinet (for cards, games, occupational therapy equipment, and so forth)

—windows for maximum light and ventilation (with control for excessive light)

—emergency call button and intercom connected to the nursing station

Storage space needs to be provided for infrequently used equipment. It should be easily accessible, but not directly in the center of the nursing unit. A stretcher alcove should be centrally located for holding stretchers and wheelchairs to be used in the unit. Public toilets can be combined with toilets for the use of handicapped patients.

Intradepartmental Relationships. The nurse control station is, ideally, located centrally in the unit with a good view of the vertical transport entrance, patient room hallways, and work area. Work areas should be located around the control station, but within easy access of all patient rooms. Patient rooms should radiate from the central core in two or more directions; this keeps the distance from the control station and work areas as short as possible. Federal guideline for maximum distance between patient room and control station is 120 feet.

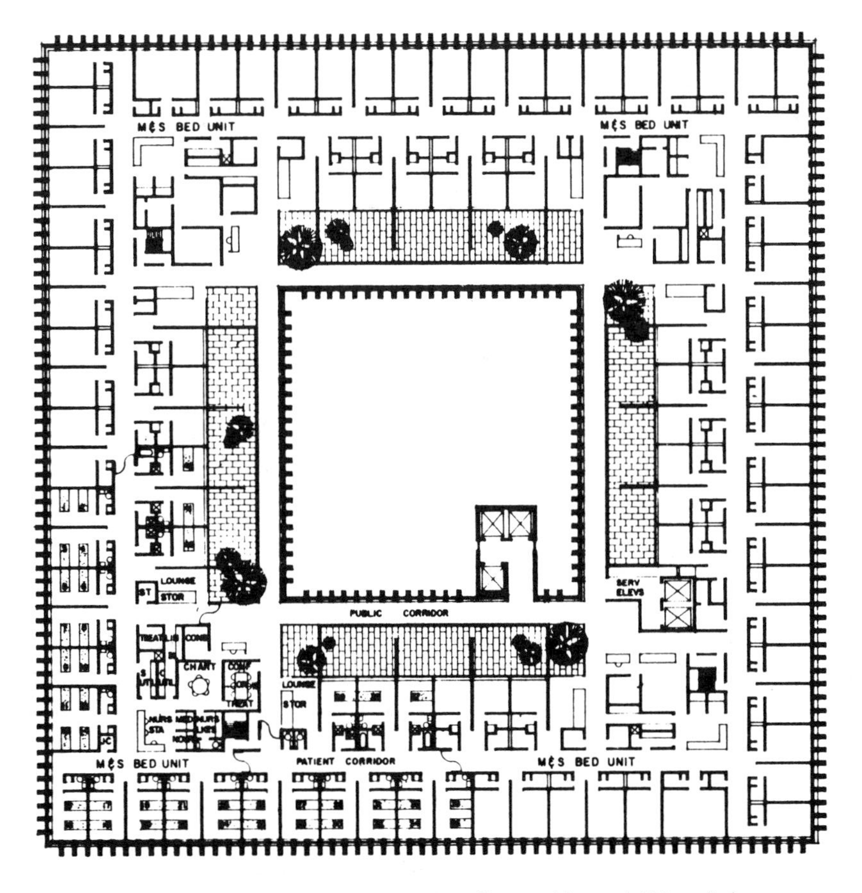

Typical nursing unit lay-out. Kent County Memorial Hospital

PEDIATRIC UNIT

The patterns of childhood illness and the requirements for services and facilities for children have changed dramatically in the past decade, and there is every indication that these changes will continue, so that innovation will continue to be necessary. The control of infectious disease and the increased use of various forms of ambulatory facilities have resulted in reduced hospitalization of children. At the same time, children who are hospitalized for acute illnesses require specialized care and services. Children with chronic conditions are living longer and, therefore, require increasing amounts of specialized types of hospitalization.

Parents, siblings, and friends are vital to the rehabilitation of the sick child. Consequently, parents are encouraged to live in with, assist in the care of, and maintain continuous contact with the child. The psychological benefit of seeing siblings and friends is now considered to over-shadow the danger of introducing infection (actually, child visitors have been found to be no greater hazard than adult visitors). In the case of older children, units designed specifically to serve the psychological and physiological needs of adolescents are being developed apart from either pediatrics or general medical-surgical services.

Location. A pediatric unit is naturally noisy. It should be located in a quiet area, removed from other hospital traffic. Natural light should be available to all bedrooms, if possible, and access to an enclosed outside terrace or play area is also desirable. The unit should be adjacent to vertical transportation in order to meet its needs for other services. Proximity, either horizontal or vertical, to the nursery is also desirable.

Design. The pediatric unit has many of the same elements and requirements as the general nursing units (nurse control station, work area, and patient units). Sick children, however, have additional needs and require an appropriate physical environment; for example, in the decor, lighting, equipment, and recreational facilities. Thus, the pediatric unit must meet unique needs and should be designed to do so. The neonatal intensive care unit (premature nursery) and isolation nursery, if part of pediatrics, should be located near the nursing station.

The number of rooms, their size, and their location should be planned to ensure efficient and effective observation and servicing by nursing personnel. A minimum of twenty to twenty-five percent of the beds on a pediatric unit should be in single rooms; they have numerous uses and add greatly to unit versatility. For instance, they are needed for critically ill patients and for those who are disturbing other patients. With appropriate equipment, they may also be used for isolation patients. It is generally accepted, however, that children adjust better to hospitalization when they are able to have the companionship of other children in the same room. Thus, with the above exceptions, efforts should be made to place children in two-bed rooms. Live-in facilities for parents should be provided, particularly for parents of infants and pre-school children. These facilities may be provided in either one-or two-bed rooms and should include space for a bed or cot for the parent and a dresser for his or her belongings.

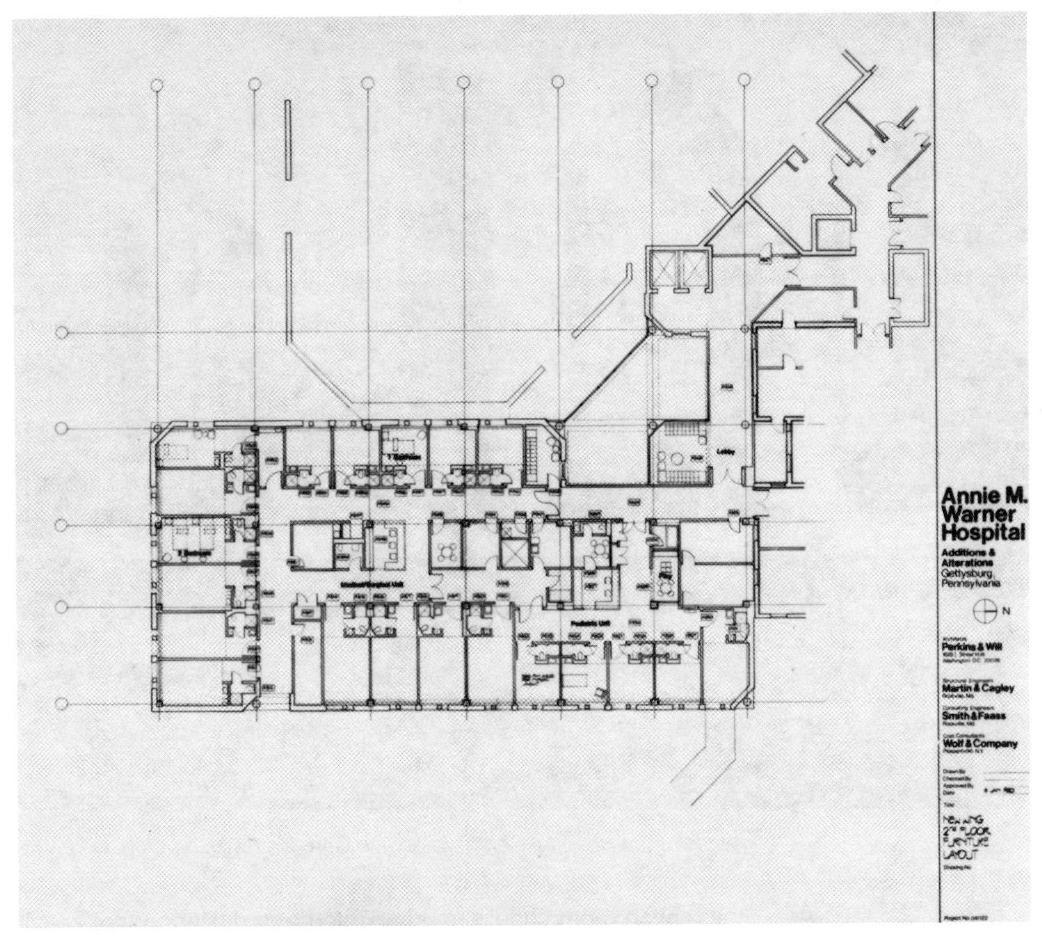

Pediatrics nursing unit. Annie M. Warner Hospital, Gettysburg, Pennsylvania

Each hospital bed should be adjustable, and youth bed, crib, or bassinet may be substituted as required. Adequate storage facilities in some part of the hospital must be provided for alternate-sized beds not currently in use. This is a problem unique to pediatric units. An overbed table for trays and toys should be provided for each bed.

Isolation rooms should have an adjoining bath equipped with shower or tub, toilet, and sink. Strict isolation techniques can be ideally met by having an anteroom between a single-bed room and the corridor. This anteroom should contain a sink; an enclosed paper towel dispenser; a soap dispenser; a linen hamper for soiled masks and gowns; a foot-operated waste receptacle with removable, waterproof liner; and a small utility case or cabinet for clean gowns, masks, and other supplies.

The special interest of adolescents in recreation and companionship with their own age group must be recognized. Rooms assigned to teenagers should be grouped together. If possible, a special social room and library, appropriately decorated and furnished, should be provided for adolescents.

The recreation room in a pediatric nursing unit varies according to the size of the unit and the age of the patients. It can be used for group activities and for recreation; for instance, as a playroom for younger children, as an occupational therapy room and classroom for older children, and as a social room and library for adolescents. It is also an ideal place for ambulatory children to dine together. The

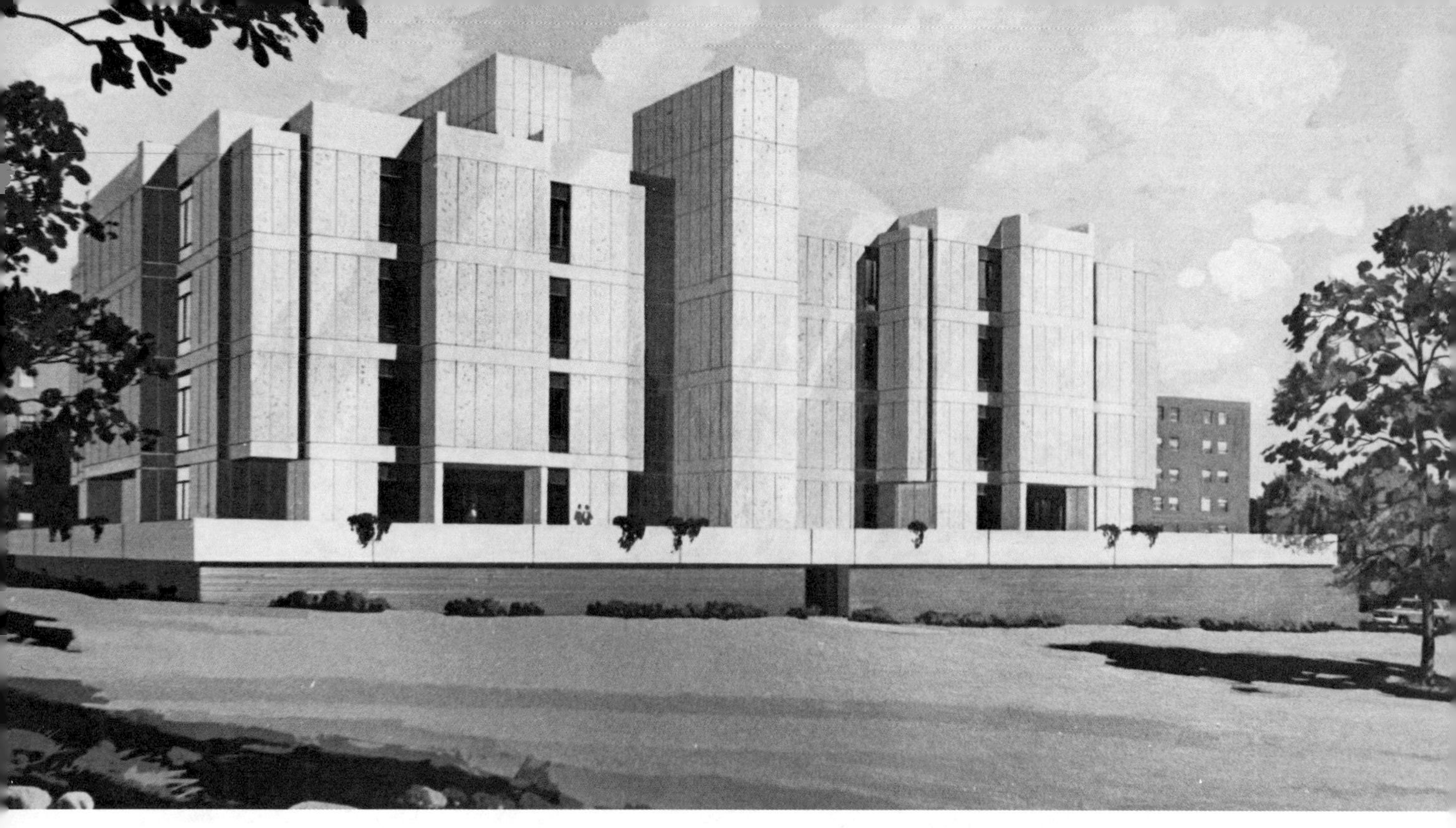

Washington Hospital Center Intensive Care Unit, Washington, D.C.

recreation room should be so located and designed that activities will not disturb patients in their bedrooms. At least half of the children may use the recreation room: if the room is used for recreation only, twelve square feet should be allowed for each patient; when it is used for dining as well, twenty-five square feet should be allowed for each child served.

The number of small children and adolescents who will be using the recreation room will also govern the amount of storage space needed. Storage closets will be required for toys, games, and other play or study materials. Bookcases, a bulletin board, and a chalkboard should be provided. Tables and chairs should be designed and sized for the anticipated use, such as dining, play, and classwork. A shuffleboard designed into the floor, a television, a rollup projection screen, and a piano could also be considered. Toilet facilities for both boys and girls should be adjoining or within the area.

At least one tub room, preferably two, should be provided on a pediatric unit. If there are two tubs, one can be a pedestal type, accessible on three sides for easier bathing of small children. Controls for the tubs should be on the wall, out of reach of the child. Toilet facilities should be provided in each tub room. The tub rooms should accommodate a wheelchair patient and should be equipped with vertical and horizontal grab-bars, emergency call, and occupancy light. Doors should have locks to give privacy, but the nurse should be able to unlock the door from outside if necessary.

Each patient shower and each dressing area should measure at least three feet by three feet to allow for a stool or wheelchair and for grab-bars. Plumbing fixtures should include a hose attachment for a sit-down shower. Shower rooms other than those in patient rooms should have an occupancy light in the corridor controlled by the same switch that controls mechanical ventilation, and emergency call buttons that can be reached from the shower and dressing area are required.

Adequate facilities should be provided for the preparation of formulas, whether they are primarily prepared in the hospital formula room or purchased from outside suppliers. A counter with sink and a small refrigerator for formula preparation should be provided within any unit that cares for infants.

A window sill height of no more than three feet is recommended to allow children to see out from their beds. Safety latches should be provided on all windows. Walls between patient rooms can have clear glass panels to allow the children to see activities around them, and to allow the nurses to see the children easily. Wire glass, safety glass, or glass of similar quality should be used to minimize injury in case of breakage. Walls and doors between the rooms and the corridors should have wire glass panels set in metal frames not exceeding 1,296 square inches. The bottom of glass panels should be mattress height to provide visibility for nurses, and draw curtains should be provided to allow for privacy when needed.

Soundproofing is desirable for the entire pediatric unit. It is required for ceilings in corridors, patient areas, nurses' stations, and dietary and dining areas. There are special standards and requirements for lighting and ventilation of elements in the pediatric unit. The architect should review these carefully. Doors to fire exits should be equipped with an alarm system arranged so it can be turned off in hours when the unit is fully staffed and reactivated at night or when the unit is only partially staffed. The services of a professional designer who is experienced in the planning of facilities for children would be beneficial.

OBSTETRICAL UNIT

Location. The obstetrical nursing unit should be adjacent to the nursery to minimize the distance of travel and consequent exposure of babies between the nursery and the mother's room. Proximity to vertical transport is necessary, but the elevator lobby should not intersect the flow of babies to mothers. Ideally, the obstetrical unit should be on the same floor as the labor–delivery suite for increased operational efficiency.

Design. The following areas are needed in the patient unit:

—private and semiprivate rooms

—patient bath

—storage area

—patient lavatory

—wardrobe

—fathers' waiting room

A rooming-in program may affect design considerations. The nurse control station requires:

—clerk-receptionist area

—nurses' charting area

—physicians' charting area (with dictation booths)

—nurses' lounge-locker room and toilet

—head nurse's office

Support areas are made up of:

—medicine room

—nourishment station

—treatment room (with toilet)

—tub room

—clean and soiled utility rooms

—conference room

—supervisor's office

—dayroom

—public toilets

—storage

—stretcher and wheelchair alcove

A conference room should also be used for patient education programs and an additional office, adjacent to the conference room, should be allocated to the supervisor. The tub room should include four sitz baths. The dayroom should be decorated cheerfully and be somewhat larger than the usual dayroom because most patients in this area are ambulatory. Many patients, it should be remembered, prefer double rooms because of the social interaction they provide.

INTENSIVE CARE COMPLEX

Specially designed intensive care facilities, an innovation of the early 1960s, are acknowledged as being essential for good medical care. Intensive care beds have increased from approximately three percent of the total bed count in the 1960s and 1970s to ten percent in the 1980s. Centralizing acutely ill patients in contiguous units, that is, an intensive care complex consisting of medical-surgical intensive care unit, coronary care unit, and specialty units such as renal and burn units, results in multidisciplinary care and economies of space and equipment.

The medical-surgical intensive care unit provides care for:

—postsurgical patients who have developed or are liable to develop complications requiring close, skilled nursing observation and care

—serious emergency patients suffering from coma, shock, hemorrhage, respiratory embarrassment, or convulsions

—patients with serious fluid or electrolyte problems

—patients who require hemodialysis due to acute renal failure from trauma or ingestion of a toxic substance (if hemodialysis unit not provided)

—other patients who meet the criteria of stated program objectives

The coronary intensive care unit is designed for:

—patients with acute cardiac conditions

—cardiac patients requiring comprehensive, continuous, individualized observation and care supplemented by electronic monitoring and therapy equipment

—other patients meeting the criteria of stated program objectives

The specialty unit provides burn treatment, renal dialysis, psychiatric care, spinal care, and so on.

Functions. The intensive care complex is set up to:

—concentrate in one geographic area the most acutely ill patients for maximum surveillance and skilled nursing care from specially trained personnel

—greatly extend the physician's capacity to treat the acutely ill through the centralization of trained support personnel and specialized equipment

—provide personal and monitor-assisted surveillance of critically ill patients so that all of their physiological parameters are instantly available to the professional staff, thus facilitating timely diagnosis, treatment, and evaluation of treatment place

—realize more effective and economical utilization of equipment and of highly trained personnel

—improve overall patient care by relieving the nursing staff on regular patient floors of the need to concentrate on a few acutely ill patients at the expense of the less ill

Location. The intensive care units should be contiguous with or readily accessible to one another. For example, patients admitted to the medical-surgical intensive care unit may have or may develop cardiac complications, often suddenly. Having all intensive care facilities in one place allows specially trained professionals almost instant access to patients in all clinical services when an emergency develops.

The intensive care complex should also be relatively close, either horizontally or vertically, to the emergency room or emergency entrance to the hospital; the operating suite and recovery room; and the special procedure room of radiology or a fluoroscopy room. Many specialty units reoccur on the related nursing unit. Most admissions to intensive care facilities are either direct emergency admissions from

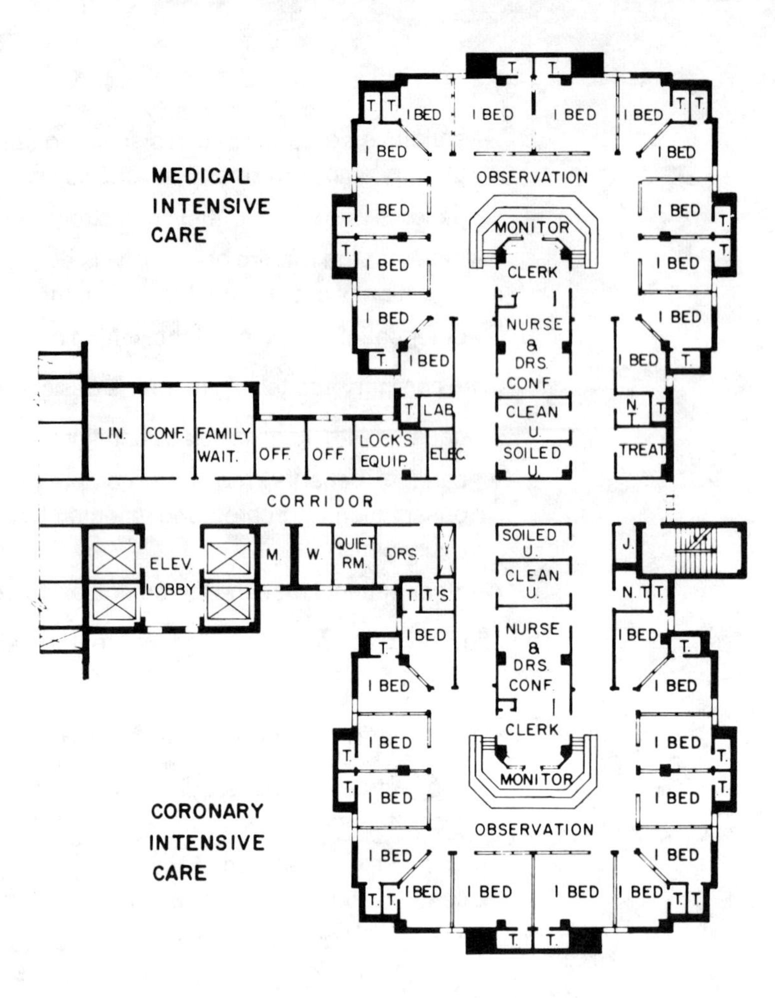

Washington Hospital Center, intensive care tower, Washington, D.C.

home or work, admissions via the emergency room, or admissions following major surgery. It is not unusual for patients following lengthy or complicated surgery or for patients following major trauma or accident to return to surgery for additional emergency care.

The intensive care facilities should also be located reasonably close to general nursing units to reduce to a minimum the movement and time required to transfer patients from general care to intensive care in an emergency. This likewise reduces transit to general care when the patient no longer requires the facilities of the intensive care unit. Considering all these factors, it is clear that the intensive care complex should have ready access to the vertical transport system for the rapid transit of patients and personnel.

Intensive care facilities should be located away from heavy traffic areas such as the main entrances and exits, visitor waiting areas, and passageways to other service areas of the hospital. It is also extremely important in determining the location of the complex to keep in mind the adverse electrical influence on the displays of the monitoring equipment of such things as elevator motors and X-ray equipment.

Design. No fewer than two emergency carts should be kept fully supplied and immediately accessible to the intensive care nursing station and all the supplies necessary to restock the emergency cart, immediately after use, should be in a clean utility room and drug-dispensing area in the unit. Adequate amounts of many items, therefore, must be maintained in the intensive care complex itself; for example, tracheostomy trays, resuscitation equipment, sterile pacemaker catheter, dressing trays, Foley catheters, catheterization kits, urinary drainage bags, sterile specimen kits, sterile gloves, syringes, needles, and intravenous solutions. This requires considerable storage space. A system of daily inventory should also be coordinated with the pharmacy to insure an adequate stock of necessary pharmaceuticals.

It is recommended that clean linen be readily available at all times on carts in the clean utility room. Soiled linen should be bagged by intensive care personnel using linen bags that disintegrate or dissolve in the wash to reduce contamination. Housekeeping supplies, cleaning equipment, and so on should also be stored in each unit.

The respiratory therapist is an extremely important member of the intensive care staff. The patient in respiratory crisis requires constant attention from the therapist and the nursing staff. Space should be allowed in the intensive care complex for storage of respiratory equipment, and it is desirable for the therapist to have an office in the area. Because therapists perform techniques such as intubation and blood gas analysis, it would be wise to utilize their services as educators when training programs for the nursing staff are presented.

Diet to intensive care patients consists chiefly of liquids, as determined by the medical and nursing staff's judgment of the patient's ability to handle oral feeding and a wide variety of such foods should be available. Nourishment should also be provided for staff who miss regular cafeteria hours because of emergencies on the unit.

It is generally accepted that for effective operation, there should be no more than twelve to sixteen beds per intensive care unit. A six-bed unit is probably the most economical to operate and requires approximately the same number of staff as do smaller units. A four-bed unit is considered the smallest unit economically feasible.

Function and accessibility are of paramount concern in intensive care unit design and direct visual contact between the patient rooms and the nurses' station is highly recommended. Patient rooms should, therefore, be as close to the station as possible. On the other hand, since the unit will serve both male and female patients, it should be designed to provide patient privacy. Individual rooms or cubicles with full-height glass walls and curtained windows between the rooms and the corridor are recommended for necessary observation and maximum flexibility of usage while providing for patient privacy as needed. Curtain or cubicle screening of beds is, however, acceptable if the construction of individual rooms is not possible.

A window to the outside is necessary for each patient cubicle or room and soundproofing of the entire area is recommended. Air conditioning, heating, and humidity control should be provided for the entire unit, with individual room controls. High-intensity lighting should be provided above each bed for examination and treatment.

The following items should be placed on the wall at the head of each bed or on a freestanding column to allow maximum circulation:

—night light switches and dimmers
—vertical wall lighting unit (mounted high enough to protect against head injuries to personnel working at the head of the bed during emergencies)
—nurses' call system
—electrical outlets, 110 and 208 volts, no lower than thirty inches off the floor
—medical gases (one compressed air, two oxygen, and three vacuum outlets per bed)
—telephone outlet
—wall-mounted manometer (swivel type) with a cuff basket for each bed
—speaker for music system
—time-recorded clock system with reset controls
—recessed plastic pan below medical gas module to hold vacuum bottles
—monitor shelf or attachment

A conduit should be available to each cubicle, in the corner of the room, for monitoring equipment. Monitor cabinet equipment should be placed at the head of the bed on the side visible from the entrance to the room. Medical gases should be located at the side of the bed and opposite the monitor cabinet. Consideration should be given to utilizing monitoring cabinets that swivel on a pole hung from the ceiling. Two beds in the medical-surgical unit should be supplied with wall-mounted dialysis machines. It is highly desirable to have a fluoroscopy room adjacent to or near the intensive care complex.

Lavatories with foot pedals and toilets with bedpan flush valves should be installed near doors of the rooms. This will allow for isolation techniques and add more flexibility.

The medical-surgical intensive care, coronary intensive care, and specialty units, while separate, should be adjacent to one another, share as many central facilities as possible, and be identical in room construction to allow maximum flexibility and expansion. The coronary care unit should be adjacent to a medical-surgical ward that has a specified number of rooms equipped for monitoring and that can function as intermediary cardiac units.

Intradepartmental Elements. Each unit should contain:

—nursing station centrally located and with visual access to each room or patient area
—medication area
—nourishment area
—utility area for clean and soiled linens and central supplies
—lockers (patient and personnel)
—staff toilets (one per unit)

—control area (including central monitoring equipment)
—equipment storage area
—janitor closet
—family waiting room
—conference area
—physician on-call rooms (with baths)

INTERMEDIATE OR STEP-DOWN UNITS

This unit contains patients who do not have intensive care needs, such as twenty-four-hour observation, but who must be monitored before progressing on into a general patient unit. Intermediate, or step-down, care beds are provided for these acutely ill patients, who may be admitted directly to this level or from the intensive care complex when they are removed from the critical list. The unit should, therefore, adjoin the intensive care complex. The design is the same as that of a general patient unit except for the monitor connection and telemetry designed into each patient space.

A twenty-two-bed intermediate unit requires one registered nurse and one practical nurse for the day shift, one registered nurse in the evening, and a practical nurse for night duty. Such units should consist of private rooms, each with its own toilet and lavatory. Privacy is especially desirable, for patients, though well enough to be aware of their surroundings, are ill enough to be particularly sensitive to them. Regardless of age, sex, or ailment, all patients in intermediate care require about the same degree of nursing attention. Thus, the single-bed room design facilitates assignment by allowing utilization of the nearest available room.

Nursing duties are lighter in the convalescent unit, and fewer nurses need be assigned to it. Convalescent units may be planned with some semiprivate rooms, for at this stage some patients will find company therapeutic. They are well enough to help each other and the nurse in small ways and to enjoy having someone to talk to. Each room should have a toilet and lavatory.

LONG-TERM CARE UNIT

In long-term and self-care units, private and semi-private bedrooms with baths and dayroom facilities should be provided. A minimum of hospital equipment and nursing supervision is required allowing the construction of economically built motel-like units rather than standard hospital rooms. This is particularly true if they can be built as pavilions independent of the main hospital structure.

The long-term care facility must compete with private nursing homes based upon need with a region. The total picture for long-term care of persons age 65 and older is one of heavy reliance on a Medicare payment structure, combined with local government social programs and government-funded facilities. The Veterans Administration offers excellent facilities and sets an industry standard for long-term care.

LOUNGE
NURSING UNIT
SOILED
ADMINISTRATIVE CONTROL CENTER
CLEAN
LOUNGE
SECOND FLOOR

NURSING UNIT

Each typical floor has 96 beds:
4-24 bed nursing units

Each 24 bed nursing unit will be served by:
1 RN-Team Leader
1 RN
2 LPN
1 Nurse Aide

The administrative control center located opposite the elevator door, except on the first floor, will serve and be responsible for 96 beds. (144 after two wings are added).

Each 48 bed unit will provide the following spaces:
2 Team Conference Rooms
1 Tub Room
1 Exam Room
1 Janitor Closet
1 Lounge Area and Public Toilets
2 Galleys
2 Drs. Conference and Exam Rooms
1 Large Janitor and Housekeeping Closet
1 Isolation and Ante Room
9 Private Rooms (21%)
19 Semi-Private Rooms (79%)
All rooms contain showers

Each 96 bed unit will include:
1 Administrative Control Center and Clerk
1 Nurse Supervisor Office
1 Clean Utility and Distribution Room
1 Soiled Utility and Distribution Room
1 Satellite Pharmacy Office
1 Therapeutic Dieticians Office
1 Supply Aide Station
1 Galley Girl

Each room provides Patient Servers for clean and soiled patient items. It contains linens, blankets, medications drug drawer, patient chart and incidential items. Narcotics will be stored in the Pharmacy satellite.

Total Stage I bed complement will be 233 beds:

First Floor	8	ICU
	8	CCU
	24	Surgical
	48	Medical/Surgical
Second Floor	96	Medical/Surgical
Third Floor	25	Pediatrics
	24	Medical/Surgical
	233	Beds

Shell space on third floor is for 48 additional beds. Lockers and Snack Shop for nurses and visitors is in the lower level of the Bed Unit.

Nursing unit lay-out. People's Community Memorial Hospital, Taylor, Michigan

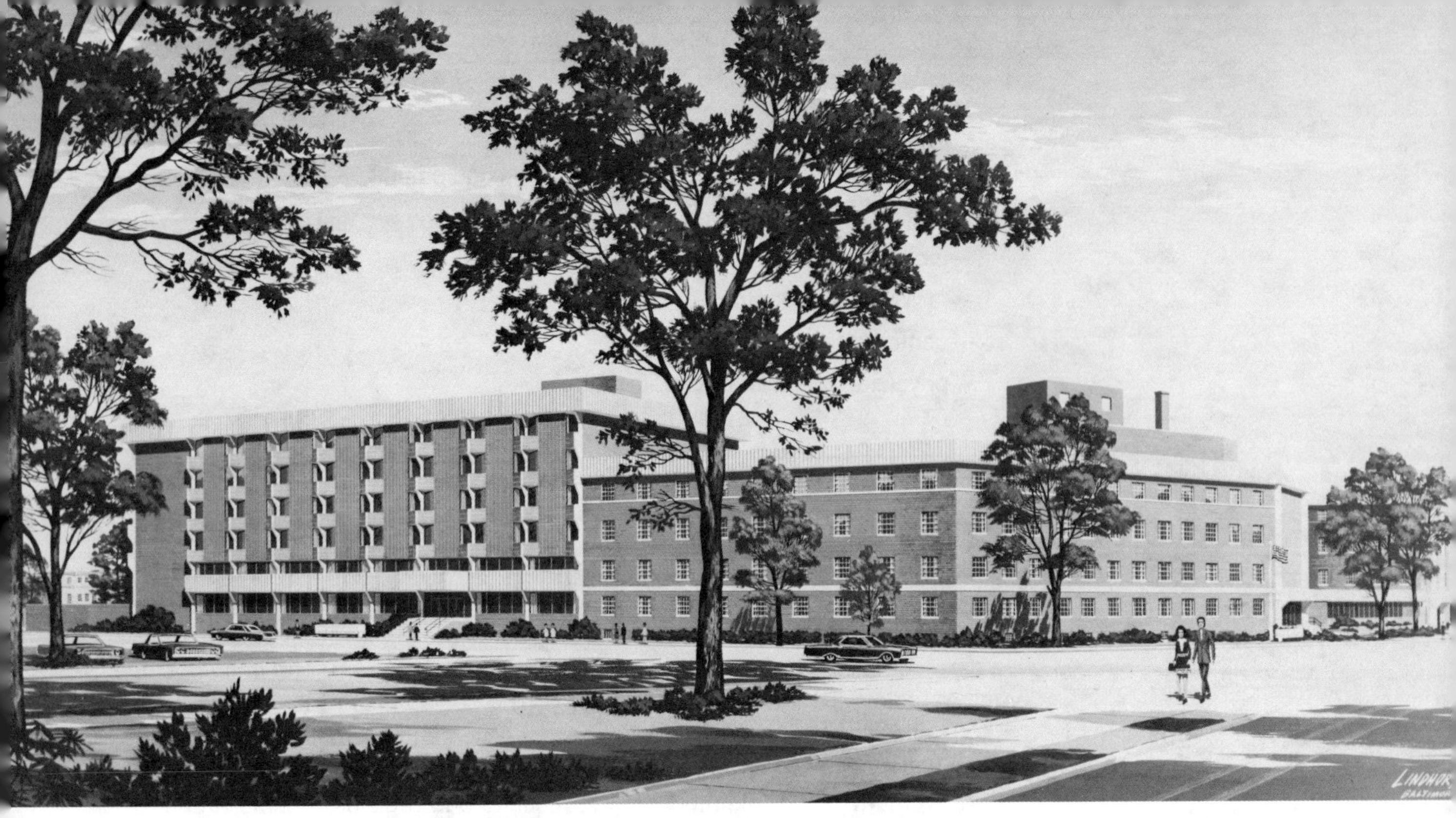

Capital Hill Hospital, Washington, D.C.

The function of long-term care facilities is to provide therapeutic or compensating environments in which patients stay weeks, months, or years rather than a few days. Because most of these populations possess as much diversity as any random group of noninstitutionalized persons, it usually is difficult to design precisely for the needs of a particular long-term care population. In theory, patients in these facilities can be classified into two groups: one requiring protracted rehabilitative therapy and the other needing supportive or custodial care. In practice, institutions may house varying proportions of each category with few environmental distinctions. For example, an effort is usually made to segregate persons with mental disabilities from those with physical ailments, but the distinction often cannot be made for geriatric or neurologically impaired patients. However, if common needs of a patient group can be identified, the design should respond to those needs, and there are environmental concerns that should be considered in the design of long-term care facilities.

Therapeutic Technology

Facilities for physical treatment require larger quantities of supplies and equipment, whereas those for psychiatric care require a greater number of office, conference, and meeting spaces. Physical treatment usually requires that the treatment staff and support spaces be integrated with the living spaces of the residents to provide assistance required on short notice. In facilities for psychiatric care, it is possible, and often desirable, to provide separate zones for living and formal therapeutic activities, although the design of the living quarters is usually influenced by therapeutic considerations.

Therapeutic Intensity

Most long-term care patients will not have acute physical illnesses; however, some of them may require a lot of care, such as physical rehabilitation services. In this case space and equipment required by the therapeutic technology may become a highly visible or even dominant feature in the design. Where a relatively high intensity of medical attention is required, the long-term care unit can be very similar to the typical hospital nursing unit in both form and content. At the other extreme, a facility that provides only custodial care or minimal assistance in routine daily activities would resemble a residential environment.

Staff Control and Patient Security

Medical and nursing staff, acutely aware of their responsibility for the physical welfare of their patients, usually demand that staff work stations be situated so as to permit direct observation of all corridors, public or shared spaces, and the door to each patient's room, if not each bed. While this organization is appropriate for most hospital nursing units, it may be neither necessary nor desirable in rehabilitation-oriented facilities. The degree of staff control, or dominance, that the design expresses should be carefully weighed against the organization's commitment to reducing the dependency of its patients. The staff control parameter also affects the design of exterior spaces and the relationship of interior to exterior spaces. The organization and details of a unit or building can influence patients either to seek or to avoid contact with the world outside the institution.

Privacy, Personal Identity, and Territoriality

Long-term care patients functioning above some minimum threshold of awareness will take an interest in and respond to their physical surroundings. The impact of environmental factors is increased precisely because residents are restricted to a particular environment for long periods of time. Denied privacy and deprived of any significant control over their environment, institutionalized persons can experience loss of dignity and decline in self-esteem, which adversely affects personal competence and social behavior. A great deal can be done to counteract this problem.

At the very least, residents must be given secure places to store personal belongings. Personalization of space should be allowed or encouraged by the details of an individual's designated territory: nameplates can contribute to his sense of identity, self-determination, and self-worth; controlling window coverings and lighting and determining the location of furnishings in personal spaces can be helpful. Within the necessary limitations of cost, and the proper degree of medical staff supervision, each resident should have maximum control over readily identifiable personal territory.

Social Opportunity

It is highly desirable that a long-term care environment provide a variety of spaces for social interaction between patients or between patients and visitors.

Ideally, the patient should be able to choose among several places suitable for an intimate conversation, a small group discussion or game, or a large group activity. The smaller social spaces are usually located near the resident's personal territories and can foster a sense of group identity, like a neighborhood, within a larger institution. Corridor alcoves, small separate rooms, or gathering space within individual suites can provide opportunities for individual and small group interactions. Dining arrangements have a major impact on social opportunity. At one extreme is the serving of meals to patients in their personal territory, while the opposite is represented by groups dining family style at a large table. The provision of social opportunity, like the provision of privacy, must be coordinated with the appropriate level of staff control.

Spatial Complexity

A complex and varied organization of space can to some extent offset the boredom that an alert patient will suffer in this restricted environment, but must be weighed against the drawbacks of increased staff effort and potential confusion of less alert patients.

Environmental Compensation

Handicapped persons in an extended care facility will benefit from a careful reevaluation of the conventional system of architectural barriers. Lowering architectural barriers compensates for the lack of personal competence of the residents, thereby giving them greater freedom and self-sufficiency. Compensation can also be made through the enrichment of sensory experiences in the environment. Purposeful design of color, texture, lighting, and graphics can assist the functioning of patients who tend to become disoriented or confused because of perceptual handicaps.

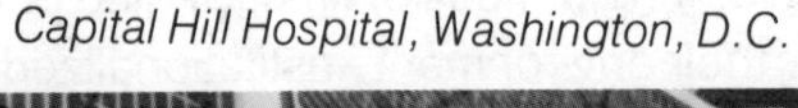

Capital Hill Hospital, Washington, D.C.

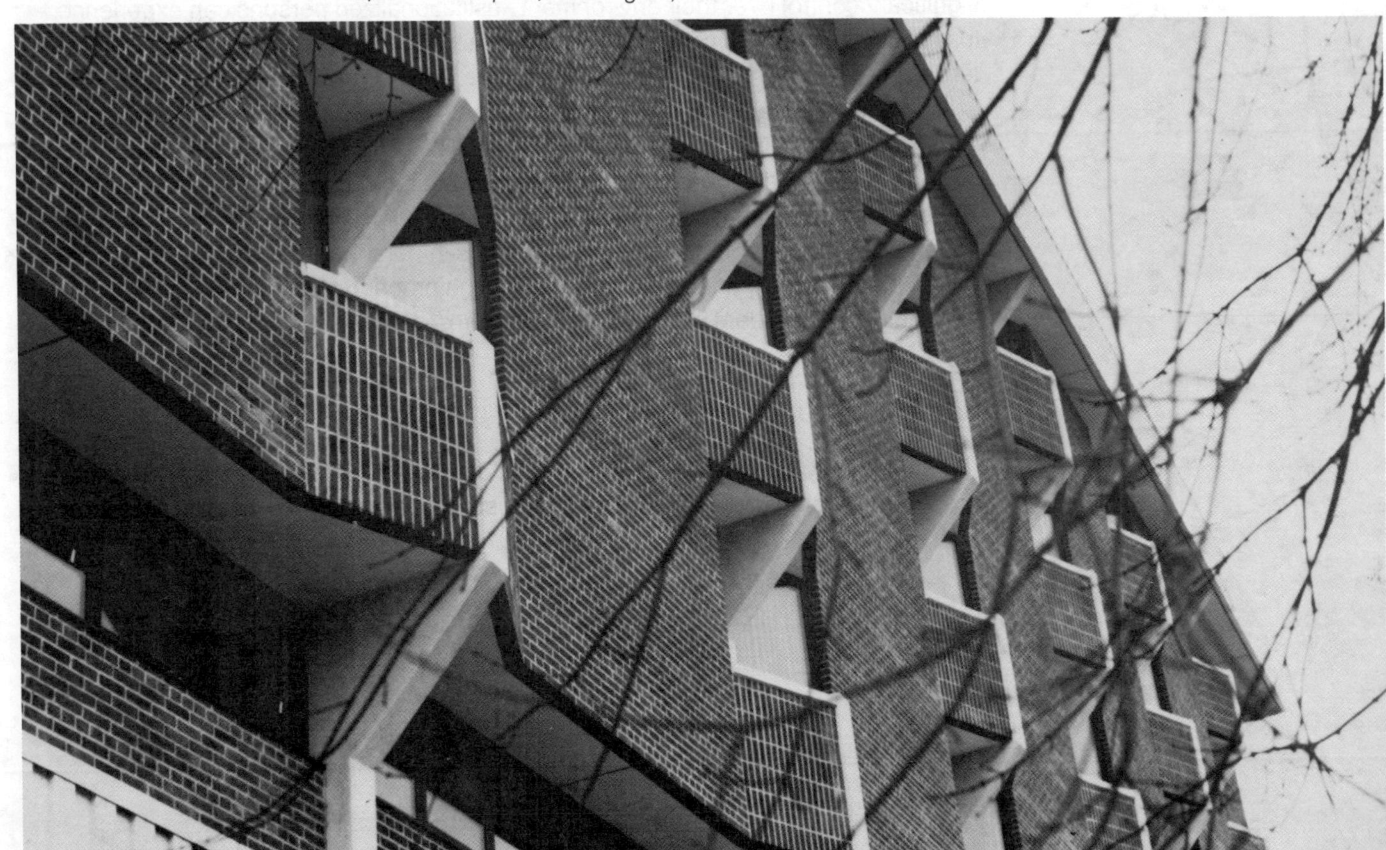

EXTENDED CARE UNIT

The broad objective of a hospital-based extended care unit is to provide post-acute care to selected patients who still need an active, medically oriented program as preparation for discharge to their own home, nursing home, or personal care facility by developing a discharge program which assures continuity of care. Although this is an important program for patients of all ages, it is especially significant for the older patient, who may need a variety of continuing therapeutic, rehabilitative, and personal services. Environment design should be based on an average patient stay of twenty days.

HOLISTIC MEDICINE

Several hospitals have announced a philosophy of establishing and maintaining holistic health care programs. A holistic health center focuses on wellness, in addition to elimination of illness, and incorporates Eastern as well as Western concepts of medicine. In that wellness and the maintenance of good health are central, the patient is seen as a learner and as a recipient of care, and the health care team sees itself as teachers and as a force for alleviating illness.

Much more consideration is given to nutrition in a holistic center than in the average hospital. Recognizing and reducing stress are also a part of the wellness instruction, since most ailments are suspected of having a significant basis in abnormal stress.

A holistic health center requires space for:

—diagnosis and blood workup

—office for a staff physician

—examination room

—office and two treatment rooms for an acupuncturist

—room for weight and stress reduction classes

—room for kilation therapy

MENTAL HEALTH UNIT

Mental illness has been called the nation's foremost health problem. Statistics show that, in addition to the number who are treated in clinics and by private psychiatrists, more than a million patients are treated yearly in mental hospitals. These same statistics indicate that an additional million people are in need of psychiatric diagnosis and treatment. Furthermore, many of the patients actually hospitalized need more treatment than can now be provided. There is little doubt that the problems in delivery of health services to this large segment of our population are enormous and that delivery systems of the past are unequal to the task. The delivery of psychiatric services must be innovative and include philosophies and concepts that recognize the increased enlightenment of the community toward mental illness, as well as the incorporation of new treatments and medications and, thus, will have little resemblance to the isolated facility of the past.

The community hospital has steadily increased its role as the hub of health services. Preventive care, ambulatory care, rehabilitative care, and extended care, as well as acute care, are now among the services available from an increasingly complex physical facility. It seems logical for the community to turn to this facility for the diagnosis, treatment, and care of the psychological components of their illness. This is similarly true of an alcohol detoxification unit, which would resemble a mental health unit.

Functions. The basic functions of a mental health unit include:

—diagnostic and treatment services

—hospitalization and partial hospitalization

—consultation for physicians and community members

—education of staff, personnel, patients, and community members

Design. There are several general considerations for the design of a mental health unit. In general, the unit will be an open unit, requiring minimum security, and have a separate entrance from the rest of the hospital. Design should avoid the typical general hospital look. Light, paint, decor, and so forth affect mood and attitude and must be chosen for a desirable therapeutic effect. Room furniture should be of the motel type rather than of the acute care type. Patients here will be predominantly ambulatory, and design of facilities such as lounge areas, occupational therapy, visiting areas, and dietary facilities should reflect this.

The ideal nursing unit is twenty to twenty-four beds. This gives the best opportunity for close observation of patients by medical and nursing staff and seems to work best from the therapeutic point of view. Private accommodations are desirable, and as many as possible should be planned within the allocated space. The unit should contain at least one secure, sound-proof, air conditioned room for management of acute toxic reactions and acute behavioral disturbances. Two rooms, adjacent to the nursing station and thus allowing direct observation and care, should be planned and equipped for handling physically ill patients or patients receiving treatment requiring bed rest or skilled nursing care.

Design of the unit should consider the total space as correlated, with subunits sharing as many common facilities as possible, yet allowing for separate functions. Space requirements for family-oriented care are greater than those for individually-oriented therapy. The mental health unit is divided into four broad subunits: the treatment-consultative area is composed predominantly of staff offices for use in individual or family care sessions for both inpatients and outpatients. These offices also form the administrative center for the unit. The conference-therapy area is designed for group therapy sessions and for observation of these sessions by staff. The inpatient area is designed to accommodate patients who have been admitted to the hospital by the mental health unit. The activities' areas are centrally located and accessible to both inpatients and outpatients for therapeutic activities such as dining, occupational and recreational therapy, and "rap" sessions.

Mental Health Unit, Intradepartmental Relationships

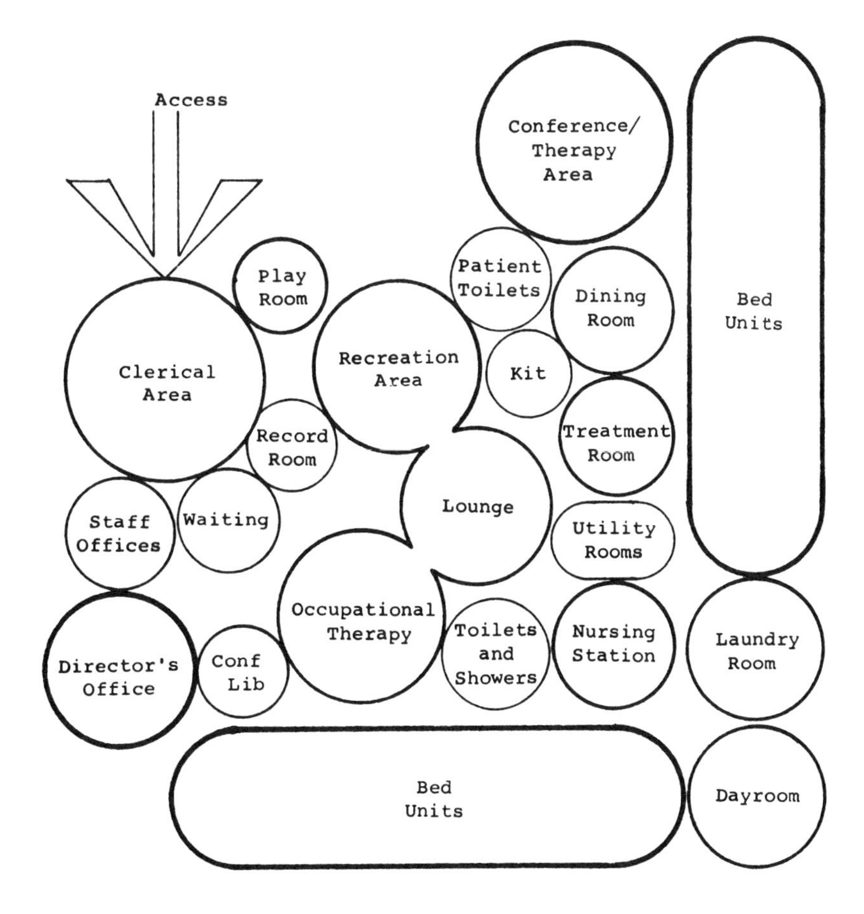

Intradepartmental Relationships. The administrative, therapy, and consulting area should be located to one side of the unit with direct access to the front entrance and inpatient bed area. There should be easy access to conference and activities' areas. The following elements are contained in the administrative, therapy, and consulting area.

The director's office provides for carrying out administrative and therapeutic responsibilities and should be located farthest from the entrance to the unit and close to the inpatient area. The conference room–library should be adjacent to the director's office for staff meetings, teaching, and so on. Staff offices provide space for consultation, family therapy sessions, and so on and should be soundproofed and contain dictating equipment. The waiting area is designed for individuals waiting to see staff members and should be adjacent to the clerical area.

A clerical area is needed for typing dictation, observing waiting patients, control, reception, and directing clients to treatment and consultation areas and must be, therefore, centrally located. The records room provides filing space for outpatient records. It should be centrally located adjacent to the clerical space and contain a copying machine. Toilet facilities are adjacent to the waiting area; there should be two for employees and two for waiting patients.

The inpatient beds should be located farthest away from the main entrance to the facility, adjacent to the conference room and the administrative areas. They must be close to the main hallway of the hospital, allowing access to supportive and diagnostic services. The following elements should be included.

The nursing station, central to the beds in the unit, should be separated from the central hall by a counter and have good visibility of the area. It should contain a medicine closet, charting space, communications equipment, and so on. There should be one soiled and one clean utility room adjacent to the nursing station. The nursing station should also have equal access to outpatient facilities. The treatment room should be easily accessible to both inpatients and outpatients and close to the nursing station for control.

The dayroom and a laundry room (for inpatient use) should be convenient. Toilets and showers should be in a central location for use by inpatients (the object being to eliminate individual facilities adjacent to rooms).

The dining room is accessible to both inpatients and outpatients and should be adjacent to a kitchen equipped with home-like fixtures for therapeutic use by both. The bed units should consist of twenty rooms for thirty inpatients and must include one security room and two for bed-ridden patients; these should be opposite the nursing station. The remainder should be divided into two units of single and double rooms on each side of the central nursing area.

The lounge and recreation area are large open rooms that can be converted into a large meeting room and should be arranged with comfortable furniture, magazine racks, card tables, and so forth. Patient toilets, for use by outpatients, should be located off the central lounge-recreation area. The occupational therapy room should be adjacent to and visible from the lounge area. It should equipped to maintain an occupational therapy program, containing, for example, a kiln for ceramics, work tables and chairs, and storage cabinets.

The conference-therapy area, located on one side of the central-common area, is to be used for group therapy sessions and observation of treatment by staff and students. Six rooms are recommended, one of which should be a play area for children. The outpatient area should be located centrally to other components with easy access from the main entrance into the unit.

PSYCHIATRIC INPATIENT UNIT

A unit for acutely ill patients has replaced the padded cells of the 1950s and 1960s. It contains patients who are capable of harming themselves and those who need daily consultation. This unit would have the same design as the long-term care unit in that a premium is placed upon lounge areas and privacy. In addition, professional staff office needs must be programmed into this space, including a consulting office for each five or six patients.

REHABILITATION UNIT

This unit is designed for an average twenty-day stay, without regard to patient age. Spinal cord injuries, hip replacements, quadriplegics, and neurosurgery patients fill these units. In keeping with the rehabilitation program, the design of this

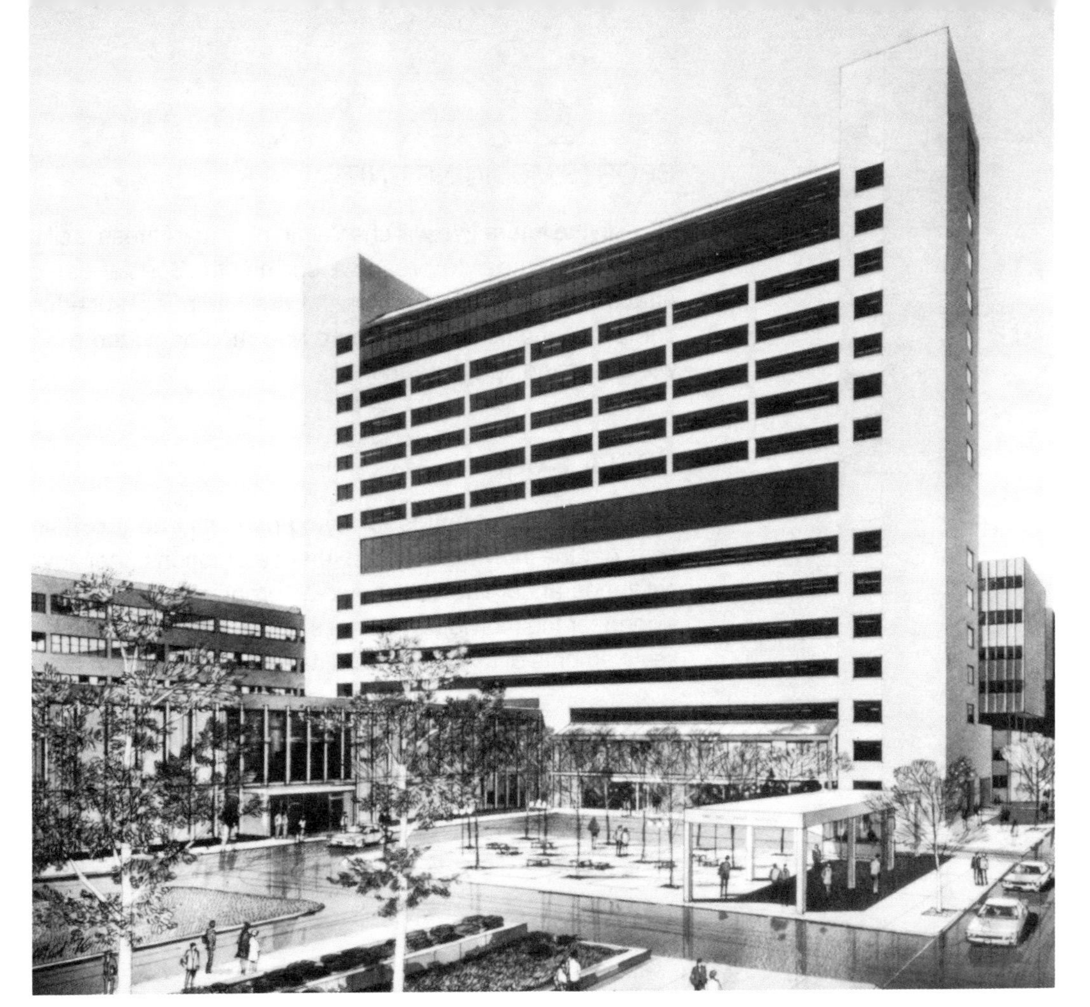

This page:
New York University Medical Center Cooperative—Ambulatory Care Pavilion

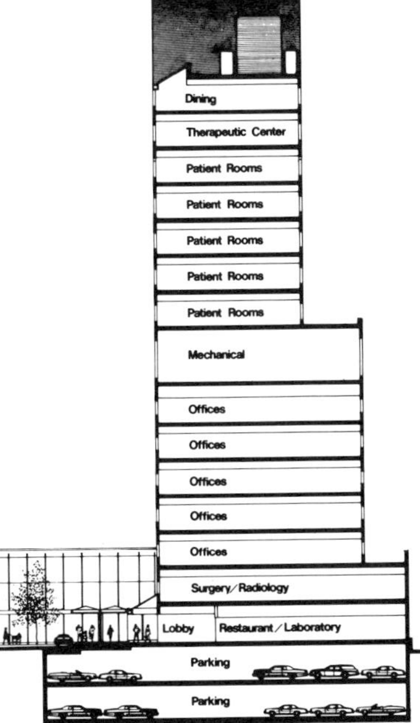

unit calls for hotel-type rooms directed at the comfort and dignity of the patient. The unit's layout will resemble that of long-term care, with additional active public areas for the patients. The ultimate design would include an area for wheelchair races.

COOPERATIVE CARE

Cooperative care may be either for ambulatory patients, at the end of their acute stay, or for patients still requiring acute care. The cooperative care concept combines the patient and a family member into a team in the final days of stay. This allows training in continuing care techniques used at home and reduces staff hours of care during the inpatient stay. The team shares a patient room and attends training classes in procedures for home care.

PSYCHOGERIATRIC UNIT

This unit deals with the total mental and physical concerns of the elderly patient. Nutrition programs, exercise, and counseling play a major role in space planning. General design is similar to that of a long-term care unit.

SPORTS MEDICINE UNIT

In the future, we will check into physical fitness facilities, be tested, rested, and observed in order to preserve our health. Special day or night care units will be attached to or within the health care campus. Procedures such as screening by computer, monitored swimming and running, video weight loss, and biofeedback will determine space needs.

HOSPICE UNIT

The hospice unit is for dying patients and their families and its design must consider the individual's most intense emotions, their level of pain, and their physical appearance. The unit should be programmed as a patient service facility and designed for the individual patient's needs. Privacy, comfort, and atmosphere are the key elements of this facility and its design.

XII

interiors and graphics

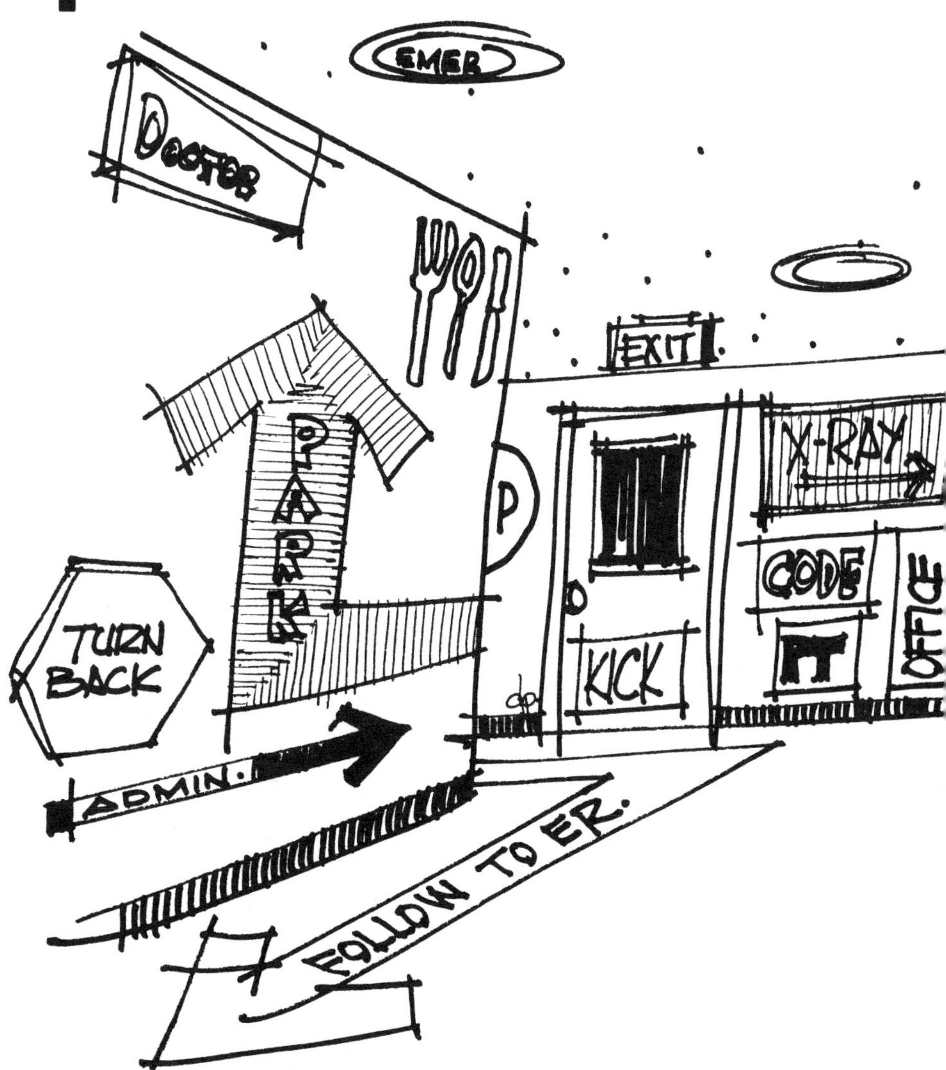

We are in an era in which interior architectural design has become an integral part of the architectural process; it begins with the earliest architectural concepts and ends with the client occupying the completed space. What does this mean to the administrator and his committee, who have been charged with the responsibility of completing the interior of their hospital? The subject of interior design is a vastly involved and complicated one; thus, we must look into many of its aspects from many directions.

Before the early 1950s, the design and furnishings of a new hospital were usually not considered until after the building had been started. A committee would be formed to search for a supplier of equipment and furniture, one who would provide the hospital with a "turnkey job" (that is, a completed interior). If the equipment supplier could do this, he was usually asked to "decorate the hospital." If he did not provide this service, a local decorator, or the volunteer committee, might be called upon to judge color coordination. If this procedure sounds rather loose and sketchy, it was. It shows the lack of care exercised in making these seemingly simple judgments that are actually crucial to the effective functioning of a hospital.

All the while, however, some very important things were brewing. There were tremendous changes in the attitudes toward, and the technology of, health care; these had a dramatic effect on health care facilities. The new and greater demands fell mainly upon the hospital architect. The professional hospital consultant also came into the picture to aid in sifting out and advising on these new advancements in medical technology. At this stage, one can perhaps begin to read between the lines and see the emergence of a strong position on the subject of hospital interior design. Before a conclusion can be drawn as to what is best, an investigation of all the avenues open to the administrator should be thoroughly investigated.

Sources of Interior Design Services

Unlike architecture and engineering, interior design suffers from dramatically varying definitions. Almost anyone can print a card and call himself a "decorator-designer." Only a few states require licensing, which assures the client of professional schooling, training, and practices. Thus, one can see why there is so much confusion in this area and why it is so difficult to select and judge interior design services. Not only is the profession difficult to evaluate, but design services are available from varying sources, all calling themselves the same thing.

Medical Supply Companies. There are local, regional, and national supply companies. Their primary function is to fill all the hospital's needs on a day-to-day basis. Because of their daily contact with hospital personnel, medical supply companies are in an ideal position to handle the supply of new furniture and equipment. Historically, national as well as most regional and local firms have offered a "free" design service if purchases are made from them. However, with the increased involvement of the architect and the independent interior designer, the role of the medical supply company has become more and more that of supplying rather than designing. Fees vary with the size of the job and the scope of involvement; they are

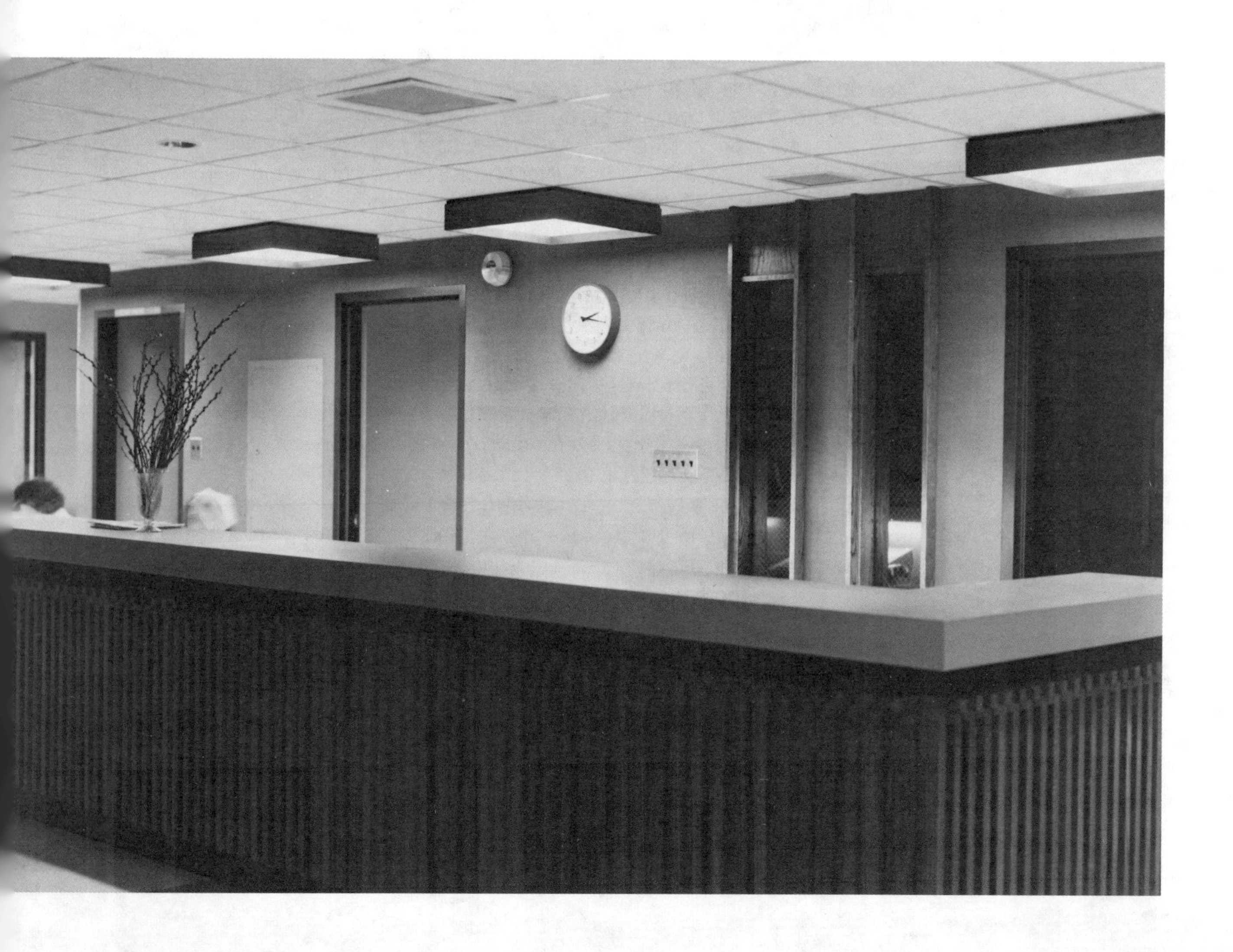

generally a percentage of the equipment bought. If the company is hired to design, it generally reserves the right to bid its own specifications. If the deal is a negotiated package (to design and supply) a total price is usually agreed upon in the beginning, thus implying that the design is free. The main factor to be considered here is that the supply company's reason for being is to serve as a total supply source rather than as an interior designer of the medical facility.

Manufacturers. In an effort to compete, a few manufacturers are offering "free" design services when their products are purchased on a negotiated basis. These manufacturers imply that bidding is not necessary because they have set prices to all clients, a questionable premise. The disadvantages and unknowns far outweigh the implied advantages. Their sole interest is in the sale of their product. Their design interest is generally only in the public spaces rather than in the down-to-earth working areas. The elimination of competition against their products also has many ramifications.

The Hospital. It is physically possible for a hospital to provide its own interior design services. This may be accomplished by administrative staff, purchasing department, appointed committee, board members, and so on. An entire chapter could be devoted to this approach, its whys and wherefores. However, present trends are definitely heading away from this procedure. Time demands upon the administrator and his staff are increasing every day; meanwhile, the increasing technological nature of equipment, the lack of intimate knowledge of the market, and the ongoing appearance of new products and methods are reducing the effectiveness of this procedure. A hospital cannot be built without highly skilled professional architects and engineers, nor should its interior be designed without skilled professional help.

The Architect. The architect has taken a new and stronger position in favor of interior design. Many large firms offer in-house interior design services equal to those of independent design firms. The architect's main concerns are that the interior, the reason for the construction of the facility, is as well designed as the building, and that the color and equipment are completely coordinated. The architect is more concerned with how well the design is done than by whom. In firms that include interior designers, the fee for design is usually an extension of the regular architectural fee or a slightly higher percentage, depending on the size of the job and the scope of work.

Design-Building Firms. If the hospital has chosen this route, the package deal may or may not include interior design. The firm may insist on interiors as part of the total services or be indifferent; or the hospital may insist from the beginning on its right to select an outside source.

Interior Decorators. The term "interior decorator" is used primarily in connection with residential design. The term "decorator" is not used by a person with professional schooling and training. The difference becomes clear when one compares the scope of the service supplied by a designer to that supplied by a decorator. The American Institute of Decorators has changed its name to the American Institute of

Designers. Decorators are still being retained to do color work in the selection of cosmetic items such as draperies, carpets, and walls, but more detailed building services are done by others. Decorators usually lack comprehensive understanding of architecture, engineering, lighting, heating, ventilation, and air conditioning; this automatically restricts their involvement. Compensation of a decorator is generally tied to the buying of furniture and furnishings; that is, the decorator buys them at a discount and sells them to the client with a markup.

Interior Designers. The interior designer is a trained professional with specific, detailed knowledge in the field in which he offers professional services. His sole source of compensation is his fee. His fees vary, but they are always based on the scope of services. He has no connection with any manufacturer and is therefore likely to be more completely objective. He is philosophically geared to cooperate with the architect in completing the interior of the facility.

Interior Architectural Designers. This is a relatively new term and reflects an extension of professional services beyond interior design. The interior architectural designer is generally hired at the same time as the architect, or shortly thereafter, to insure maximum coordination between the two. Accordingly, the interior architectural designer is uniquely able to work as a direct extension of the architect and is often hired directly by the architect to perform work included in the basic architectural contract. Such designers are the best qualified to perform the total range of services needed to complete any medical facility including basic design and functional considerations, durability and maintenance of product, and control of costs. Fees vary, based on scope.

Scope of Services

The extent of outside services used should be in direct proportion to the size of the project, type of building, and in-house capability. Another extremely important factor is timing: the earlier the consultant is retained, the better. Listed below in chronological order are some of the interior design services available.

Preliminary Consultation, Analysis of Scope, and Architectural Review. Before beginning the project, it is essential to establish the procedures and respective areas of responsibility between the client, interior designer, and architect. All architectural documents and the architectural program should be reviewed by the interior designer with the architect to ensure complete architectural coordination.

Interior Architectural Materials and Color Coordination. Earlier in the design process, and in coordination with the architects, general contractor, and client, all interior architectural material and colors are selected and submitted to the client in a graphic presentation.

Environmental Programming. When applicable, research is conducted to secure information based on social and behavioral factors; this information is used in the overall operational programming.

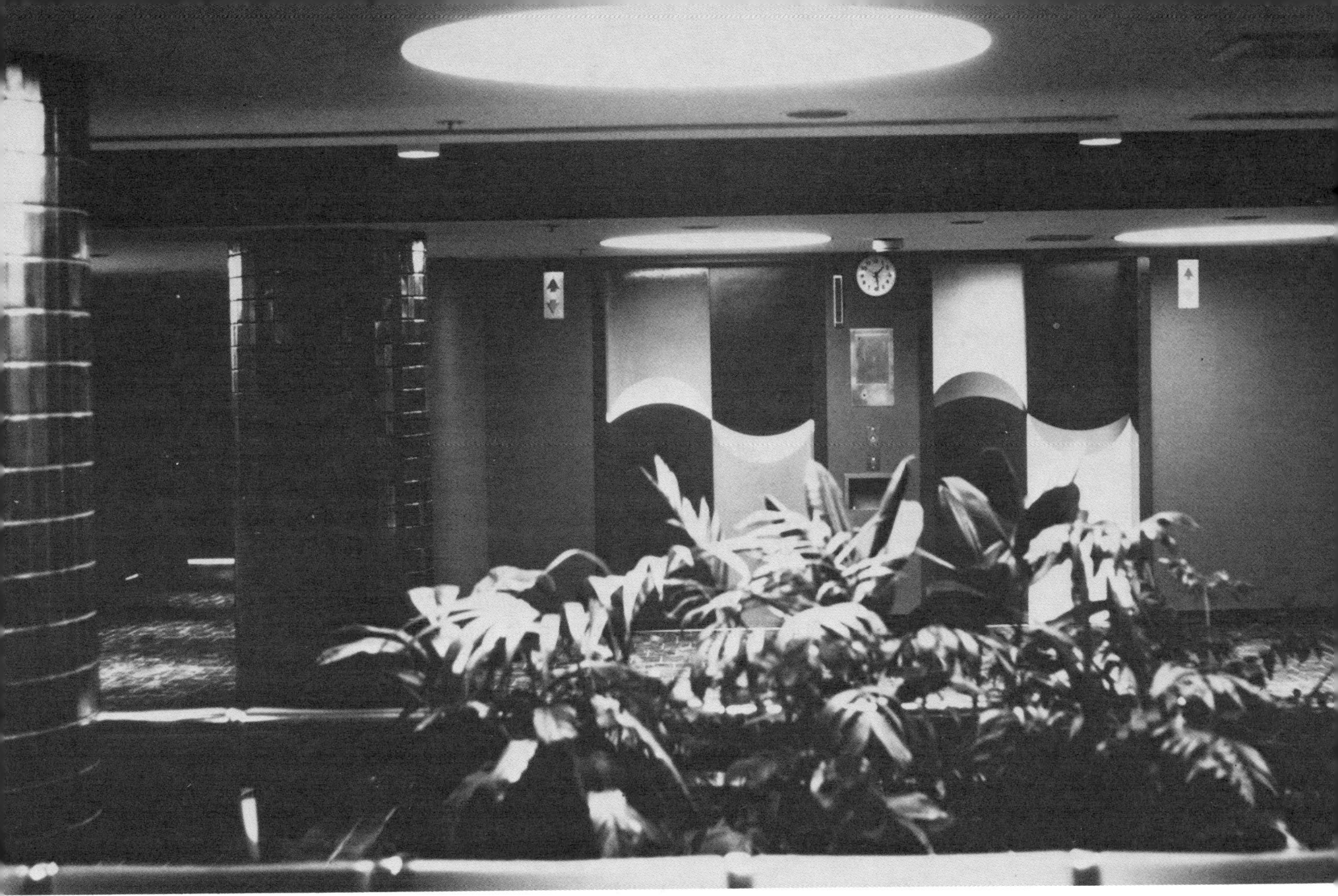

Public lobby. Capital Hill Hospital Center, Washington, D.C.

Operational Programming. Through research, interviews, observation, and consultation with key personnel, a program is developed to determine the most efficient use of space, the optimum organization of functions, the amount and types of furniture and equipment required, and costs.

Inventory Analysis and Evaluation. Existing furniture and equipment are evaluated for possible reuse and relative costs.

Preliminary Budget. To provide for the establishment and control of funds for the project, a complete preliminary budget should be prepared, evaluated, and reconciled with the available money.

Space Allocation. Based on the programming data, block space plans are prepared. These establish special departmental relationships and the total square footage required for both current needs and projected growth.

Engineering Review. Before proceeding further with the planning and design of space, there should be a review of all engineering systems to ensure complete understanding and coordination and to indicate any problems or new considerations identified during the programming phase.

Space Planning. Upon evaluation and approval of the block plans, detailed space plans are prepared, indicating partition layouts, interdepartmental and personnel space assignments, furniture and equipment layouts, and coordination with electrical and telephone outlets.

Lighting Design, Coordination, and Review. Concurrent with the space planning phase, the design and development of lighting concepts are reviewed, including light sources, fixture layout, and types of fixtures.

Interior Architectural Design—Special Design Areas. If it is determined that there are special areas that need design treatment not originally planned by the architect, the design consultant takes care of all estimating, planning, detailing, drawing, specifications, bidding, site coordination, and inspection; this is done in coordination with the architect and consulting engineers.

Furniture Selection, Budget, and Specifications. The next step is to design, select, document, and graphically present for approval all interior finishes, materials, furniture and furnishings, equipment, graphics, and accessories. Before preparing the final specifications and beginning the bidding phase, a detailed cost estimate of furniture and other related items is submitted to the client for approval. Final specifications of all approved furniture, equipment, and accessories are then prepared.

Optional Direct Procurement Management

The interior designer can extend his or her services to include the following procurement management functions:

—acting as the agent for the client and purchasing at the prices indicated on the approved specifications, unless acknowledged to the contrary at the time of procurement

—processing purchase orders with approved sources and forwarding copies of all orders to the client

—making certain that the client receives invoices from the various sources and separate invoices to cover freight in local delivery, warehousing (when necessary), installation, labor, and sales tax (where applicable), all of which have been included in the budget estimate

—processing, approving, and forwarding all invoices to the client for payment (noting any amounts to be withheld pending conformance to specifications)

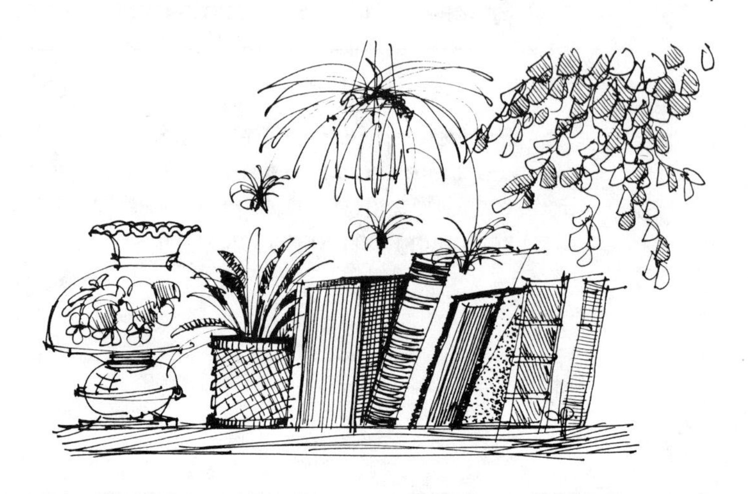

—advising when final payments should be made to each contractor

—processing and forwarding all checks in payment of invoices (checks are made payable to each source directly and are sent to the interior designer firm for forwarding)

—helping the client determine whether an item is unsatisfactory due to manufacturer's defective workmanship (otherwise, the client is responsible for the prompt payment of all invoices in strict accordance with the terms of the contract)

—consulting with the client (after award of the contract) about contractual problems caused by vendors; procurement problems initiated by the client due to change in price, manufacturer's specifications, or discontinuance of items; and expediting and delivery problems

—coordinating, scheduling, and expediting delivery of all items to the site and directing and coordinating the installation of all items in their designated area

—inspecting the installation with the client or his representative to review the entire facility and each contractor's performance

—after inspection, consulting with the client about problems arising from situations such as deviation from or nonconformance to specifications by manufacturers or contractors, manufacturing defects, freight damages uncovered during final inspection, errors or omissions by the contractors, and any other problems causing less than complete satisfaction to the client

Public lobby. Hurley Medical Center, Flint, Michigan

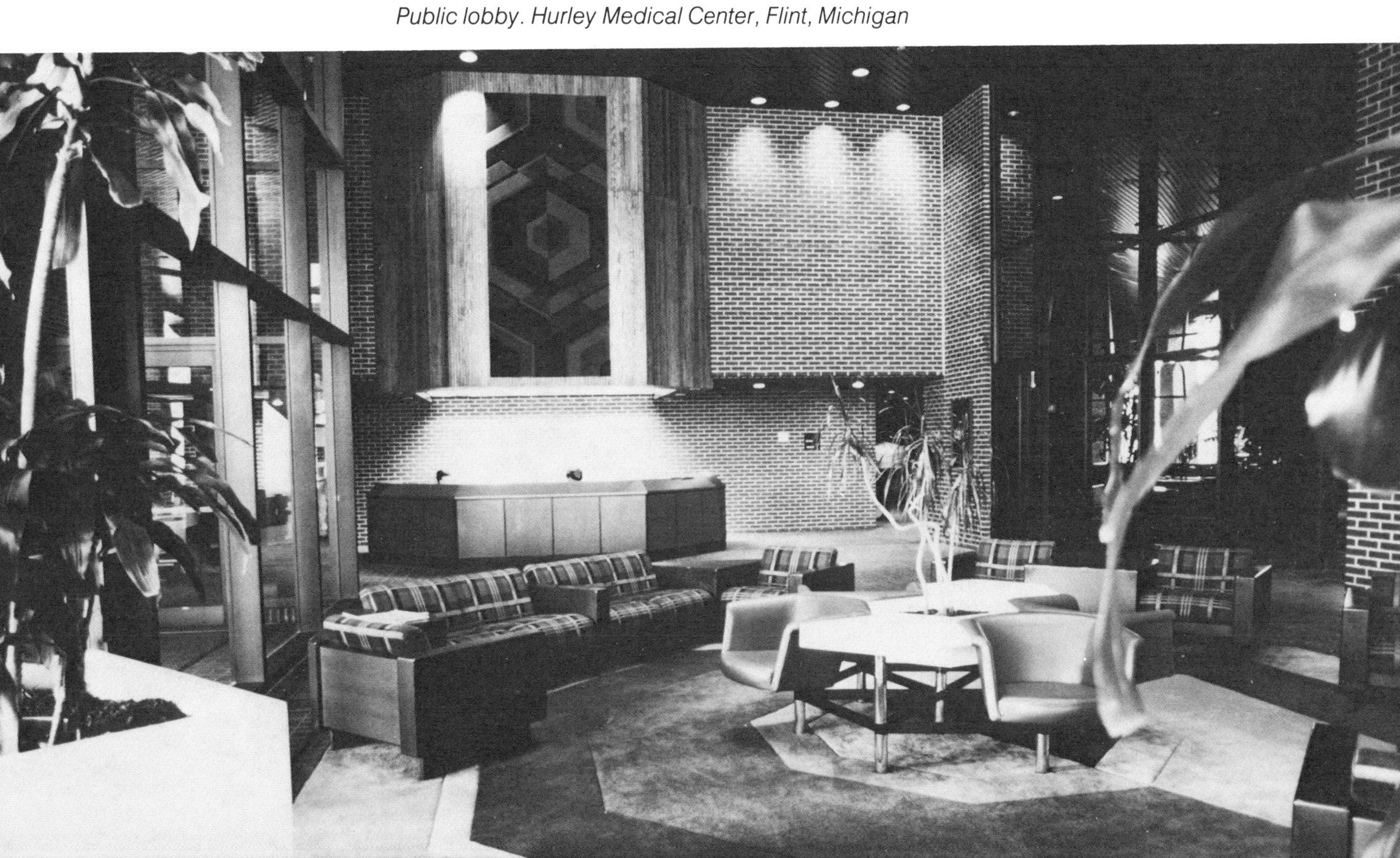

Competitive Bidding

The following steps are taken in the process of competitive bidding:

Bid Data. The interior designer will assist in the legal portion of the specifications, including bid bonds and bidding forms, that are affixed to the previously approved specifications. In addition, the interior designer will notify all manufacturers or their representatives that bids will be requested on their items. In consultation with the client, the interior designer will determine the list of competent bidders for each group of items in the specifications and forward the specifications to all approved bidders. The interior designer will administer the bidding procedure and work with the bidders concerning problems that may arise.

Bid Analyzation. Upon receipt of the bids, the interior designer will assist in the tabulation of all submissions. The interior designer will also assist in the evaluation of various bids, considering the bidder's quotation, compliance with specifications, size of his organization, financial rating, and ability to supply the items within the time specified: in general, the interior designer will be looking out for the client's best interest. A report listing recommended awards and the reasons for them is then prepared.

Bid Award. The bid analysis and recommendations are presented to the client for final evaluation and award of contracts. Purchase orders are then prepared by the client and forwarded to each successful bidder.

Consultation after Award of Contract. The interior designer will consult with the client during the delivery and installation phase about problems caused by vendors, procurement problems initiated by the client, changes in the manufacturers' specifications, discontinuance of items, expediting and delivery problems, and recommended solutions.

Inspection of Installation and Follow-up. An inspection of the installation will be made with the client or his representative to review the entire facility and each contractor's performance. The interior designer will also consult with the client concerning any problems encountered during this inspection and recommend solutions.

FINAL INSTALLATION AND FOLLOW-THROUGH

Regardless of the procurement method, the interior designer will inspect the installation and consult with the client about problems uncovered during the first year of operation.

Fee Structure

Within the profession of interior design there are many established methods of determining fees. Notice should be taken of three general points: the amount of the fee should be in direct relationship to the scope of the services required; regardless of the method, the fee should be the sole source of compensation; and the client should select the specific fee procedure. The following are commonly used fee structures:

—*Fixed fee*: a predetermined figure, based on a specific scope of services

—*Hourly fee*: a method used when the scope of work is undetermined and based on the number of hours reported on a weekly basis, multiplied by individual rates of those people working on the project

—*Hourly maximum fee*: a method based on the number of hours reported weekly, multiplied by the individual rates of those people working on the project, and with a previously agreed-upon maximum figure

— *Percentage fee*: a percentage of the total furniture and equipment cost or five to six percent of the building construction estimate multiplied by ten percent of the cost of interior furnishings only (not including technical hospital movable equipment)

—*Square footage*: a common guideline is one dollar per gross square foot of the building

GRAPHICS

"Corporate image" does not sound like a term that should be applied to design and construction, but it is an area of design that can greatly affect a hospital. Hospital promotional staffs are becoming quite common, even in small community hospitals, and the whole area of groundbreaking ceremonies, public dedications, hospital events, and public image are very important to a hospital's market success. The overall concept of hospital image includes graphic art and design. The massive amount of literature and other paper that goes from the hospital to the public and the image of the hospital that the patient carries out of the hospital are largely influenced by hospital graphics.

Reception-control desk. Phoenix Baptist Hospital

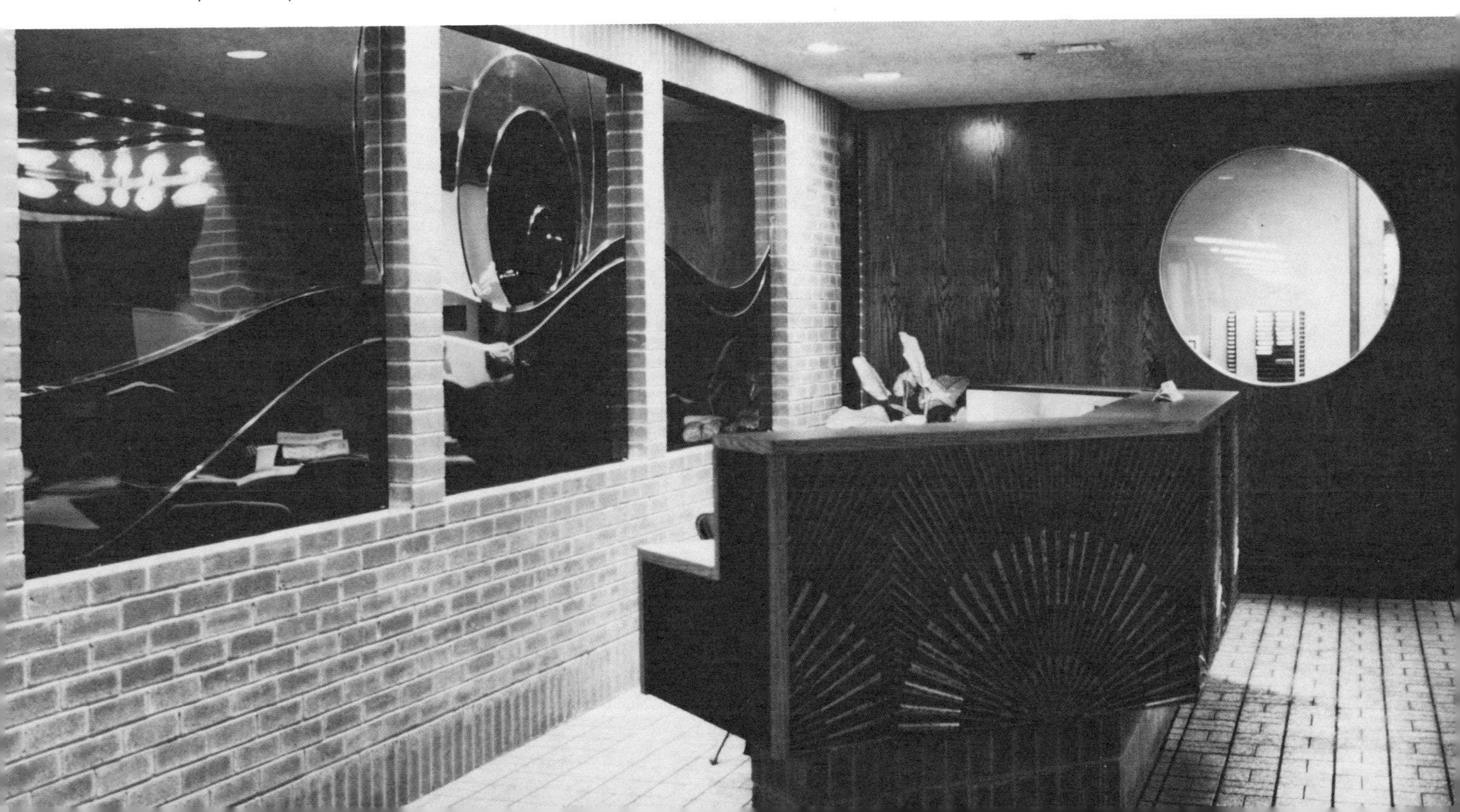

The interior of the hospital lacks something else unless it is tied to a graphics program. Two types interest the hospital designer: one is that of directional graphics, a signing program. A mass of information must be transmitted visually to the patient, visitor, and staff so that time and motion are not wasted. A signing program not only produces the directional signs inside and outside of the hospital, but also develops a consistent lettering style and directional program. Letter style and size are outlined with the design, placement, and color code of the entire hospital. This is done on a fixed fee or hourly basis by a graphics firm and can run thirty dollars per hour, or as high as $10,000 per 100 beds. Need must be determined by the administrator, but if industry trend serves as an example in the particular case, a graphics program should always be part of the budget.

The second type of graphics design used by hospitals is the corporate image as a hospital logo and master program for all printed data. Logo design can cost from $1,500–$10,000, depending on corporate complexity and the master program. This is important to the design team, as it may carry over into the physical form and color makeup. Work is usually done on an hourly basis.

Usually by the time graphics are needed, it is too late to develop them. Graphic design should be thought through early in the design stage, thus allowing the graphic designer to participate in the total design concept.

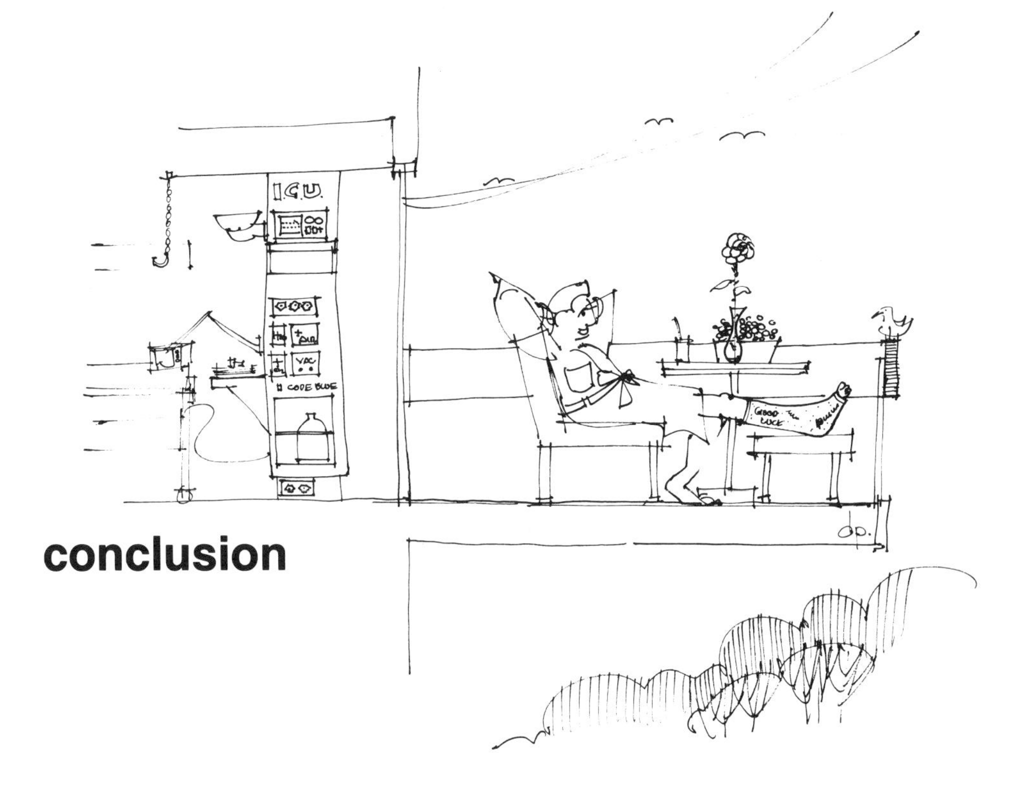

conclusion

This book has attempted to devise a common language for hospital planning, programming, architecture, engineering, and construction. A complete hospital project should be based upon a series of clear tasks and a straightforward schedule that is understood by the hospital, consultant, architect, engineer, and contractor.

An important feature of this book is the presentation of operational programming ratios. These ratios were developed through various consultants, federal agencies, and my own experience. The use of these ratios as a basis for sizing hospital department would give all of us a common method of reviewing hospital utilization. Enormous differences in size, ranging from 600 to 1,200 gross square feet per bed, of hospitals in the same community should not exist. A baseline measurement is needed for all hospitals in order to assure quality space for the patient and to contain excessive facility cost based upon department wish-lists.

The health care system must also reach out to meet the overlooked areas of our society's health. Health programs in our schools, health concerns of the changing family structure, physical exercise as habit, correct nutritional education for teenagers, and proper care and understanding of the elderly are a leadership responsibility of the health care system. The planning issues of health are clear to all of us: they involve the whole person and the entire family. I will end this book by stressing again what it's all about—patients. To understand that a single flower can mean as much to a cancer patient's progress as a series of toxic drugs is the essence of all design.

glossary

Air conditioning: The process of treating air so as to control simultaneously its temperature, cleanliness, humidity, and distribution to meet the requirements of the conditioned space.

Air-handling unit: An assembly of components used to cool or heat, filter, humidify or dehumidify, and circulate air to occupied spaces to maintain a controlled environment.

Alcoholism and detoxification: Treatment of and education in alcoholism.

American Institute of Architects: Professional society that does not license architects.

Anesthesiology: The suspending and restoring of consciousness, depending upon the patient's mental and physical status; it is used to maintain circulation, respiration, and vital signs during surgery.

Architectural registration: State licensing procedure based upon testing and application.

Average daily census: Patient days divided by 365.

Average length of stay: Number of days spent in hospital bed service divided by number of patients.

Average patient days: Number of beds divided by 365.

BTU monitoring: A system of instrumentation to determine the total amount of energy being used.

Cardiology: Diagnosis and treatment of heart, artery, and vein disease; it makes use of surgery, electrical heart monitoring, radioactive tracing, high frequency sound study, and cardiac catheterization and angiography.

Central plant: A central grouping of mechanical, heating and ventilation, and electrical equipment designed to provide maximum flexibility, maintainability, and operating efficiency over the useful life of the facility.

Centrex: A type of central telephone system which permits direct dialing between telephones in that system.

Chiller: A mechanical device used to chill water that is circulated throughout a building to terminal cooling coils; it consists of a compressor to compress vapor refrigerant, a condenser to convert the pressurized refrigerant into a liquid, and an evaporator to chill the supply.

Circuit breaker: A device designed to automatically open an electrical circuit at a predetermined overload.

Condenser: A device in which refrigerant vapor is condensed in a closed shell with a cooling medium circulated through an assembly of tubes within the shell.

Constant volume system: An air conditioning system designed to deliver air to occupied spaces at a fixed, predetermined flow rate.

Converter: A device designed to transfer heat from steam to water; used to generate hot water for heating with steam from a steam boiler.

Cooling tower: An enclosed device for cooling water by contact with air that is moved through the unit by one or more fans.

Critical path method: Type of scheduling using a computer input that maps various desirable inputs to time.

Cystoscopy: A procedure in which the physician looks into the bladder through a lighted tube.

Dermatology: The treatment of skin disorders; it uses various treatments and procedures such as cryotherapy (freezing cancerous tissues) and photochemotherapy (a combination of light and drugs).

Domestic water heater: A piece of mechanical equipment used to heat potable water for delivery to plumbing fixtures such as sinks, showers, or laundry equipment.

Ductwork: A system of sheet metal conduits used to convey conditioned air to and from occupied spaces.

Electric distribution: A general term used to describe the building's electrical system from the main building electrical service to the loads which it serves, including wiring, controls and protective devices.

Electric resistance heating: A radiation heating unit in which the heat is generated by passing an electrical current through a resistance-type wire.

Emergency generator: An engine-driven device that generates electrical power to serve essential needs when the normal power supply is out of service.

Endocrinology: The study of tiny endocrine glands that control growth, maturation, and reproduction, including the pituitary, thyroid, adrenals, parathyroids, ovaries, and testes glands; hormonal disorders such as hyper- and hypothyroidism, diabetes mellitus, and severe hypoglycemia are treated, and patient education and counsel are given.

Endoscopy: The internal examination of hollow areas of the body using a long, flexible periscope-type instrument.

Energy audit: Breaking down total energy consumption so it can be analyzed.

Extended care facility: One designed for long patient stays.

Fan coil unit: A prefabricated assembly including heat transfer coils, a fan driven by an electric motor, air filter, controls, and air outlet; it is located in occupied spaces to provide a controlled environment within that space.

Fast-tracking: Advanced construction phases (such as building utilities and foundation) before construction drawings have been completed.

Feeders: Sets of electrical conductors extending from the main service to the panelboard.

Fire alarm system: A system designed to detect the presence of fire or smoke in a building and to automatically transmit signals which are used to initiate certain automatic and manual procedures in a fire emergency.

Fire detection system: A system of devices within occupied and unoccupied spaces and within the air conditioning system to provide an early warning that fire is present.

Fire protection: A term loosely used to describe a system of sprinklers, hose outlets, fire extinguishers, fire and smoke detectors, and alarms designed to detect smoke or fire, extinguish a fire, and warn personnel.

Fire zone: An area separated from other areas by walls and doors having a high resistance to fire, designed to prevent the spread of fire to or from adjacent fire zones.

Four-pipe system: A system that utilizes two heat transfer coils, one for heating and one for cooling. Heating or cooling is available at any time.

Gastroenterology: Problems affecting the organs of the digestive tract—esophagus, stomach, intestines, liver, pancreas, and biliary duct system.

General surgery: The beginning of all surgical subspecialties and still the most extensive range of procedures.

Ground fault: A type of short circuit caused by an electrical contact between an energized electrical conductor and any part of the grounding system which results in a flow of currents in grounding conductors.

Health maintenance organization: Group formed to supply health care insurance services on a prepaid plan.

Hematology: The study of blood, including nutrients, proteins, hormones, white blood cells, platelets, and bone marrow, to aid in diagnosing a medical condition or disease.

Hot water coils: A component of an air-handling unit consisting of pipe with metal fins on the outside; designed to transfer heat from hot water within the pipe to the air contacting the fins.

Incremental units: A prefabricated assembly that includes a refrigeration system, steam, or air filters, electric motor-driven fan, heater, and controls. The heater can be either hot water, steam, or electric resistance. The unit is located on an exterior wall within the occupied space.

Induction unit: A prefabricated assembly, including heat transfer coils, air filters, controls, and a connection to a central, conditioned, primary air supply; room air is induced into the unit by primary air, they mix, and the mixture is delivered to the room to provide a controlled environment.

Interstitial space: Unoccupied space between floors, approximately six to ten feet high, enabling mechanics to work on air conditioning and equipment without disturbing the occupied floors.

Laboratory and pathology: The performing of tests to confirm (or not) diagnoses, tracing and identifying microbes that cause infectious diseases, running the blood bank and hematology test section, and studying chromosomal abnormalities (cytogenetics), tropical diseases, and parasites (parasitology).

Life-cycle costs: Process by which total costs are determined over a selected period of years; included are yearly maintenance costs, yearly energy costs, and the initial purchase price, including installation costs. The process is effective in determining the most economical system by comparing their life-cycle costs over the normal life expectancy.

Lightning protection: A special wiring system designed to intercept atmospheric lightning and cause it to flow to the ground, thereby preventing damage to structure or building.

Load shedding: A process of shutting down electrically operated equipment in a predetermined sequence to limit the maximum demand and thereby reduce electrical costs.

Medical gases: Gases used in medical treatment and laboratory procedures; they include air, gas, oxygen, nitrous oxide, and vacuum.

Medicine: The general category of subspecialties include cardiac, endoscope, pulmonary, and internal medicine.

Nephrology: Study of the kidneys; kidney dialysis (artificial kidney machine) and kidney transplant depend on this service.

Neurology and neurosurgery: The study and treatment of brain, spinal cord, and nervous system disorders or injuries, including seizures, tumors, multiple sclerosis, and headache; stroke, vision, cancer complications, and blood pressure are all related to neurology.

Nuclear medicine: The application of internally administered radiopharmaceuticals to diagnose or to treat conditions.

Obstetrics and gynecology: Obstetrics is the specialty dealing with pregnancy, labor, delivery, and postpartum care; gynecology deals with disorders of the female reproductive tract. Patients with high-risk pregnancies are now referred to specialists in fetology and perinatal-neonatal services.

Ophthalmology: Treatment of diseases of the eye; programs with visual aids and eye-wear clinics.

Oral surgery: Correction of facial deformities, removal of cysts and tumors from the jaws, and joint dysfunction.

Orthopedics: Surgical and nonsurgical care of patients with problems of the musculoskeletal system, such as back problems, fractures, torn ligaments, and torn tendons.

Otorhinolaryngology: Specialty dealing with the ear (otology), nose (rhinology), and throat (laryngology).

Oxygen system: A large central supply and piping to locations where oxygen is used in treatment.

Panelboard: A unit designed for control of a number of individual lighting and other electrical loads, including automatic overload protection devices.

Passive solar energy: The use of a building's exposures to the sun to absorb heat.

Patient days: Admissions multiplied by length of stay; average daily census divided by target occupancy.

Perinatal and neonatal pediatrics: Intensive care nurseries, constant care, and transitional nurseries for twins, jaundiced infants, breech birth or cesarean section infants, and infants who are underweight or overweight at birth; neonatologists and fetologists become involved in high-risk pregnancies long before delivery.

Physical medicine and rehabilitation: Treating disabled patients; a rehabilitation team involves physical and occupational therapists, rehabilitation nurses, speech pathologists, recreational therapists, social workers, a psychiatrist, a psychologist, and vocational rehabilitation counselors.

Plastic surgery: Reconstructive work to restore body function and appearance.

Pneumatic controls: A system of controls for regulating system functions, operated by air pressure from a central air system.

Power factor: The ratio of the true power, or watts, to the product of current and voltage in an alternating current electrical circuit.

Pressure differential: The difference in pressure across a device, expressed in pounds per square inch or inches of water.

Primary care: Deals with minor illnesses and injuries and includes family practice physicians, outpatient facility, or primary care center.

Psychiatry: Inpatients who become physical threats to themselves and outpatients with mental conditions.

Pulmonary medicine and respiratory therapy: The treatment of lung and breathing disorders, including chronic bronchitis, emphysema, asthma, sarcoidosis, and lung cancer, as well as respiratory failure accompanying shock, trauma, burns, surgery, and various medical diseases.

Radiant heat: A heating unit located in occupied spaces; heating is provided by a combination of radiation to objects within the space and conduction to surrounding air, which is circulated by natural convection.

Radiation therapy: A tissue-destroying procedure primarily directed toward diseases characterized by tumor or new growth, using cobalt gamma rays and radiation of varying intensities.

Radiology: The use of radiant energy in treatment; also brain scanning by computerized tomography.

Reheat: A process related to control of space humidity during the cooling season. Air is cooled to the dew point to remove excess humidity and then reheated to the temperature which, when delivered to the space, will provide the proper space temperature.

Retrofit: Existing building space remodeled for a different function.

Rheumatology: The treatment of rheumatoid arthritis and related disorders.

Secondary care: More specialized services such as maternity, general surgery, and diagnostics; usually involves hospitalization.

Shock and trauma: Subspecialty of emergency with advanced diagnostic, resuscitative, and monitoring techniques.

Short list: Reducing the number of professional firms down from many to a few for final selection.

Smoke damper: An automatic damper in an air duct system designed to close and prevent the spread of smoke to occupied spaces.

Smoke-purging mode: A particular arrangement of equipment components and controls which causes smoke removal from within a space or spaces without circulating it to other spaces.

Smoke zone: An area separated from other areas by walls and doors to prevent the spread of smoke to or from adjacent smoke zones.

Speech and hearing: Speech and language pathologists work with patients who have difficulty in speaking because of stroke, disease, or injury; audiology provides tests for diagnosing the cause of hearing loss.

Sprinklers: A system of piping containing water under pressure and sprinkler heads designed to automatically trip at the presence of heat, thus spraying water on a fire.

Standpipes: Vertical piping containing water under pressure with valved hose outlets at strategic locations for use by personnel in fighting fires.

Step-down: Care for patients who need monitoring but not intensive, direct viewing.

Tertiary care: Most specialized medical care available, including open-heart surgery, burn centers, kidney transplants, and microsurgery; receives referred patients from primary and secondary care facilities and includes a teaching program or major affiliation; examples are University medical school hospitals and large private institutions.

Thoracic and vascular surgery: Surgery on vital organs of the chest and vascular system.

Two-pipe system: A system that utilizes one heat transfer coil for both heating and cooling. Chilled water is supplied to the coil during hot weather, and hot water is supplied during cold weather. The water is changed over from cold to hot in the fall and from hot to cold in late spring. The disadvantage is that one cannot switch back and forth between heating and cooling; only one is available at any time.

Unit heater: A direct heating, prefabricated assembly including a heating element, a fan driven by an electric motor, and an air outlet.

Urology: Diagnosis and treatment of the urinary system and the male reproductive system; subspecialties include fertility, sterility, reconstructive surgery, oncology, infectious diseases, and renal (kidney) surgery.

Utility services: A term used to describe the main utility services to a building from a larger system owned by a municipality or utility company. These services include electrical power, water, sanitary sewer, storm drainage, natural gas, and telephone.

Vacuum system: One or more vacuum pumps and piping to locations where a vacuum is used in medical procedures such as aspiration.

Water treatment: Chemical treatment of water to prevent corrosion or the growth of bacteria and algae in mechanical equipment and piping.

about the author

DAVID R. PORTER is principal in the Rockville, Maryland, architectural firm David R. Porter and Associates, Architects, and has been prime or consulting architect for 160 health care facilities. He has specialized in health care architecture for twenty years. His previous book, *Health Design Administration* (George Washington University, 1973), was published during his five-year lecture series at the George Washington University Graduate School of Health Care Administration, where he established a course in architectural design. His credits include: project manager for the new ambulatory care research facility of the National Institutes of Health; consultant to various equipment manufacturers; and consulting architect for the first institute-specific bed need study in the country. His professional commitments include partnership in an international construction management firm; vice-presidency in the architectural-engineering firm of KZF, Inc., Cincinnati, Ohio; partnership in the architectural firm Porter-Nash, Baltimore, Maryland; member of a national value management team; and a practicing principal of his own prime architectural firm.

The author and Health Administration Press gratefully acknowledge the following sources of illustrations.

CHAPTER I

9: Good Samaritan Hospital, Cincinnati, Ohio. Robert von Otto, consulting engineer. Gallagher/Craig & Assoc., architects. O'Conner and Engel & Assoc., engineers. David R. Porter, consulting architect.

10: St. Luke Hospital, Fort Thomas, Kentucky. David R. Porter, consulting architect.

CHAPTER II

37: Annie M. Warner Hospital, Gettysburg, Pennsylvania. Perkins and Will, architect. David R. Porter, project manager.

CHAPTER III

43: People's Community Hospital, Taylor, Michigan. Perkins and Will, architect. Photo by Hedrich-Blessing.

44: People's Community Hospital, Taylor, Michigan. Perkins and Will, architect. Photo by Hedrich-Blessing (top).

52: Medical Center of Beaver County, Pennsylvania. Perkins and Will, architect.

53: Children's Memorial Hospital, Chicago. Perkins and Will, architect.

54: Children's Memorial Hospital, Chicago. Perkins and Will, architect.

55 and 56 (top): National Institute of Health Ambulatory Care Research Facility, Washington, D.C. David R. Porter, consulting architect. Robert Nash; Henningson, Durham and Richardson; and Curtis & Davis, architects/engineers.

56: Washington Hospital Center, Washington, D.C. David R. Porter, architect. Block, McGibony & Assoc., hospital consultants. Robert von Otto, consulting engineer.

CHAPTER IV

75: Rogers Memorial Hospital, Washington, D.C. David R. Porter, architect. Block, McGibony & Associates, hospital consultants.

87: Annie M. Warner Hospital physicians' office building. David R. Porter, project manager; Perkins & Will, architect.

88: Group Health Association, Rockville, Maryland. David R. Porter, architect.

89: Hurley Medical Center, Flint, Michigan. Henningson, Durham & Richardson, architect/engineer. Fugard, Orth & Associates, Inc., JV Firm. Herman Smith, Associates, consultant. McBro Planning & Development Co., construction manager.

91: Medical University of South Carolina, Charleston. Perkins and Will, consulting architect.

92: Charity Hospital, Mecca, Saudi Arabia. Perkins and Will, architect.

92: King Abdulaziz University Health Sciences Center, Jeddah, Saudi Arabia. David R. Porter, hospital designer. Henningson, Durham and Richardson, architect/engineer. Warnecke & Associates, associate engineers. Herman Smith Associates and Stanford Research Institute consultants.

95: Northwest General Osteopathic Hospital, Milwaukee, Wisconsin. David R. Porter, architect. Block, McGibony and Associates, consultant.

95: Kent County Memorial Hospital. Perkins and Will, architects.

96-97: Heart House, American College of Cardiology, Bethesda, Maryland. Perkins and Will, architects. Photo bottom p. 96 by Lautman, Washington, D.C. Photo top right p. 97 by Jaime Ardilles-Arce, New York.

99: Kent County Memorial Hospital. Perkins and Will, architect.

100-102: Annie M. Warner Hospital, Gettysburg, Pennsylvania. David R. Porter, project manager. Perkins and Will, architect.

CHAPTER V

125-126: Marcus J. Bless Building, Georgetown University Hospital. Perkins and Will, architect.

CHAPTER VI

139: Houston Memorial Baptist Hospital. S.I. Morris Associates, architect. David R. Porter, consulting architect. Block, McGibony and Associates, hospital consultants.

141: Tucson Medical Center, Tucson, Arizona. Perkins and Will, architect.

CHAPTER VII

150, 154: New York University Medical Center Cooperative Care Center. Perkins and Will, architect. David R. Porter, architect.

CHAPTER VIII

161: Annie M. Warner Hospital, Gettysburg, Pennsylvania. David R. Porter, project manager. Perkins and Will, architect.

CHAPTER IX

184: People's Community Hospital, Taylor, Michigan. Perkins & Will, architect.

187: Medical Center of Beaver County, Pennsylvania. Perkins and Will, architect.

207: St. Luke Hospital, Fort Thomas, Kentucky. David R. Porter, architect. KZF, Inc., engineer.

CHAPTER X

217: Washington Hospital Center, Washington, D.C. David R. Porter, architect. Block, McGibony & Associates, hospital consultants. Robert von Otto, engineer.

229: St. Luke's Medical Center, Sioux City, Iowa. Henningson, Durham and Richardson, architect/engineer. Herman Smith Associates, consultant.

234: Searle Research Pavilion, Children's Memorial Hospital, Chicago. Perkins and Will, architect.

245: San Pedro Sula Hospital, Honduras. David R. Porter, consulting architect.

CHAPTER XI

265: Marcus J. Bless Building, Georgetown University Hospital. Perkins and Will, architect.

268: Capital Hill Hospital, Washington, D.C. David R. Porter, architect.

270: Medical Center of Beaver County, Pennsylvania. Perkins and Will, architect.

273: Annie M. Warner Hospital. Gettysburg, Pennsylvania. David R. Porter, project manager. Perkins and Will, architect.

274, 278: Washington Hospital Center, Washington, D.C. David R. Porter, architect. Robert von Otto, engineer. Block, McGibony & Associates, consultant.

281: People's Community Memorial Hospital, Taylor, Michigan. Perkins and Will, architect.

282, 284: Capital Hill Hospital, Washington, D.C. David R. Porter, architects. Block, McGibony & Associates, consultant.

289: New York University Medical Center Cooperative. Perkins and Will, architect.

CHAPTER XII

297: Capital Hill Hospital Center, Washington, D.C. David R. Porter, architect. Perkins and Will, architect.

299: Hurley Medical Center, Flint, Michigan. Henningson, Durham and Richardson, architect/engineer. Fugard, Orth and Associates, Inc., JV Firm. Herman Smith Associates, consultant. McBro Planning & Development Co., construction manager.

301: Phoenix Baptist Hospital. Henningson, Durham and Richardson, architect/engineers. Booz, Allen and Hamilton, Inc., consultants.

83 099

Text cartoons by David R. Porter.

Book design and layout by Don Ross.